Contents

Acknowledgements

Photographs

The authors and publisher would like to thank the following organisations and individuals for permission to reproduce photographs:

Comstock Images – Pages 72, 73, 207
Corbis – Pages 19, 106
Getty Images/PhotoDisc – Page 254
Harcourt Education Ltd – Pages 40 (Gareth Boden), 70 (Rob Judges), 96 (Martin Sookias/Mencap), 106 (Gareth Boden), 278 (Jules Selmes), 285 (Gareth Boden), 343 (Arnos Design)
Harcourt Education Ltd/Tudor Photography – Pages 151, 189 (AAF), 205, 263t, 263b
iStockphoto – Page 328
Jupiterimages.Photos.com – Page 188
PhotoDisc – Pages 66 (Siede Preis), 67, 90

Text

The authors and publisher would like to thank the following individuals and organisations for permission to reproduce copyright material:

Chatto & Windus – Page 193
Elsevier Inc – Pages 99, 100
EMIS and PiP 2007 (chart distributed on www.patient.co.uk) – Page 307
Lee Glendinning, the *Guardian* (article copyright © Guardian News & Media Ltd 2007) – Page 327
Mind – Page 194
Gaylan Ritchie, All About Multiple Sclerosis website (www.mult-sclerosis.org) – Pages 299, 300

Every effort has been made to contact copyright holders of material reproduced in this book. Any omissions will be rectified in subsequent printings if notice is given to the publishers.

The units in this product have been written by the following authors:

Marilyn Billingham – Unit 7
Karon Chewter – Units 1, 2, 9
Sue Ford – Units 3, 10, 11
Diane Goff – Unit 12
Jo Hatton – Units 4, 8, 22, 29
Pam Lang – Units 6, 44
Pamela Lloyd – Units 19, 20
Saloua Wach – Units 5, 13, 14

Health & Social Care

Assessment and Delivery Resource

Series editor: Karon Chewter

www.harcourt.co.uk

✓ Free online support
✓ Useful weblinks
✓ 24 hour online ordering

01865 888058

Heinemann

Heinemann is an imprint of Harcourt Education Limited, a company incorporated in England and Wales, having its registered office: Halley Court, Jordan Hill, Oxford OX2 8EJ. Registered company number: 3099304

www.harcourt.co.uk

Heinemann is the registered trademark of Harcourt Education Limited

Produced for Harcourt Education by
White-Thomson Publishing Ltd,
Bridgewater Business Centre
210 High Street, Lewes,
East Sussex, BN7 2NH

Text © Marilyn Billingham, Karon Chewter, Sue Ford, Diane Goff, Jo Hatton, Pam Lang, Pamela Lloyd, Saloua Wach 2007. The moral rights of the authors have been asserted.

First published 2007

12 11 10 09 08 07
10 9 8 7 6 5 4 3 2 1

British Library Cataloguing in Publication Data is available from the British Library on request.

ISBN 978 0 435499 17 4

Edited by Kelly Davis
Typeset by Tech-Set Limited
Original illustrations © Harcourt Education Limited 2007
Illustrated by Tech-Set Limited and Tek-Art
Picture research by Kelly Davis and Sian Salmon
Printed by Athenaeum Press Ltd.

Every effort has been made to contact copyright holders of material reproduced in this book. Any omissions will be rectified in subsequent printings if notice is given to the publishers.

Websites
The websites used in this book were correct and up-to-date at the time of publication. It is essential for tutors to preview each website before using it in class so as to ensure that the URL is still accurate, relevant and appropriate. We suggest that tutors bookmark useful websites and consider enabling students to access them through the school/college intranet.

Introduction

Welcome to the new Heinemann BTEC National Diploma in Health and Social Care Assessment and Delivery Resource.

The health and social care sector is constantly changing. In recent years, the Skills for Health and Skills for Care development organisations have placed the education and training needs of both the current and the future workforce high on their list of priorities for improving service provision.

Now the new BTEC National Diploma in Health and Social Care offers learners an opportunity to gain both theoretical and practical knowledge through a range of core and specialist units. This training offers an excellent basis for a future career, and successful progression, in the health and social care sector.

Using the Assessment and Delivery Resource

This Assessment and Delivery Resource (ADR) has been designed to complement the Student Books. It should also make the core units, and a selection of specialist units, as easy as possible for you to deliver and assess.

The Holistic Grid (see pages vii–xii) will help you plan your BTEC National Diploma in Health and Social Care. Within the diploma, there are the eight core units, which must be delivered and together provide for 480 guided learning hours. There are also 31 other specialist units, which can be selected according to your requirements, as long as they cover 600 guided learning hours.

Experience has shown that selection of the specialist units is dependent on a number of factors, such as appropriately qualified teaching staff, availability of resources and placement opportunities. If units are not carefully selected this can result in duplication, too much work, and boredom – not only for the teaching staff but also for the learners!

The grid will help you to plan your course, making the most of the experience of the teaching staff and providing an interesting and enjoyable experience for the learners. This should also have a positive impact on your retention and achievement data, as learners will not be put off early in the course by too much repetition and tedium.

The Assessment and Delivery Resource content

This ADR contains a range of activities and supporting PowerPoint® presentations for each unit, which aim to engage students of different learning styles and abilities. Each activity is clearly cross-referenced to the Student Book, and many of them include practical examples that encourage learners to apply theory to practice. There is also advice on inviting guest speakers from the health and social care sector in to talk to the learners and appropriate topics for them to cover.

Activities include:

- Case studies
- Gapped handouts
- Research tasks
- Problem-solving exercises
- Role plays
- Debates
- Plenary games and quizzes
- Video clips
- PowerPoint® presentations

Each unit includes a Scheme of Work, which clearly shows:

- Learning outcomes
- Tutor preparation

- Learner activity
- Resources
- Links to grading criteria
- Tasks for placement

This is cross-referenced to the At-a-Glance Activity Grid included in each unit, which provides more detailed advice on delivery.

The CD Rom

The accompanying CD Rom contains all the pages from the ADR in PDF format. The activities can be adjusted to reflect local situations or for the specific needs of particular groups of students. The worksheet activities and PowerPoint® presentations are also included, along with the answers to worksheets and answers to the questions in the Student Book.

Legislation on the web

There is also an Appendix to this ADR which summarises key aspects of legislation that apply across several units. Learners should look at these summaries whenever a piece of legislation is mentioned in the text of any of the units. This will help reinforce their learning about the key features of each Act and how the legislation relates to the theory and practice being discussed in the units. They will find this Appendix on our website: www.harcourt.co.uk/btechsc

Holistic overview

Unit number, title, year group, and guided learning hours (GLH)	Cross-referenced areas	Cross-referenced with: Unit number and name
Unit 1: Developing effective communication in health and social care **Year 1 – 60 GLH**	Communication skills Barriers to communication Managing behaviour Legislation Policies Codes of Practice Confidentiality Ethical practice	**Unit 2:** Equality, diversity and rights in health and social care **Unit 6:** Personal and professional development in health and social care **Unit 9:** Values and planning in social care **Unit 24:** Introduction to Counselling Skills for health and social care
Unit 2: Equality, diversity and rights in health and social care **Year 1 – 60 GLH**	Active promotion of individual rights Individual rights Anti-discriminatory practice Care Value Base Legislation Understanding of own responsibilities Awareness of own attitudes and beliefs Confidentiality	**Unit 6:** Personal and professional development in health and social care **Unit 9: Values and planning** (Follows on from this unit very well. The same teacher should deliver Unit 1 in year 1 and Unit 9 in year 2.)
Unit 3: Health, safety and security in health and social care **Year 1 – 60 GLH**	Understanding own responsibilities Legislation Policies and procedures Risk assessment Preventing infection Improving health through education Storage and disposal of waste Storage and disposal of substances Storage and disposal of equipment	**Unit 6:** Personal and professional development in health and social care **Unit 12:** Public health **Unit 20:** Health education (Follows on from this unit very well. The same teacher could deliver this unit in year 2 for the Health pathway.) **Unit 39:** Infection prevention and control (Follows on from this unit well for the Social Care pathway in year 2.)
Unit 4: Development through the life stages **Year 1 – 60 GLH**	Life factors Major life events Theories of ageing Biological theory – understanding developmental norms Theories of transition Stress Application of theories to development	**Unit 8:** Psychological perspectives for health and social care **Unit 24:** Introduction to counselling skills for health and social care **Unit 25:** Coping with change in a health and social care context **Unit 29:** Applied psychological perspectives for health and social care
Unit 5: Fundamentals of anatomy and physiology **Year 1 – 60 GLH**	Understanding the human body in terms of body systems	**Unit 14:** Physiological disorders **Unit 21:** Nutrition for health and social care
Unit 6: Personal and professional development in health and social care **Year 1 and 2 – 120 GLH plus 100 hours in placement**	Reflective practice Communication skills Barriers to communication Learning styles Understanding own attitudes Applying theory to practice Legislation Teamwork Personal development plan Recommendations Structure of placement	**Unit 1:** Developing effective communication in health and social care **Unit 2:** Equality, diversity and rights in health and social care **Unit 44:** Vocational experience for health and social care **Unit 46:** Independent learning in health and social care **Unit 47:** Academic literacy in health and social care
Unit 7: Sociological perspectives for health and social care **Year 1 first semester – 30 GLH**	Concepts of health and illness Patterns and trends in health and illness Models of health Understanding inequalities in health	**Unit 20:** Health education (Follows on from this unit very well.) **Unit 22:** Research methodology for health and social care **Unit 19:** Applied sociological perspectives for health and social care
Unit 8: Psychological perspectives for health and social care **Year 2 second semester – 30 GLH**	Life factors Major life events Theories of ageing Biological theory – understanding developmental norms Theories of transition Stress Application of theories to development	**Unit 29:** Applied psychological perspectives **Unit 30:** Health psychology (Follows on from this unit for the Health pathway.) **Unit 4:** Development through the life stages

Unit number, title, year group, and guided learning hours (GLH)	Cross-referenced areas	Cross-referenced with: Unit number and name
Unit 9: Values and planning in health and social care **Year 2 – 60 GLH**	Active promotion of individual rights Individual rights Anti-discriminatory practice Care Value Base Legislation Confidentiality Understanding of own responsibilities Awareness of own attitudes and beliefs Reflective practice Multi-disciplinary working Ethical issues Person-centred approach Communication skills Barriers to communication	**Unit 1:** Developing effective communication in health and social care **Unit 2:** Equality, diversity and rights in health and social care **Unit 6:** Personal and professional development in health and social care
Unit 10: Caring for children and young people **Year 2 – 60 GLH**	Reflective practice Communication skills Barriers to communication Understanding own attitudes Applying theory to practice Legislation Nutritional health of babies and children Therapeutic practices e.g. family therapy Child abuse Confidentiality Individual rights	**Unit 1:** Developing effective communication in health and social care **Unit 2:** Equality, diversity and rights in health and social care **Unit 6:** Personal and professional development in health and social care **Unit 8:** Psychological perspectives for health and social care **Unit 21:** Nutrition for health and social care **Unit 29:** Applied psychological perspectives for health and social care
Unit 11: Supporting and protecting adults **Year 2 – 60 GLH**	Reflective practice Communication skills Barriers to communication Understanding own attitudes Applying theory to practice Legislation Nutritional health of adults Individual rights	**Unit 1:** Developing effective communication in health and social care **Unit 2:** Equality, diversity and rights in health and social care **Unit 6:** Personal and professional development in health and social care **Unit 8:** Psychological perspectives for health and social care **Unit 21:** Nutrition for health and social care **Unit 28:** Caring for older people **Unit 29:** Applied psychological perspectives for health and social care
Unit 12: Public health **Year 1 – 60 GLH**	Historical perspective Patterns of ill health Health promotion activities Health strategies Factors affecting ill health e.g. root causes Pressure groups (e.g. Greenpeace, World Health Organisation) Legislation	**Unit 20:** Health education **Unit 38:** Environmental health **Unit 48:** Social policy for health and social care
Unit 14: Physiological disorders **Year 2 – 60 GLH**	Understanding the human body in terms of body systems	**Unit 5:** Fundamentals of anatomy and physiology for health and social care
Unit 17: Working in the social care sector **Year 1 (for Social Care pathway) – 60 GLH**	Reflective practice Communication skills Barriers to communication Understanding own attitudes Legislation Teamwork Multidisciplinary working Making recommendations Confidentiality Sharing of information	**Unit 1:** Developing effective communication in health and social care **Unit 6:** Personal and professional development in health and social care **Unit 44:** Vocational experience for health and social care **Unit 45:** Competence based vocational experience for health and social care

Unit number, title, year group, and guided learning hours (GLH)	Cross-referenced areas	Cross-referenced with: Unit number and name
Unit 18: Working in the health sector **Year 1 – for Health pathway – 60 GLH**	Reflective practice Communication skills Barriers to communication Understanding own attitudes Legislation Teamwork Multidisciplinary working Making recommendations Confidentiality Sharing of information Application of theory to practice Making recommendations	**Unit 1:** Developing effective communication in health and social care **Unit 6:** Personal and professional development in health and social care **Unit 44:** Vocational experience for health and social care **Unit 45:** Competence based vocational experience for health and social care
Unit 19: Applied sociological perspectives for health and social care **Year 2 – 60 GLH**	Concepts of health and illness Patterns and trends in health and illness Models of health Understanding inequalities in health	**Unit 2:** Equality, diversity and rights in health and social care **Unit 7:** Sociological perspectives **Unit 20:** Health education **Unit 22:** Research methodology for health and social care
Unit 20: Health education **Year 2 – 60 GLH**	Historical perspective Patterns of ill health Health promotion activities Health strategies Factors affecting ill health e.g. root causes Pressure groups (e.g. Greenpeace, World Health Organisation) Influence of health-related beliefs and behaviours Legislation	**Unit 12:** Public health **Unit 30:** Health psychology **Unit 38:** Environmental health **Unit 48:** Social policy for health and social care
Unit 21: Nutrition for health and social care **Year 2 – 60 GLH**	Function of nutrients in body Nutritional health of adults Nutritional health of babies and children Improving health Identifying research need	**Unit 5:** Fundamentals of anatomy and physiology for health and social care **Unit 10:** Caring for children and young people **Unit 11:** Supporting and protecting adults **Unit 14:** Physiological disorders **Unit 20:** Health education **Unit 22:** Research methodology for health and social care
Unit 22: Research methodology for health and social care **Years 1 and 2 – 90 GLH (second semester of year 1 and both semesters of year 2)**	Identifying research need Conducting research Implications of research Effects on policy Patterns and trends in health and illness Ethical issues	**Unit 7:** Sociological perspectives for health and social care **Unit 8:** Psychological perspectives for health and social care **Unit 12:** Public health **Unit 19:** Applied sociological perspectives for health and social care **Unit 29:** Applied psychological perspectives for health and social care **Unit 30:** Health psychology **Unit 38:** Environmental health
Unit 23: Complementary therapies for health and social care **Year 2 – 60 GLH**	Communication skills Barriers to communication Identifying research need Understanding own attitudes Applying theory to practice Legislation Ethical issues	**Unit 1:** Developing effective communication in health and social care **Unit 6:** Personal and professional development in health and social care **Unit 22:** Research methodology for health and social care
Unit 24: Introduction to counselling skills for health and social care **Year 2 – 60 GLH**	Communication skills Barriers to communication Understanding own attitudes Applying theory to practice Legislation Confidentiality Ethical issues	**Unit 1:** Developing effective communication in health and social care **Unit 6:** Personal and professional development in health and social care

Unit 25: Coping with change in a health and social care context **Year 2 – 30 GLH (one semester)**	Life factors Major life events Theories of ageing Biological theory – understanding developmental norms Theories of transition Stress Application of theories to development Support services Understanding the impact of chronic and terminal illness	**Unit 1:** Developing effective communication in health and social care **Unit 4:** Development through the life stages **Unit 8:** Psychological perspectives for health and social care **Unit 28:** Caring for older people **Unit 30:** Health psychology
Unit 26: Caring for individuals with additional needs **Year 2 – 30 GLH (one semester)**	Communication skills Barriers to communication Reflective practice Discrimination Inequality Legislation Empowerment Person-centred planning Models of disability	**Unit 2:** Equality, diversity and rights in health and social care **Unit 6:** Personal and professional development in health and social care **Unit 9:** Values and planning in health and social care **Unit 30:** Health psychology
Unit 27: Dealing with challenging behaviour **Year 2 – 30 GLH (one semester)**	Communication skills Barriers to communication Reflective practice Understanding own attitudes Understanding behaviour of individuals Interventions Effects of residential care on individuals Promoting independence Empowerment	**Unit 1:** Developing effective communication in health and social care **Unit 6:** Personal and professional development in health and social care **Unit 29:** Applied psychological perspectives for health and social care
Unit 28: Caring for older people **Year 2 – 30 GLH (one semester) Could be combined with Unit 40: Dementia Care – 30 GLH (second semester)**	Major life events Theories of ageing Biological theory – understanding developmental norms Theories of transition Stress Application of theories to development Support services Understanding the impact of chronic and terminal illness Nutritional health of older people Person centred approach Legislation Reflective practice Communication skills Barriers to communication Understanding own attitudes Applying theory to practice Individual rights	**Unit 9:** Values and planning in health and social care **Unit 11:** Supporting and protecting adults **Unit 21:** Nutrition for health and social care **Unit 40:** Dementia care
Unit 29: Applied psychological perspectives for health and social care **Year 2 – 60 GLH**	Life factors Major life events Theories of ageing Biological theory – understanding developmental norms Theories of transition Stress Application of theories to development Understanding own attitudes Understanding behaviour of individuals Interventions Effects of residential care on individuals	**Unit 8:** Psychological perspectives for health and social care **Unit 25:** Coping with change in a health and social care context **Unit 27:** Dealing with challenging behaviour **Unit 30:** Health psychology
Unit 30: Health psychology **Year 2 – 60 GLH for Health pathway**	Biological theory – understanding developmental norms Theories of transition Stress Application of theories to development Understanding own attitudes Understanding behaviour of individuals Interventions Effects of residential care on individuals Models of disability	**Unit 8:** Psychological perspectives for health and social care **Unit 25:** Coping with change in a health and social care context **Unit 26:** Caring for individuals with additional needs **Unit 27:** Dealing with challenging behaviour
Unit 34: Human inheritance for health and social care **Year 2 – 60 GLH**	Ethical considerations Health belief model Individual rights and responsibilities Regulation and legislation Societal values	**Unit 8:** Psychological perspectives for health and social care **Unit 20:** Health education **Unit 29:** Applied psychological perspectives for health and social care **Unit 30:** Health psychology

Unit number, title, year group, and guided learning hours (GLH)	Cross-referenced areas	Cross-referenced with: Unit number and name
Unit 38: Environmental health **Year 2 – 60 GLH**	Historical perspective Patterns of ill health Health promotion activities Health strategies Factors affecting ill health, e.g. root causes Pressure groups (e.g. Greenpeace, World Health Organisation) Influence of health-related beliefs and behaviours Legislation	**Unit 12:** Public health **Unit 20:** Health education
Unit 39: Infection prevention and control **Year 2 – 30 GLH (one semester)**	Understanding own responsibilities Legislation Policies and procedures Risk assessment Preventing infection Improving health through education Storage and disposal of waste Storage and disposal of substances Storage and disposal of equipment	**Unit 3:** Health, safety and security in health and social care **Unit 6:** Personal and professional development in health and social care **Unit 12:** Public health
Unit 40: Dementia care **Year 2 – 30 GLH (one semester) Could be combined with Unit 28: Caring for older people – 30 GLH (first semester)**	Major life events Theories of ageing Biological theory – understanding developmental norms Theories of transition Stress Application of theories to development Support services Understanding the impact of chronic and terminal illness Nutritional health of older people Person-centred approach Reflective practice Communication skills Barriers to communication Understanding own attitudes Applying theory to practice Legislation Individual rights	**Unit 4:** Development through the life stages **Unit 6:** Personal and professional development in health and social care **Unit 9:** Values and planning in health and social care **Unit 11:** Supporting and protecting adults **Unit 28:** Caring for older people
Unit 41: Working with medication in health and social care **Year 2 – 30 GLH (one semester)**	Communication skills Legislation Recording and reporting Safe handling of medicines Confidentiality	**Unit 1:** Developing effective communication in health and social care **Unit 3:** Health, safety and security in health and social care **Unit 6:** Personal and professional development in health and social care
Unit 42: Support work in health and social care **Year 2 – 30 GLH (one semester)**	Communication skills Barriers to communication Discrimination Inequality Legislation Empowerment Person centred planning Confidentiality Reflective practice Understanding own attitudes Storage and disposal of waste Storage and disposal of substances Storage and disposal of equipment	**Unit 1:** Developing effective communication in health and social care **Unit 2:** Equality, diversity and rights in health and social care **Unit 3:** Health, safety and security in health and social care **Unit 6:** Personal and professional development in health and social care **Unit 9:** Values and planning in health and social care
Unit 43: Technology in health and social care **Year 2 – 60 GLH**	Communication Overcoming barriers to communication Autonomy Empowerment Care planning Person-centred approach	**Unit 1:** Developing effective communication in health and social care **Unit 2:** Equality, diversity and rights in health and social care **Unit 9:** Values and planning in health and social care

Unit number, title, year group, and guided learning hours (GLH)	Cross-referenced areas	Cross-referenced with: Unit number and name
Unit 44: Vocational experience for health and social care **Year 2 – 60 GLH, plus 200 hours of placement, in addition to 100 hours required for Unit 6: Personal and professional development in health and social care**	Reflective practice Communication skills Barriers to communication Confidentiality Understanding own attitudes Applying theory to practice Legislation Teamwork Personal development plan Recommendations Structure of placement	**Unit 6:** Personal and professional development in health and social care
Unit 45: Competence based vocational experience for health and social care **Year 2 – 60 GLH, plus 200 hours of placement, in addition to 100 hours required for Unit 6: Personal and professional development in health and social care**	Reflective practice Communication skills Barriers to communication Understanding own attitudes Applying theory to practice Legislation Teamwork Confidentiality Personal development plan Recommendations Structure of placement	**Unit 6:** Personal and professional development in health and social care
Unit 46: Independent learning in health and social care **Year 1 – 60 GLH**	Learning styles Reflective practice Personal development plan	**Unit 6:** Personal and professional development in health and social care
Unit 47: Academic literacy in the health and social care sectors **Year 1 – 60 GLH**	Learning styles Reflective practice Personal development plan	**Unit 6:** Personal and professional development in health and social care
Unit 48: Social policy for health and social care **Year 2 – 30 GLH (one semester)**	Concepts of health and illness Patterns and trends in health and illness Models of health Understanding inequalities in health Influence of pressure groups Legislation Policy-making process	**Unit 2:** Equality, diversity and rights in health and social care **Unit 7:** Sociological perspectives for health and social care **Unit 9:** Values and planning in social care **Unit 19:** Applied sociological perspectives for health and social care **Unit 20:** Health education **Unit 38:** Environmental health

1

Developing effective communication in health and social care

unit overview

This unit explores the importance of communication and interpersonal interaction in health and social care. It has strong links with Unit 2 (Equality, diversity and rights in health and social care) and Unit 6 (Personal and professional development in health and social care). The unit is split into four Learning outcomes.

Learning outcomes

On completion of this unit learners should:

1.1 understand the importance of effective communication and interpersonal interaction in health and social care

1.2 understand the factors that influence communication and interpersonal interaction in health and social care

1.3 understand how service users can be assisted by effective communication

1.4 understand how to demonstrate communication skills in a caring role.

Suggested activities

The At-a-glance activity grid shows how the activities in the Assessment and Delivery Resource (ADR) relate to the content of the unit. The activities include introductory and plenary activities and a variety of case studies, research tasks, discussions and presentations, using written, verbal and presentation skills. The activities may help learners prepare for assessment, and the grid indicates which assessment criteria are relevant for each activity. Copies of activity sheets can be given to learners.

Teaching Unit 1

I am fortunate enough to teach Units 1, 2 and 6. If it is possible for you to do likewise, I think you will find it more rewarding and the learners will have a more productive learning experience. Rather than repeating information, you can deliver the underpinning knowledge in one unit and build on this in the other units. I have also found this the best way to facilitate learners' achievement of the merit and distinction criteria for all three units, as I have been able to move them on to analytical and evaluative tasks more quickly. If you are unable to deliver all three units, I would urge you to work closely with your colleagues who are delivering the others, in order to ensure continuity and avoid repetition.

Where possible, Unit 1 and Unit 2 should be delivered in year one of the two-year programme, and Unit 6 should be taught across both years. This will give learners underpinning knowledge and skills early on, before they begin their first placement. Ideally, your learners should not go out to their first placement until around week 6 of Unit 1. The first placement is always a nerve-racking time. However, focusing on communication skills will help to prepare even the most timid learners for their first placement experience. Setting tasks for learners to complete while they are on placement will help them to see the links between theory and practice more clearly. You will see a range of suggested placement activities included in the At-a-glance activity grid, and all learners should be encouraged to keep a reflective journal of their experiences in placement. These reflective journals can be used as material for class discussion.

Role play is an invaluable tool when learning about communication – learners usually enjoy pretending to be angry service users or very professional health or social care workers. It is useful to video these interactions and play them back so that learners can assess their own communication skills and make plans for improvement. (Always remember to follow college protocols concerning recording images of learners, and make sure that any peer evaluation of role play takes place in a positive and supportive atmosphere.) You should encourage learners to draw on their own life experiences when evaluating role plays, as this enables them to see the relevance of reflective practice in their future learning.

Learners also need to understand group dynamics and the effect they can have on communication. An excellent tool for this is *Big Brother*. If you can obtain video clips at various stages of the contest, you will be able to generate fantastic discussion about the norming, forming, storming and conforming stages that can be seen in the *Big Brother* house. Learners will be engaged by this reference to popular culture, particularly if there is currently a new series of *Big Brother* on TV!

Unit 1 is an extremely rewarding unit to teach and one that helps you and your learners get to know each other well. This unit not only enables learners to become effective health and social care professionals but also encourages them to develop their confidence and self-esteem.

The content of each Learning outcome

Learning outcome 1: Understand the importance of effective communication and interpersonal interaction in health and social care (relevant criteria: P1, P2, M1)

The first Learning outcome begins with a PowerPoint® presentation introducing the importance of effective communication skills in health and social care. The Activity 1.12 worksheet is an excellent way to encourage learners to start thinking about how they communicate. This can be followed by the case studies in Activity 1.1, which will help learners formulate more complex ideas about strategies for effective communication. Activity 1.2 (a miming/drawing team game) familiarises learners with different types of communication. This fun activity embeds learning about different types of communication. It also requires learners to practise their own non-verbal skills, and enables them to see the difficulties in communicating without spoken language.

Activity 1.3 (a role play) engages learners for the first time in role play scenarios. You might find that learners are initially unwilling to participate, but it is my experience that most if not all learners will participate and actually enjoy it! I try to include role plays as often as possible so that learners can gradually build their confidence. Activity 1.4 (a PowerPoint Presentation®) and Activity 1.5 (a gapped handout) introduce the idea of the communication cycle and provide an opportunity for learners to understand how the communication cycle works in practice.

Learning outcome 2: Understand the factors that influence communication and interpersonal interaction in health and social care (relevant criteria: P3)

This Learning outcome underpins the other three Learning outcomes, providing the 'backbone' for achievement of all the criteria for Unit 1. The factors that influence effective communication are first introduced in a PowerPoint® presentation and Activity 1.12. These factors are then explored in Activity1.6 (a case study that requires learners to consider how doctor/patient interactions can be improved by overcoming barriers to effective communication). Activity 1.7 is a fun way of embedding learning by pairing communication barriers with strategies to overcome them.

Activity 1.8 is a PowerPoint® presentation that introduces learners to the importance of assertiveness in managing difficult or sensitive situations, and helps them distinguish between assertiveness, aggression and passivity. Activity 1.9 is a reflective exercise designed to make learners think about how open, direct and honest they are in their own interactions. The students' understanding of assertiveness is put to the test in Activity 1.10 (two case studies looking at difficult behaviour). One case study (Lennie) is more complex than the other (Sylvia and Mary) which should help you differentiate the task, according to students' abilities. Learners should read their case study in pairs and consider the strategies they would use to manage the situation and support the individuals involved.

Learning outcome 3: Understand how service users can be assisted by effective communication (relevant criteria: P4, M2, D1)

This Learning outcome introduces support services and aids to communication with a PowerPoint® presentation. Activity 1.11 is a long task requiring learners to research support services, prepare a presentation and present it to the rest of the class, while you and their peers complete witness statements. There are three separate research tasks of varying complexity, focusing on support services, technology or preferred languages, that can be allocated to each group of learners. This activity may take up to three sessions to complete, but it should prove to be extremely rewarding in terms of the learners' development of their own communication skills. I suggest that you ask each group to print copies of their presentation to distribute to the other groups.

Learning outcome 4: Understand how to demonstrate communication skills in a caring role (relevant criteria: P5, P6, M3, D2)

In this Learning outcome the focus is directly on the learner's own communication skills. By this stage, learners should be comfortable reflecting on their own development. They must be able to use their own communication skills effectively in a caring role, and this can be demonstrated by reflective writing and witness statements. All these criteria can be achieved using Activity 1.12 (a reflective writing task/action plan). More space will be required than is provided on the form itself. Activity 1.13 gives learners an opportunity to evaluate their communication skills, based on their experiences in placement. Finally, Activity 1.14 (a quiz game) is a light-hearted way to end the unit, while consolidating learners' knowledge and communication skills!

How this unit will be assessed

To reach Pass level, the evidence must show that the learner is able to:

P1 describe different types of communication and interpersonal interaction, using examples relevant to health and social care settings

P2 describe the stages of the communication cycle

P3 describe factors that may influence communication and interpersonal interactions with particular reference to health and social care settings

P4 identify how the communication needs of patients/service users may be assisted, including non-verbal communication

P5 describe two interactions that you have participated in, in the role of a carer, using communication skills to assist patients/service users

P6 review the effectiveness of own communication skills in the two interactions undertaken.

To reach Merit level, the evidence must show that, in addition to the Pass criteria, the learner is able to:

M1 explain how the communication cycle may be used to communicate difficult, complex and sensitive issues

M2 explain the specific communication needs patients/service users may have that require support, including the use of technology

M3 explain how own communication skills could have been used to make the interactions more effective.

To reach Distinction level, the evidence must show that, in addition to the Pass and Merit criteria, the learner is able to:

D1 analyse how communication in health and social care settings assists patients/service users and other key people

D2 analyse the factors that influenced the interactions undertaken.

The importance of evidence gained during placement experience

It will be easier for learners to achieve all the grading criteria for this unit if they continually record examples of interactions during placement in their reflective journals and obtain as many witness statements as possible. (Witness statements will also be needed as resources for Unit 6.)

The pass and merit criteria are targeted by Learning outcome 1. They are also integrated into Assessment task 1: Create an information booklet. These criteria require learners to provide examples of the specific communication needs of service users (including language needs and preferences, barriers, the influence of behaviour and the effects of the environment). Learners will also be expected to explain how these particular communication needs can be met. Students can achieve the pass and merit criteria using information gained from their research tasks and reflective journals. Creating an information booklet should engage learners in a way that writing essays may not. This task also targets criteria relevant to Learning outcomes 2 and 3. The merit criteria require learners to explain how the communication cycle can be used to communicate complex, difficult and sensitive issues. Again, learners will be able to draw upon examples from their reflective journals and witness statements to achieve these criteria.

Assessment task 2 requires learners to describe two interactions they have participated in during placement, where they have used their communication skills to assist service users. One must be with an individual, the other with a group of individuals. Learners are expected to explore their verbal and non-verbal skills, and the effectiveness of their personal interaction in supporting service users and other key people such as families, friends and staff. To meet the merit and distinction criteria, learners need to explain how they could have used their communication skills to improve the effectiveness of their interactions. They also need to analyse the factors that influence the interaction and make plans for improvement.

Achievement of the distinction criteria for Learning outcome 3 requires a more general approach to the importance of effective communication in health and social care settings. This includes not only communication with service users but also with other key people such as families, friends and staff. Learners should evaluate the use of communication skills in providing a caring and safe environment, which supports the individual.

Assessment tasks

Assessment tasks need to be carefully timed to give learners the best chance of achieving at the highest level. Assuming that learners will undertake at least 50 hours of placement in two different settings in year one of the programme, Task 1 should ideally be set at the end of the first placement, and Task 2 should be set at the end of the second placement.

Task 1 (relevant criteria: P1, P2, P3, P4, M1, M2, D1)

For this task, you should refer to your reflective journal and witness statements from your placement(s). Please remember to maintain the confidentiality of all individuals, whether service users, staff, friends or relatives, by making sure that no one can identify the people you write about.

Create a detailed information booklet (approximately 2000–2500 words) for health and social care workers, giving advice on effective communication and interpersonal interactions.

Describe the stages of the communication cycle and include images and examples of different types of communication and interactions between service users and staff, members of a small group of service users, and service users/staff and you. **(P1, P2)**

Choose at least three of the following types of communication and interpersonal interaction.

Types of communication:

- one to one
- group communication
- formal
- informal
- text
- visual
- music and drama
- arts and crafts
- use of technology.

Types of interpersonal interaction:

- non-verbal
- verbal
- variations between cultures
- listening and reflecting back.

Describe factors that may influence communication and interpersonal interactions (i.e. needs and preferences, environment, behaviour and barriers) in health and social care settings. **(P3)**

Using examples from your placement, explain how the communication cycle may be used to communicate difficult, complex and sensitive issues. **(M1)**

Identify ways in which service users can be assisted in communicating. These methods may include preferred spoken language, non-verbal ways of communicating (e.g. sign language, symbols, pictures, communication passports, objects of reference), use of interpreters and advocates and technological aids. **(P4)**

Using examples from your placement, explain the specific communication needs service users may have that could require support, including the use of technology. **(M2)**

Analyse how communication in health and social care settings can assist service users and other key people. **(D1)**

Task 2 (relevant criteria: P5, P6, M3, D2)

Ask your placement supervisor to observe you undertaking two separate interactions. Ask him/her to complete a witness statement for each. This statement should detail your use of communication skills, both verbal and non-verbal, in supporting the service users. **(P5)**

1   An interaction with an individual service user where, in the role of carer, you used your communication skills to assist him/her (e.g. assisting with eating).

2   An interaction with a group of service users where, in the role of carer, you used your communication skills to assist them (e.g. in a group activity such as a game of cards or bingo).

You should consider whether the communication cycle could be seen working, how you overcame any barriers to the interaction, and whether your verbal and non-verbal communication skills were appropriate. Using the reflective writing/action plan form, one for each interaction, review the effectiveness of your own communication skills in the two interactions undertaken. **(P6)**

Explain how your communication skills could have been used to make the two interactions more effective. **(M3)**

Analyse the factors that influenced the two interactions undertaken and make plans for improvement. **(D2)**

Scheme of work

BTEC National Health and Social Care
Unit 1 Developing effective communication in health and social care

Broad aim: Successful completion of the unit

Teacher(s): ....

Academic year: ....

Number of weeks: 35

Duration of session: 2 hours

Guided learning hours: 70

Week/s	Topic/outcome	Tutor preparation	Student activity	Resources	Links to grading criteria
1	Introduction to Unit 1: The importance of effective communication in health and social care	Use PowerPoint® 1 as an introduction to the themes. For Activity 1.1, distribute both case studies to the class and give them five minutes to read them	Direct and indirect questions are used to generate discussion with Activity 1.1	PowerPoint® 1, Activity 1.1, Activity 1.12 (optional)	All
2–3	Types of communication (team game)	Prepare the cards in advance	Group work can be used to get learners thinking about communication	Activity 1.2	P1, P2, M1
3–4	Types of interpersonal interaction (role play)	Record the learners' interactions on video and play them back so that they can evaluate their communication skills	Discussion in pairs; role playing will encourage learners to empathise with the situations in the case studies. Group discussion of each role play allows learners to think in more depth about issues raised. **Activity for placement: Identify different types of interaction in placement**	Activity 1.3	P1, P2, M1
4–6	The communication cycle	Activity 1.4 is a PowerPoint® and can be used as an introduction to the themes. For Activity 1.5 a scenario is provided to assist learners	Learners complete the cycle by working through the stages. Learners can either work in pairs or larger groups on this activity, or discuss their answers with the rest of the group on completion	Activity 1.4, Activity 1.5	P1, P2, M1
7–8	How do I communicate?	The worksheet from Activity 1.12 forms the basis of an action plan to improve communication skills. This activity can be used one or more times (e.g. in weeks 1, 7–8, 29–30, 31–34)	Students should work individually to complete the form **Activity for placement: Write a reflective account of how you used your communication skills in one interaction**	Activity 1.12	P5, P6, M3, D2
9–12	Verbal and non-verbal communication	Use PowerPoint® 2 as an introduction to the themes	Encourage learners to discuss the themes and relate them back to the earlier topics	PowerPoint® 2	P5, P6, M3, D2
12–13	Factors that influence communication	For Activity 1.6, distribute the case study to the whole class and encourage them to write their answers to the questions	Use answers from individual students to generate discussion	Activity 1.6	P3

Unit 1 Developing effective communication in health and social care

Week/s	Topic/outcome	Tutor preparation	Student activity	Resources	Links to grading criteria
14–15	Overcoming barriers to communication (pairing game)	You need thin card cut into sets of 35	In small groups of two or three, learners pair up ways of overcoming barriers with the barrier to be overcome. Learners can also create their own cards. **Activity for placement: Identify and describe an example of an interaction where barriers to communication have been managed successfully**	Activity 1.7	P3
16–17	Assertiveness	Activity 1.8 is a PowerPoint® and can be used as an introduction to the themes. Activity 1.9 enables learners to explore their own assertiveness	Learners can split into pairs and question each other on this exercise. Use learners' answers to generate discussion about strategies for developing assertiveness	Activity 1.8, Activity 1.9	P3
18–20	Case studies: Managing behaviour	One case study (Lennie) is more complex than the other (Sylvia and Mary). Put learners into pairs and allocate a case study to each pair according to ability	Each pair should decide upon their strategies. Then you should generate a class discussion so that the pairs can share their ideas with the rest of the class. **Activity for placement: Identify an example from placement where challenging behaviour has been managed effectively**	Activity 1.10	P3
21–24	Assisting effective communication; Support services (research task)	Use PowerPoint® 3 as an introduction to the themes. You could complete a witness statement based on learners' presentation skills	Learners can work in small groups to aid differentiation. Learners will use group work, discussion and presentation skills to complete this activity	PowerPoint® 3, Activity 1.11	P4, M2, D1
25–28	Demonstrating own communication skills	Use PowerPoint® 4 as an introduction to the themes		PowerPoint® 4	P5, P6, M3, D2
29–30	Effectiveness in supporting service users	The worksheet from Activity 1.12 forms the basis of an action plan to improve communication skills	Learners should work individually to complete the form. **Activity for placement: Identify an example from placement of a service user being supported with effective communication skills**	Activity 1.12	P5, P6, M3, D2
31–34	Reviewing own communication skills	Make observations of skills used by learners, and encourage them to keep a record of good examples	Learners to evaluate their own skills. This can be done by working alone	Activity 1.13	P5, P6, M3, D2
35	Review of Unit 1 content (quiz game)	Up to four teams can play this game	Group work – try and ensure an equal spread of skill levels across the teams	Activity 1.14	All

At-a-glance activity grid
Unit 1 Developing effective communication in health and social care

Activity	Title and description	Scheme of work	File/CD	Delivery notes	Additional resources	Links to grading criteria	Activities for placement / Links to other units	Links to Student Book 1
Outcome 1.1 Understand the importance of effective communication and interpersonal interaction in health and social care								
Power Point 1	Introduction to Unit 1 and Learning outcome 1	Week 1	CD	Introduce the importance of effective communication in health and social care. Use in conjunction with Activity 1.1 case studies		P1, P2, M1		pp 4–17
1.1	Effective communication: Two case studies	Week 1	File	Use in conjunction with PowerPoint 1. Distribute both case studies to class and give them five minutes to read them. Ask direct and indirect questions to generate discussion about effective communication		P1, P2, M1		pp 4–17
1.2	Types of communication	Weeks 2–3	File (Tutor information on CD)	Learners to mime or draw types of communication for the rest of their team to guess	Whiteboard, pen, cards (as in Tutor information)	P1, P2, M1		pp 4–17
1.3	Role play	Weeks 3–4	File	Four different role play scenarios for learners to work at in pairs, practising effective communication skills in supporting a service user. Once learners have practised, you should record the interactions and play back on a TV. Not only is this good fun, but learners will be able to evaluate their communication skills, both verbal and non-verbal	Video camera and TV	P1, P2, M1	Learners should look out for examples of effective communication skills being used to support service users, and record them in their reflective journals. They should also use their journals to record times when they use effective communication skills themselves	pp 4–17
1.4	Communication cycle: PowerPoint presentation	Weeks 4–6	CD	Introduces the communication cycle. Use in conjunction with Activity 1.5		P1, P2, M1		pp 4–17
1.5	The communication cycle	Weeks 4–6	File	Learners to complete the cycle by working through the stages in a gapped handout. A scenario is provided to assist learners		P1, P2, M1		pp 4–17

Activity	Title and description	Scheme of work	File/CD	Delivery notes	Additional resources	Links to grading criteria	Activities for placement / Links to other units	Links to Student Book 1
1.12	How do I communicate?	Weeks 7–8	File	Learners to complete reflective worksheet/action plan		**P1, P2, M1**	Learners to identify and record examples of times when they have communicated effectively with a service user in placement. They should ask their placement supervisor to observe them and record their observations as a witness statement. This could contribute to the assessment criteria for this unit (see Assessment task 1)	pp 4–17
Outcome 1.2 Understand the factors that influence communication and interpersonal interaction in health and social care								
Power Point® 2	Introduction to Learning outcome 2	Weeks 9–12	CD	Introduce the factors that influence effective communication. Use in conjunction with Activity 1.6		**P3**	Learners to look at the furniture in their placement. Can the layout be improved in any way to help the service users communicate more effectively?	pp 18–34
1.6	Dr Jones: Case study	Weeks 12–13	File	Case study that looks at poor communication skills in patient/doctor interactions. Distribute case study to whole class and encourage them to write their answers to the questions before you generate discussion		**P3**		pp 18–34
1.7	Overcoming barriers	Weeks 14–15	File (Tutor information on CD)	In small groups of two or three, learners pair up ways of overcoming barriers with the barrier to be overcome	Cards (as in Tutor information)	**P3**	Learners to write in their reflective journal ways in which they have overcome barriers to communication in placement. How effective was this? Links to Unit 6, Learning outcome 2	pp 18–34
1.8	Assertiveness: PowerPoint® presentation	Weeks 16–17	CD	Introduce the importance of assertiveness in health and social care. Use in conjunction with Activity 1.9		**P3**	Ask learners if there is anyone in placement who they would say is assertive. Why and what effect does this have on their communication with service users and members of staff? Learners to record this in their reflective journals	pp 18–34

Activity	Title and description	Scheme of work	File/CD	Delivery notes	Additional resources	Links to grading criteria	Activities for placement / Links to other units	Links to Student Book 1
1.9	How assertive are you?	Weeks 16–17	File	Learners explore their own assertiveness. You should generate discussion about strategies for developing assertiveness		P3	Learners to practise assertiveness skills in placement and ask their supervisor to complete a witness statement outlining how they managed the situation. Learners should reflect on the following questions: How well did you communicate? Have your communication skills improved since you started your placement? What further improvements could you make?	pp 18–34
1.10	Behaviour: case studies	Weeks 18–20	File	Two case studies for learners to decide how they would manage the situation. One case study (Lennie) is more complex than the other (Sylvia and Mary). Put learners into pairs and allocate a case study to each pair according to ability. Each pair should decide upon their strategies. Then you should generate a class discussion so that the pairs can share their ideas with the rest of the class		P3	Ask learners if they have witnessed any examples of difficult behaviour in their placement? How was it managed and by whom? They should record this in their reflective journals	pp 18–34
Outcome 1.3 Understand how service users can be assisted by effective communication								
Power Point® 3	Introduction to Learning outcome 3	Weeks 21–24	CD	Introduce support services and aids to communication. Use in conjunction with Activity 1.11		P4, M2, D1		pp 35–41
1.11	Support services	Weeks 21–24	File	Three different tasks of varying complexity for small groups to research and prepare a PowerPoint® presentation. You could complete a witness statement based on their presentation skills		P4, M2, D1	Ask learners if any of these services are used by service users in their placement? They should ask their placement supervisor if they can observe an interaction which utilises one of the support services (if appropriate). They should record this in their reflective journals	pp 35–41

Outcome 1.4 Understand how to demonstrate communication skills in a caring role

Activity	Title and description	Scheme of work	File/CD	Delivery notes	Additional resources	Links to grading criteria	Activities for placement Links to other units	Links to Student Book 1
Power Point® 4	Introduction to Learning outcome 4	Weeks 25–28	CD			**P5, P6, M3, D2**	Encourage learners to keep a reflective log of interactions from placement. They will keep a reflective journal for Unit 6 so this can be part of that. It can be used to evaluate communication skills and will contribute to Unit 6, Learning outcome 2	pp 42–43
1.12	How do I communicate?	Weeks 29–30	File	Learners to identify their own communication style and make plans for improvement. Worksheet forms the basis of an action plan regarding improving communication skills	Video clip of inappropriate communication skills. (Should be something amusing, e.g. from *Little Britain* or *The Catherine Tate Show!*)	**P5, P6, M3, D2**	Learners to identify and record examples of positive and negative communication between placement staff and service users. Links to Unit 6, Learning outcome 2	pp 42–43
1.13	How can you evaluate your own communication skills?	Weeks 31–34	File	This handout helps learners reflect on their communication skills		**P5, P6, M3, D2**		pp 42–43
1.14	Plenary activity: Communication skills quiz game	Week 35	CD (see Tutor information and Answers)	To consolidate learners' knowledge at end of unit. Up to four teams can play the game		All		pp 42–43

Unit 1 Lesson plan

Aims

- To introduce Unit 1
- To encourage learners to identify their own communication style and to make plans for improvement.

This structure may be spread over a number of lessons as required.

Learning outcomes
- be able to identify own communication style
- be able to list ways of developing communication skills
- be able to see the link between effective communication skills and supporting service users
- begin to develop first action plan.

Timing	Content	Teacher activity	Student activity	Resources	Individualised activity
5 mins	Welcome learners and register	Introduce unit: tutor to display lesson aims and objectives on flipchart		Flipchart	
10 mins	State Learning outcomes and introduce unit content by providing simplified version of Scheme of work. Relate assessment of unit to placement	Moderate use of language to ensure full understanding of all learners. Use indirect questions to check understanding		Copies of simplified version of Scheme of work	
15 mins	PowerPoint® presentation	Moderate use of language to ensure full understanding of all learners	All learners engaged and responding to direct/indirect questioning	PowerPoint® 1	
20 mins	Activity 1.12: Reflective writing task/Action plan	Explain task using different levels of language		Activity 1.12 worksheets	Circulate around class to check understanding and offer assistance or extension where needed
20 mins	Group work	Divide learners into groups of four. Give each group a sheet of flipchart paper and some pens. Ask learners to divide paper into four sections, and write one group member's name in each section. Refer them back to their Activity 1.12 worksheets and the communication style they identified as their own. Encourage each group to discuss how each member could improve these skills in preparation for placement. Offer positive feedback and praise in response to learners' suggestions. Remind them that all comments *must* be positive. You should expect to see at least four points for each learner	Responding to indirect and direct questioning. Relating to each other in groups and responding to questions	Flipchart, pens	Circulate around class to check understanding and offer assistance or extension where needed

10 mins	Each group to nominate one member to explain how each member needs to develop their communication skills		Interpreting the requirements of the task		Repeat information offered by learners in different forms (i.e. moderate language for extension and differentiation)
5 mins	Learners to complete 'Areas for development' section of their worksheet, using information on flipchart paper	Collect in partially completed Action plans for informal assessment. These should be returned to learners in next lesson	Completing 'Areas for development' section of worksheet	Activity 1.12 worksheets	Circulate around class to check understanding and offer assistance or extension where needed
5 mins	Recap learning outcomes	Ask if there are any questions. Thank you. Close	Responding to indirect and direct questioning		

1.1   Effective communication: Two case studies

Student Book 1
pp 2–17

Rachael and Miss Telford

Rachael is shy and quiet. She works in a care home for the elderly. She has been asked by her manager to help Miss Telford put on her coat. Rachael has not spoken to Miss Telford before and says to her, 'Come on, Miss Telford. You are going out, so put your coat on!' Miss Telford starts to cry. Rachael feels angry and then shouts at Miss Telford to stop being silly.

■ What should Rachael have done before going to help Miss Telford?

■ What did Rachael do wrong?

■ How would you suggest that Rachael should communicate with Miss Telford to support her?

■ What would you say and how would you say it?

Ben and Sue

Ben is a teenager with cerebral palsy and limited speech. He is a wheelchair user and is unable to feed or care for himself. However, his cognitive ability is normal. Sue is a new carer who has come to Ben's home to assist him. She does not know any details of Ben's condition, just that he needs personal care. When she first meets him she talks loudly and slowly. This annoys Ben and he shouts back. Sue assumes that, because Ben is physically disabled, he must have cognitive disabilities. She therefore ignores the fact that he is shouting at her and carries on with her tasks.

■ What should Sue have done before meeting Ben?

■ What did Sue do wrong?

■ How should Sue communicate with Ben to support him?

■ What would you say and how would you say it?

1.2   Miming and drawing game: Types of communication

Student Book 1
pp 2–17

For this activity, your tutor will divide the class into two teams. Some cards will be placed on a table at the front of the class. Each one will have a type of communication written on it. Each team member will take it in turns to come to the front, select a card and either act out the type of communication or draw it on the board (like a game of Charades or Pictionary) for their team members to guess.

When one team can't guess the answer, the other team takes a turn. Continue until you have a winner.

1.3   Four role plays

Student Book 1
pp 2–17

In pairs, practise the following role plays. Each role play will be shown to the rest of the group and recorded for your evaluation.

Role play 1
One of you is an elderly man called Alf, who is in a care home. Alf thinks someone has stolen his money from the drawer in his room. He is angry and upset. One of you is the carer who responds to Alf's shouts that his money is missing. How do you support Alf and manage the situation with effective communication skills?

Role play 2
One of you is Rosie, a young woman who is terminally ill. She tells you that she really wants to leave hospital and go home. One of you is the carer Rosie talks to. How do you support Rosie and manage the interaction with effective communication skills?

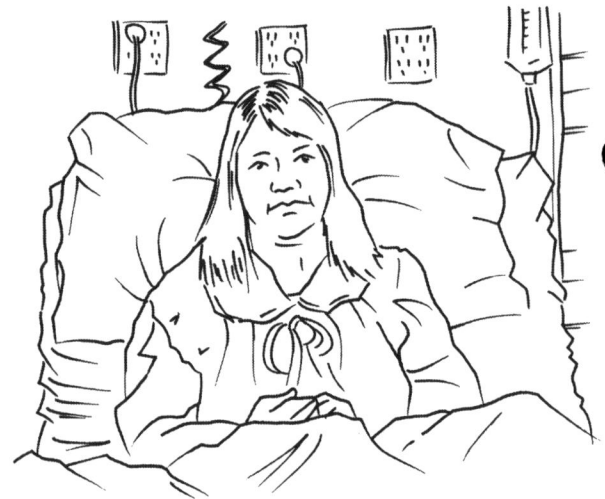

Role play 3
One of you is Helen, a teenager with a learning disability. She goes to a respite centre every weekend to give her parents a rest. It is Friday and she does not want to go; she becomes angry and aggressive. One of you is the social worker who arrives to take Helen to the respite centre. How do you use effective communication skills to support Helen and her parents, while at the same time managing the situation?

Role play 4
One of you is Austin, a middle-aged man with multiple sclerosis. He is feeling very depressed because his condition is getting worse. He says he can't see any point to life any more. One of you is the carer who cares for Austin in his home every day. How do you use effective communication skills to support Austin?

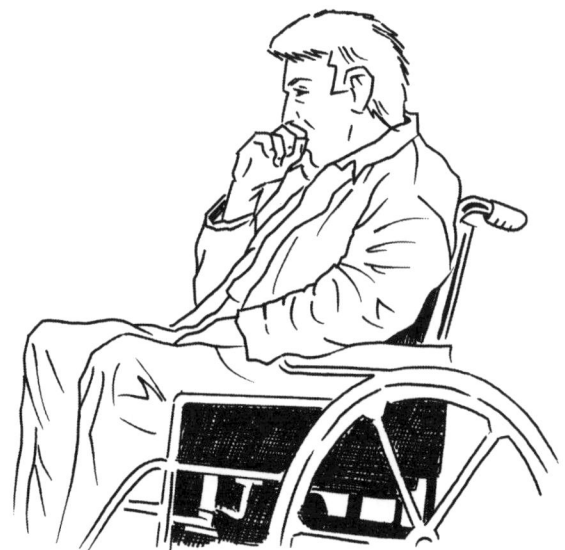

1.5   The communication cycle

Student Book 1
pp 2–17

Complete the missing information in the sentences below:

In order for me to communicate effectively with service users and staff, the

…………..……………………. must be completed.

Stage 1: The sender decides *what* they are going to say.

Stage 2: The sender decides *how* they are going to say it. This can be by using

……………………………, …………………………………,

…………………………………, or …………………………………….

Stage 3: The information is sent to the other person.

Stage 4: The other person receives the information.

Stage 5: The other person makes sense of the information or ……………………………it.

Stage 6: The other person shows a reaction, which can be …………………………….

if the communication is taking place face to face.

Stage 7: The other person may send a ……………………………………, which

completes the communication cycle.

There are many factors which act as ………………………… and may interrupt the

communication cycle. These include:

L……………….D……………..………

D……………………….

E……………………….

T………… **of V**…………….

B……………………….

T………….

E……… C………………..

B…………… L……………………..

Continued overleaf

1.5 The communication cycle (*contd*)

The communication cycle in practice

Imagine you are serving afternoon tea and biscuits in Rose View Elderly Care home. Ethel is 96 years old and a wheelchair user. You ask her if she would like a cup of tea and she says 'Yes please'. Complete the communication cycle to show each stage of the interaction:

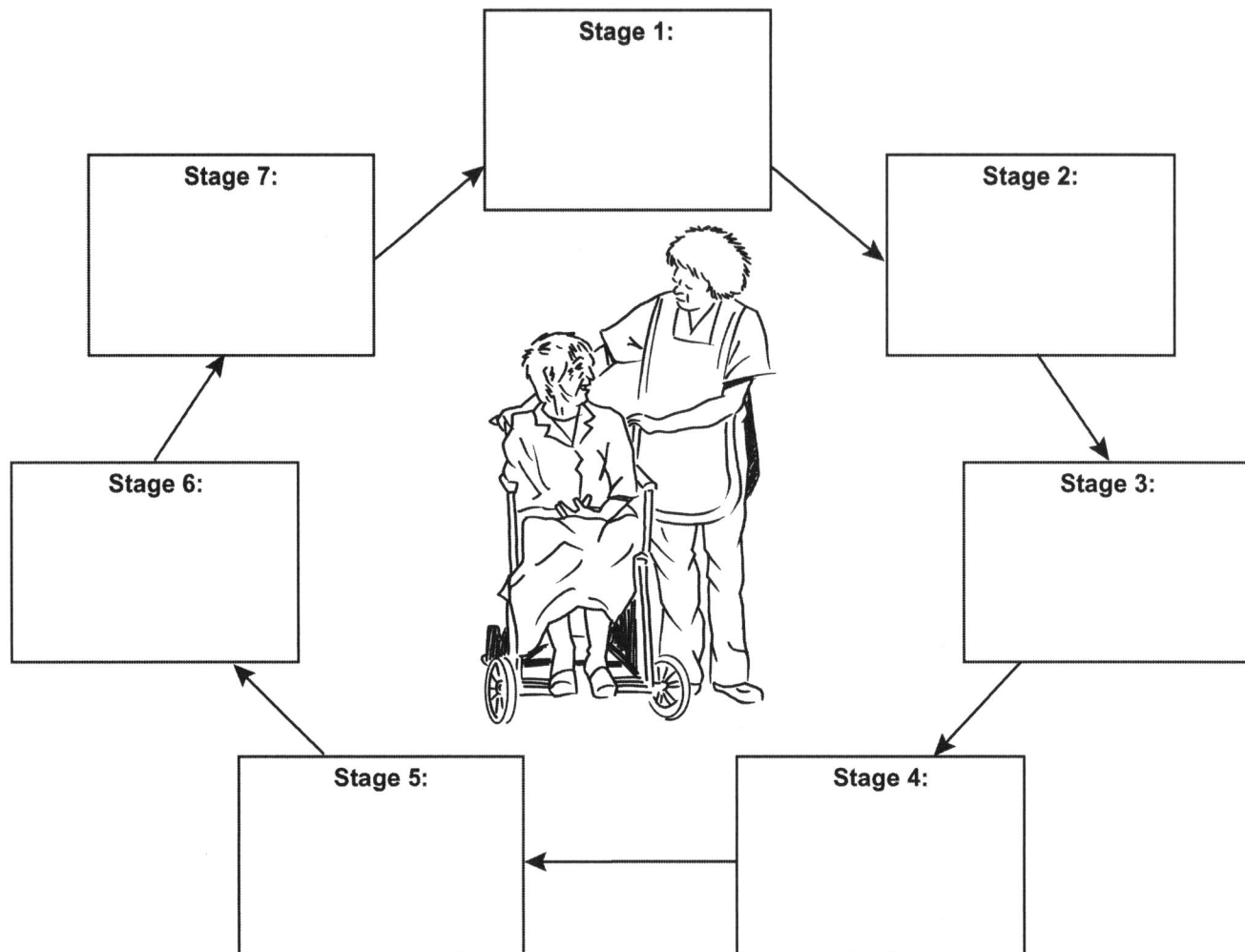

Stage 1:

Stage 2:

Stage 3:

Stage 4:

Stage 5:

Stage 6:

Stage 7:

1.6 Case study: Dr Jones

Student Book 1
pp 18–34

Dr Jones is a GP. He has been working at Cherry Hill Surgery for over 30 years and is retiring in two years' time. He describes himself as a 'traditional family doctor' and has old-fashioned views about the doctor/patient relationship:

- He insists that his consulting room is laid out in a traditional way, with his chair behind a large oak desk.

- He has the radio on, tuned to Radio 4.

- He refuses to use a computer to access patient notes or information about medication so his desk is always piled high with files, notes and other items.

- He insists on sticking to the 'five-minute rule'. (Patients never get longer than five minutes with him.)

- He does not encourage patients to describe any personal concerns and asks them to stick to the physical symptoms.

- He sits behind his desk and looks at the patient with raised eyebrows.

- He does not comment on the physical symptoms until he has made his diagnosis. Then he writes out a prescription.

- Patients leave the surgery with very little information about their symptoms.

Discuss the following questions:

- How do you think Dr Jones makes his patients feel?

- Do you think some patients might prefer this style of communication?

- What improvements could Dr Jones make to his consulting room and to his personal communication style?

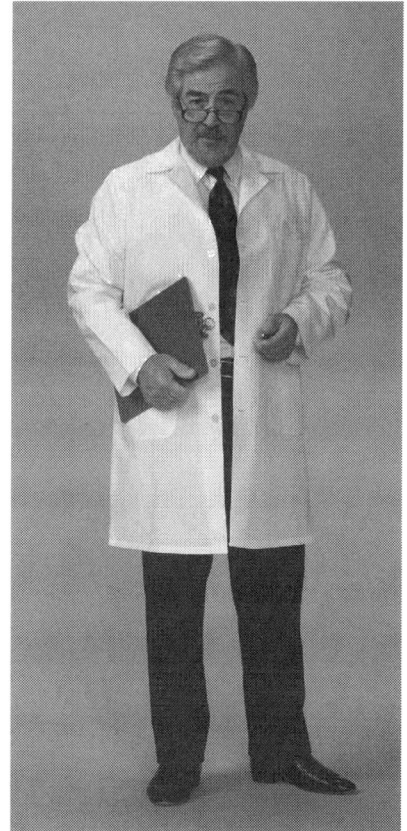

1.7   Pairing game: Overcoming barriers

For this activity, your tutor will put you into groups of two or three, and give you a set of 35 cards.

Six of the cards will show the following headings:

- Visual disability

- Hearing disability

- Environmental barriers

- Language barriers

- Physical disabilities

- Cognitive difficulties.

The remaining cards will show ways of overcoming these barriers to communication. In your groups, you need to pair up the ways of overcoming barriers with the appropriate headings. You will have about 15–20 minutes for this activity.

1.9   Worksheet: How assertive are you?

Student Book 1
pp 18–34

Do you agree with the following statements?

1 I have the right to state my own needs.

2 I have the right to be treated with respect as an intelligent human being.

3 I have the right to express my feelings.

4 I have the right to express my opinions and values.

5 I have the right to say 'YES' or 'NO'.

6 I have the right to make mistakes.

7 I have the right to change my mind.

8 I have the right to say 'I don't understand'.

9 I have the right to ask for what I want.

10 I have the right to decline responsibility for other people's problems.

Now think about the people in your life and how you relate to them. Look at the table below and tick the boxes that apply to you and your relationships with these other people. By looking across the table you will be able to see which skills you need to develop.

	Parents	Partner	Brothers/sisters	Friends	Teachers
Tell them I appreciate them					
Offer my opinion					
Feel embarrassed					
Ask for things					
Get angry					
Show I feel hurt					
Say no					
Refuse to be put down					
Become aggressive					
Complain					
Try to get my own way					
Say the right thing so as not to upset them					

Who are you most assertive with? Why do you think this is?

How will you develop your assertiveness to prepare yourself for working in health and social care?

[21]

1.10 Case studies: Managing behaviour

Student Book 1
pp 18–34

Lennie

Lennie is 36 years old. He attends a day centre for people with brain injuries. You are working there for your placement and you are playing a game of pool with Lennie. When you win, Lennie becomes angry and aggressive. He throws the pool cue down on the floor and moves towards you.

What do you do, and how do you manage the situation?

Sylvia and Mary

Sylvia is 54 years old and has lived in institutional care all her life. She has learning difficulties and can find it hard to communicate with other service users. Mary lives in the same residential home as Sylvia and they are friends. Sylvia and Mary are sitting together in the lounge when they start to argue about something on the TV. The argument gets louder and Sylvia starts to swear. One of the other service users becomes upset, as he does not like shouting.

What do you do, and how do you manage the situation?

1.11   Group task: Researching support services

Student Book 1
pp 35–41

In groups of two or three, research the following subjects. At the end of each task, prepare a PowerPoint® presentation in order to share your group's findings with the rest of the class.

Task 1: Support services

- Advocates
- Interpreters
- Translators
- Signers
- Speech therapists
- Counsellors
- Mentors
- Befrienders
- Psychologists

For each of these services, investigate the following questions:

- Who is the service for?
- What does the service offer?
- How can this service help people with communication difficulties?
- How do people access the service?
- Is it free or do people have to pay for it?

Task 2: Preferred languages

- Makaton
- Signalong
- Braille

For each of these languages, investigate the following questions:

- Who is likely to use this language?
- Where is it used?
- How does it help people to communicate effectively?

Task 3: Technological aids

Investigate the following questions:

- What technological aids are available?
- What does each one do?
- Who would use them?
- How can people access them?
- Are they free?
- Are there any amazing advances in technology that have not yet reached the general public?

1.12   Worksheet/Action plan: How do you communicate?

Student Book 1
pp 2–17

Think about how you communicate with other people. Tick one characteristic from the following list:

- Quiet
- Shy
- Loud
- Chatty
- Argumentative
- Aggressive
- Silly
- Immature
- Rude.

Write a couple of lines to explain why you think you are:

Why do you think your communication style is sometimes like this?

Areas for development

What will you need to change about the way you communicate in order to work effectively in health or social care?

How do you think you will do this? What will you actually do?

Continued overleaf

1.12 Worksheet/Action plan: How do you communicate? (*contd*)

Reflective writing/action plan

Consider one of the interactions you have been involved in during placement. This may have been with a service user, a group of service users, a service user's family and friends, or members of staff.

What happened?

Think about how effective your communication was. Did you use appropriate communication skills?

Is there anything you can improve?

How did I communicate and do I need to make improvements?

What strategies will you use to make these improvements?

How can I improve my communication skills?

When will you achieve this?

When will I achieve this?

Student name..   **Date**..

Date of next review..   **Tutor signature**..

1.13   How can you evaluate your own communication skills?

Student Book 1
pp 42–43

While you are on placement, it is important to evaluate your own communication skills.

Listening is one of the most important communication skills and you can learn a lot about your own skills by monitoring:

- the quality of your contribution to an interaction

- your improvement compared with a previous occasion

- your knowledge and understanding.

This listening and monitoring can be done using a variety of methods:

- Verbal feedback can be obtained from the person with whom you are interacting.

- Verbal feedback can be obtained from an observer.

- Written feedback, in the form of a witness statement, can be obtained from an observer (usually the placement supervisor).

- The interaction can be filmed. Video observation is useful, because you can actually see your own behaviour. You may see things that you had not noticed while you were engaged in the interaction.

Why do you need to reflect on your communication skills?

Reflecting on your experiences is vital for both understanding and improvement. Learning to use effective communication skills in all situations requires reflective practice. It is important for you to observe and reflect not only on your own communication skills but also on other people's communication skills. Even the most advanced health and social care professionals undertake a process of continual reflective practice.

Practice makes perfect

You should consider regularly recording interactions from your placement and considering ways in which you could improve them. This will help you with the distinction criteria for Unit 1 and Unit 4.

2

Equality, diversity and rights in health and social care

unit overview

This unit explores equality, diversity and rights in health and social care. Some tutors might expect this subject to be a bit dry – because of the conventions, legislation and charters detailed in the specification. But I love it! The unit is split into four Learning outcomes.

Learning outcomes

On completion of this unit learners should:

2.1 understand concepts of equality, diversity and rights in relation to health and social care

2.2 understand discriminatory practice in health and social care

2.3 understand how national initiatives promote anti-discriminatory practice in health and social care

2.4 understand how anti-discriminatory practice is promoted in health and social care settings.

Suggested activities

The At-a-glance activity grid shows how the activities in the Assessment and Delivery Resource (ADR) relate to the content of the unit. The activities include introductory and plenary activities and a variety of case studies, research tasks, discussions and presentations, using written, verbal and presentation skills. The activities may help learners prepare for assessment, and the grid indicates which assessment criteria are relevant for each activity. Copies of activity sheets can be given to learners.

Teaching Unit 2

Health and social care learners are drawn to a caring profession, and therefore usually respect other people's values and beliefs. Yet I have had some of the most exciting, amusing and moving moments with learners during this unit as they have started to understand the causes of discrimination and begun to make huge changes to their own attitudes and beliefs. The practical effects of these changes can be seen not just in placement but also in their relationships with other learners and with college staff.

A few years ago I had a learner who was fairly 'fixed' in her attitudes towards other people. This led to a great deal of hard work and sometimes confrontation with myself and other learners. But by the end of the course she had become an equality, diversity and rights ambassador for the college. She even spoke on the subject in public, at an event attended by local dignitaries. I can't tell you how proud I felt!

It is not difficult to make this unit interesting, but you do need to have a passion for the subject. It is important to continually relate the four Learning outcomes to learners' personal experience. You also need to encourage them to see the relevance of the 'boring bits' to things they are interested in, such as the attitudes and views of Jade, Jo and Danielle in *Big Brother 2007*! This will have benefits later on, when they come to reflect on their own practice.

I also like to use other types of real-life material. For instance, you will notice that I have included case studies about David 'Rocky' Bennett, abuse of the elderly, and abuse of children and young people with disabilities.

When discussing discrimination it is important to use real examples, as this helps learners to grasp the horrendous impact that discrimination can have. Learners are more likely to become outraged at the treatment of these people if they are *real* people.

Unit 2 will give you perhaps the best opportunity of any unit to really get to know your learners. Providing you make them feel safe, and assure them that all discussion is completely confidential, they will open up to you and their fellow learners. The knowledge you gain about your learners will enable you to help them make major changes in their lives, and thereby increase the positive impact they will have when working in health and social care services. I hope you will enjoy teaching this unit and will see your learners grow and mature, into open-minded, tolerant and effective anti-discriminatory practitioners.

The content of each Learning outcome

Learning outcome 1: Understand concepts of equality, diversity and rights in relation to health and social care (relevant criteria: P1, P2)

The first Learning outcome introduces the idea that diversity is important to our society with a PowerPoint® presentation. This may be the first time that learners have been expected to formulate their own views on diversity. Some of them may have very 'fixed' opinions on subjects such as immigration and homosexuality but it is very important that there is no condemnation of them for their views. If learners don't feel free to express their ideas openly, there is little possibility of the unit content being able to effect any change for the better!

This Learning outcome also looks at the new terminology relating to diversity and equality, which learners may not have come across before. They will be more confident about expressing their thoughts and ideas if they are familiar with the terminology. They will also need to use the correct terminology in order to meet the P2 criterion. I have included a pairing task (Activity 2.1), which should help you deliver this rather dull topic!

The benefits of diversity can be explored using Activity 2.2 (a PowerPoint® presentation), 2.3 (a gapped handout) and 2.4 (a poster task). These activities will provide learners with relevant information and the opportunity to formulate their own opinions on the subject. At the same time, they will be working towards achievement of the P1 criterion (Explain the benefits of diversity to society). Activity 2.6 (a group task) encourages learners to consider an individual's rights within a health and social care setting. It also gives learners a chance to consider whether they have different rights from service users. This task, together with the Care Value Base activities (2.7 and 2.8) and the complaints activities (2.9 and 2.10), should enable learners to achieve the P2 criterion (Use recognised terminology to explain the importance of promoting equality, recognising diversity and respecting rights in health and social care).

Learning outcome 2: Understand discriminatory practice in health and social care (relevant criterion: P3)

Although the Assessment tasks for the second Learning outcome only relate to one criterion (P3), there is a lot of information to cover. I have included a PowerPoint® presentation which explores the roots of discrimination and its potential effects on service users within health and social care settings, together with the cycle of disadvantage. This can be used in conjunction with the Activity 2.11 gapped handout. Activity 2.12 uses some real-life examples of the effects of discrimination, focusing on some extreme cases of abuse. In their groups, learners should discuss the bases of discrimination in their particular article. You can then lead a class discussion exploring these difficult issues, but you need to remain vigilant in case any learner becomes overly distressed. You may be unaware of similar events that have occurred in a learner's own life.

By the end of Learning outcome 2, learners' attitudes and beliefs will undoubtedly have changed. It would be a good idea to use Activity 2.17 at the beginning of this Learning outcome and again at the end, just to see how different their views are!

Learning outcome 3: Understand how national initiatives promote anti-discriminatory practice in health and social care (relevant criteria: P4, M1, D1)

Now we come to the really dull bit – legislation and codes of practice. This is an example of why it is so important to work closely with your colleagues who are teaching other units on the course. I have known learners cover the Human Rights Act in three different units! Please don't make them go over it more than once. If you do, they will let you know (loud and clear) how boring they find this topic.

A PowerPoint® presentation introduces the relevant legislation, conventions and codes of practice. Then Activity 2.13 (a handout) helps learners make the link between legislation and organisational policies. Activity 2.14 (Understanding legislation) is a group task that engages learners' research skills as well as their creativity. Each group of learners is required to design a display board, and you will need to find enough display boards for each group to have one. There are huge benefits to this activity. Learners will be able to clarify important points from the main pieces of legislation, while presenting this information to the rest of the college (depending on the location of the display boards). In my experience, these displays generate lots of interest, mostly positive and sometimes controversial. The controversial comments can then provide good material for further discussion! This task is followed by Activity 2.15, in which learners investigate how a particular piece of legislation supports service users' rights. Finally, Activity 2.16 is a PowerPoint® presentation and task on the issue of service users' right to privacy and confidentiality.

By the end of Learning outcome 3, learners should be familiar with the main conventions, legislation, codes of practice and charters relating to health and social care. They should understand the links between national initiatives and organisational policies, and they should be able to explain their practical applications in health and social care settings.

Learning outcome 4: Understand how anti-discriminatory practice is promoted in health and social care settings (relevant criteria: P5, P6, M2, M3, D2)

In the fourth Learning outcome, a PowerPoint® presentation introduces the idea that the individual has a direct influence on anti-discriminatory practice. In Activity 2.17 (Reflective practice/Action plan worksheet) learners are encouraged to reflect on their own practice regarding anti-discriminatory practice. Activity 2.18, a crossword on equality, diversity and rights in health and social care, is a light-hearted way to finish this unit and consolidate learners' knowledge.

By the end of Learning outcome 4, learners should understand the importance of individuals taking responsibility for their own anti-discriminatory practice. They should also be prepared to actively promote inclusion in their day-to-day practice.

How this unit will be assessed

To reach Pass level, the evidence must show that the learner is able to:

P1   explain the benefits of diversity to society
P2   use recognised terminology to explain the importance of promoting equality, recognising diversity and respecting rights in health and social care settings
P3   explain the potential effects of discriminatory practice on those who use health and social care services
P4   explain how legislation, codes of practice, rules of conduct, charters and organisational policies are used to promote anti-discriminatory practice
P5   explain how those working in health and social care settings can actively promote anti-discriminatory practice.

To reach Merit level, the evidence must show that, in addition to the Pass criteria, the learner is able to:

M1   explain the influences of a recent or emerging national policy with regard to anti-discriminatory practice
M2   explain difficulties that may be encountered when implementing anti-discriminatory practice
M3   analyse how personal beliefs and value systems may influence own anti-discriminatory practice.

To reach Distinction level, the evidence must show that, in addition to the Pass and Merit criteria, the learner is able to:

D1   evaluate how a recent or emerging policy development influences organisational and personal practice in relation to anti-discriminatory practice
D2   evaluate practical strategies to reconcile own beliefs and values with anti-discriminatory practice in health and social care.

The importance of evidence gained during placement experience

Throughout Unit 2, I have included a range of suggested activities for placement that should help learners make the connection between theory and practice. There will be numerous opportunities in placement for learners to gain and demonstrate the skills necessary for effective practice. This will also help them develop the skills needed to achieve Unit 6, Learning outcome 2 (Be able to plan for, monitor and reflect on own development).

In Unit 2, Learning outcome 2, learners will need to draw heavily on examples from placement to achieve the P3 criteria. I have included suggested placement activities that involve collecting copies of policies and procedures and reflecting on their practical applications. These will enable learners to collect some examples even before they begin Assessment task 3.

The Learning outcome 3 activities, together with examples from placement, will help facilitate learners' achievement of the P4 criteria.

The merit criteria require learners to explain how a fairly new or emerging national policy has influenced organisational policies on anti-discriminatory practice. To meet these criteria, learners need to research the national initiative and apply their findings to examples from their own placement. As long as learners write in their reflective journals regularly, such examples should be readily available.

Once learners have researched and formulated the material for the merit criteria, they should be able to achieve the distinction criteria fairly easily. They should evaluate the national policy by looking at the strengths and weaknesses of its influence on organisational policy. What benefits or difficulties have there been, or are there likely to be, for organisations that are trying to incorporate the new initiative into their anti-discriminatory policies?

One of the suggested placement activities provides an extension of Activity 2.17. Learners are asked to record in their reflective journals examples of times when they have actively promoted anti-discriminatory practice. They should also note the strengths and weaknesses of their strategies on each occasion. These notes will form a basis for repeated and regular use of Activity 2.17. This activity also links directly to Unit 6, Learning outcome 2 (Be able to plan for, monitor and reflect on own development).

Assessment tasks

Assessment tasks need to be carefully timed to give learners the best chance of achieving at the highest level. Assuming that learners will undertake at least 50 hours of placement in two different settings in year one of the programme, Task 1 should ideally be set at the end of the first placement, and Task 2 should be set at the end of the second placement.

Task 1 (relevant criteria: P1, P2)

Write an essay (approximately 1500–2000 words) explaining the benefits of diversity to society. You should consider factors such as: cultural enrichment, social cohesion, economic benefits, tolerance, education and language. **(P1)**

Go on to explain the importance of promoting equality, diversity and rights in health and social care settings. Make sure that you use recognised terminology in your explanation such as: equity, overt discrimination, labelling, prejudice, empowerment, interdependence and disadvantage. **(P2)**

Task 2 (relevant criteria: P3)

Write an essay (approximately 700–1000 words) explaining the potential effects of discriminatory practice on those who use health or social care services. You should consider the bases of discrimination (e.g. class, race, gender, sexuality, cognitive ability, etc) and how discrimination can be seen in practice (e.g. prejudice, stereotyping, labelling, bullying, infringement of rights, etc). You should also consider the impact on service users of loss of rights.

How do these factors affect service users (e.g. marginalisation, low self-esteem, restricted opportunities, etc)? These can all lead to the cycle of disadvantage. **(P3)**

Task 3 (relevant criteria: P4, M1, D1)

Create an information booklet (approximately 2000–2500 words) that explains how legislation, codes of practice, rules of conduct, charters and organisational policies are used to promote anti-discriminatory practice in health and social care services.

You should consider how specific pieces of legislation are used in health and social care settings. These pieces of legislation might be, for example, the Human Rights Act 1989, the Race Relations Act (Amendment) 2000, the

Care Standards Act 2000, the Disability Discrimination Act 1995, or the Data Protection Act 1998. You should also consider the codes of conduct and charters established by professional bodies (e.g. the Social Care Council) as the legal framework for creation of their own organisational policies and procedures on staff development, quality issues, complaints procedures, confidentiality, human rights, etc.

You should provide an example of the practical implementation of an organisational policy or code of practice from your placement experience (remember to maintain staff and service users' confidentiality). **(P4)**

Include a section in your booklet that explains the influence of a recent national anti-discriminatory policy development on organisational policy. Evaluate the strengths and weaknesses of this national policy's influence on organisational and personal practice in relation to anti-discriminatory practice. Use examples from your placement to support your evaluation. **(M1, D1)**

Task 4 (relevant criteria: P5, M2)

Write an essay (approximately 1000–1500 words), explaining how the individual health and social care worker can actively promote anti-discriminatory practice. Use examples from your own placement. These may include:

- following ethical principles
- challenging discrimination
- acting as a role model
- being familiar with and applying the care value base
- putting the service user at the heart of service provision
- treating service users as individuals with dignity
- providing active support, consistent with beliefs, culture and preferences
- respecting service users' views by promoting the individual's rights, choices and well-being
- empowering individuals
- allowing privacy
- protecting from danger and harm
- maintaining confidentiality. **(P5)**

Explain the difficulties that may be encountered when implementing anti-discriminatory practice. You should consider: staff development and training, quality issues, balancing the rights of individual service users with the rights of others and potential conflicts. **(M2)**

Task 5 (relevant criteria: P6, M3, D2)

Write an essay (approximately 1500–2000 words) describing ways of reflecting on and challenging discriminatory issues in health and social care. Using examples from your reflective journal and reflective writing/action plans, you should consider the need to develop greater self-awareness by exploring your own attitudes and beliefs in order to address any potential areas of prejudice. You should also describe the importance of the individual's commitment to the care value base, use of language and working within legal, ethical and policy guidelines. **(P6)**

Analyse the ways in which your personal beliefs and value systems may influence your own anti-discriminatory practice. How could your own upbringing, culture and past events affect your promotion of anti-discriminatory practice, if these factors have not been addressed through greater self-awareness? **(M3)**

Evaluate practical strategies to reconcile your own beliefs and values with anti-discriminatory practice in health and social care. Describe practical strategies that you have used to address areas of potential prejudice in your practice and to increase your personal awareness. What are the strengths and weaknesses of these strategies? Are there any areas for further development? **(D2)**

Scheme of work

BTEC National Health and Social Care
Unit 2 Equality, diversity and rights in health and social care

Broad aim: Successful completion of the unit

Teacher(s): ....

Academic year: ....

Number of weeks: 35

Duration of session: 2 hours

Guided learning hours: 70

Week/s	Topic/outcome	Tutor preparation	Student activity	Resources	Links to grading criteria
1	Introduction to Unit 2: Understanding terminology	Use the PowerPoint® in conjunction with the Activity 2.1 group task pairing game	Learners can discuss the themes raised. Small group work for Activity 2.1. Groups can then present their answers to the rest of the class	PowerPoint® 1, Activity 2.1	P1, P2
2–3	The benefits of diversity: What does a diverse society have to offer?	Activity 2.2 is a PowerPoint® and can be used as an introduction to the themes; use this in conjunction with Activity 2.3	The PowerPoint® and Activity 2.3 can be used to generate discussion. Small group work can be used for Activity 2.4, with learners presenting their poster to the class. Learners can be encouraged to evaluate the strengths and weaknesses of the posters	Activity 2.2, Activity 2.3, Activity 2.4	P1, P2
3–4	Exploring attitudes: Labelling people	This activity will encourage learners to explore how we label people based on their appearance	Small group work in creating the person, followed by a class presentation and discussion of the results	Activity 2.5	P1, P2
5–8	Empowering individuals: Individual rights	Encourage learners to decide on their own priorities regarding simple rights, and priorities for service users	Learners to work in small groups of three or four; this should lead to effective discussion of different expectations, values, etc	Activity 2.6	P1, P2
9–11	The care value base (CVB)	Activity 2.7 is a PowerPoint® and can be used as an introduction to the themes. Use this in conjunction with Activity 2.8	The PowerPoint® and Activity 2.8 can be used to generate discussion. Encourage learners to work in groups or pairs to discuss and complete the grid. **Activity for placement: Explore the setting's policies and procedures to see how they promote the care value base**	Activity 2.7, Activity 2.8	P1, P2
11–12	Complaints procedures	Activity 2.9 is a PowerPoint® and can be used as an introduction to the rights of service users, their families and staff to complain about services.	Learners work in groups of three or four, and assess how they would manage the situation when a service user wishes to complain. **Activity for placement: Ask your placement supervisor how complaints are dealt with**	Activity 2.9, Activity 2.10	P1, P2
13–15	Bases of discrimination and discriminatory practice	Use the PowerPoint® in conjunction with the Activity 2.11 gapped handout. This should introduce learners to the themes of the outcome	Learners can complete the gapped handout alone or in pairs, but encourage them to discuss their answers before completion	PowerPoint® 2, Activity 2.11	P3

Unit 2 Equality, diversity and rights in health and social care

Week/s	Topic/outcome	Tutor preparation	Student activity	Resources	Links to grading criteria
16–19	The effects of discrimination and loss of rights	This may be a highly charged session, as the case studies can provoke anger and upset in the learners. Excellent basis for discussion!	In small groups of three or four, learners explore the bases of discrimination and its effects through case studies. Learners then discuss the issues raised. Learners can use these examples as a basis for researching their own examples from recent news. **Activity for placement: Have you seen any examples of discrimination in your placement? Give examples**	Activity 2.12	P3
20–24	How national and organisational policies promote anti-discriminatory practice	This PowerPoint® introduces the legal framework for health and social care services. Use in conjunction with the Activity 2.13 handout	For Activity 2.14, learners research a specific piece of legislation and create a display board. For the Activity 2.15 group task, learners research how legislation supports service users' rights. For both activities, learners can work in small groups and present their results to the rest of the class. **Activity for placement: Identify and explain examples of anti-discriminatory practice in your placements**	PowerPoint® 3, Activity 2.13, Activity 2.14, Activity 2.15	P4, M1, D1
25	The right to confidentiality	This PowerPoint® introduces every person's right to have information about them kept confidential	**Activity for placement: How does your placement setting manage confidentiality? Is there a confidentiality policy? What instructions have you been given as a 'trainee' about upholding confidentiality whilst in that placement?**	Activity 2.16	P4, M1, D1
26–27	Active promotion of anti-discriminatory practice	This PowerPoint® introduces the themes of the outcome	**Activity for placement: Has there been a difference in the quality of anti-discriminatory practice between placements? Give examples**	PowerPoint® 4	P5, P6, M2, M3, D2
28–32	Exploring own attitudes and beliefs: Have personal attitudes and beliefs changed?	Encourage learners to draw on examples of how they have promoted anti-discriminatory practice, and make plans for improvement	Learners should work individually to complete the form	Activity 2.17	P5, P6, M2, M3, D2
33–35	Review of Unit 2 content	Activity 2.18 is a light-hearted crossword to consolidate learners' knowledge and review the unit	Learners complete crossword	Activity 2.18	All

At-a-glance activity grid
Unit 2 Equality, diversity and rights in health and social care

Activity	Title and description	Scheme of work	File/CD	Delivery notes	Additional resources	Links to grading criteria	Activities for placement Links to other units	Links to Student Book 1
Outcome 2.1 Understand concepts of equality, diversity and rights in relation to health and social care								
Power Point® 1	Introduction to Unit 2 and Learning outcome 1	Week 1	CD	This PPT will help you to generate discussion. Use in conjunction with the Activity 2.1 pairing game		**P1, P2**		pp 50–75
2.1	Understanding terminology	Week 1	File (Tutor information and Answers on CD)	Group task: learners to identify meanings of terminology and pair with correct word	A1 sheets of paper, thin card	**P1, P2**		pp 50–75
2.2	The benefits of a diverse society	Weeks 2–3	CD	This PPT will help you to generate discussion. Use in conjunction with the Activity 2.3 gapped handout		**P1, P2**		pp 50–75
2.3	What are the benefits of diversity?	Weeks 2–3	File	Use this gapped handout in conjunction with the Activity 2.2 PPT		**P1, P2**		pp 50–75
2.4	Celebrate diversity	Weeks 2–3	File	Learners create a poster which shows images that celebrate diversity	Large sheets of paper	**P1, P2**		pp 50–75
2.5	Labelling people	Weeks 3–4	File (Tutor information on CD)	This group task will encourage learners to explore how we label people based on their appearance	Small pieces of card, A3 paper, glue or sticky tack, pens	**P1, P2**		pp 50–75
2.6	Individual rights	Weeks 5–8	File (Tutor information on CD)	In small groups of three or four, learners decide on their own priorities regarding simple rights and priorities for service users. Should lead to effective discussion of different expectations, values, etc	Thin card, wall charts or flipcharts	**P1, P2**	What evidence is there, in placement, that service users' rights are being respected? Learners to record examples in their reflective journals	pp 50–75
2.7	Introduction of the care value base (CVB)	Weeks 9–11	CD	This PPT introduces the CVB. Use in conjunction with the Activity 2.8 gapped handout		**P1, P2**	Is there evidence of the CVB working in placement? Learners to record examples in their reflective journals	pp 50–75

Activity	Title and description	Scheme of work	File/CD	Delivery notes	Additional resources	Links to grading criteria	Activities for placement / Links to other units	Links to Student Book 1
2.8	Care value base	Weeks 9–11	File (Answers on CD)	Learners to complete blank sections to embed concepts of CVB		**P1, P2**		pp 50–75
2.9	The right to complain	Weeks 11–12	CD	This PPT introduces the right of service users, their families and staff to complain about services. Use in conjunction with the Activity 2.10 Complaints case studies		**P1, P2**	Is there a complaints procedure in placement? Learners to investigate how complaints are dealt with and record these examples in their reflective journals	pp 50–75
2.10	Complaints case studies	Weeks 11–12	File	In small groups of three or four, learners assess how they would manage the situation when a service user wishes to complain. There is an opportunity for discussion at the end of this activity				pp 50–75
Outcome 2.2 Understand discriminatory practice in health and social care								
Power Point 2	Introduction to Learning outcome 2	Weeks 13–15	CD	This PPT introduces the bases of discrimination and its potential effects on service users and their families. Use in conjunction with the Activity 2.11 gapped handout		**P3**		pp 75–82
2.11	The cycle of disadvantage	Weeks 13–15	File (Answers on CD)			**P3**		pp 75–82
2.12	The effects of discrimination	Weeks 16–19	CD	In small groups of three or four, learners explore the bases of discrimination and its effects through case studies. This may be a highly charged session, as the case studies and related issues can provoke anger and upset in the learners. Excellent basis for discussion!		**P1, P2**		pp 75–82

Outcome 2.3 Understand how national initiatives promote anti-discriminatory practice in health and social care

Activity	Title and description	Scheme of work	File/CD	Delivery notes	Additional resources	Links to grading criteria	Activities for placement Links to other units	Links to Student Book 1
PowerPoint® 3	Introduction to Learning outcome 3	Weeks 20–24	CD	This PPT introduces legislation as the legal framework for health and social care services. Use in conjunction with the Activity 2.13 handout		P4, M1, D1	Learners to investigate the policies, codes of practice and procedures in their placements. They should ask if they can see the setting's policies and take copies, then record in their reflective journals how they see these policies in action. Are policies (e.g. the Health and Safety policy) adhered to all the time?	pp 82–91
2.13	Organisational policies	Weeks 20–24	File	Use this handout in conjunction with PowerPoint® 3		P4, M1, D1		pp 82–91
2.14	Understanding legislation	Weeks 20–24	File	Learners research a piece of legislation (e.g. the Human Rights Act, Sex Discrimination Act, Children's Act or Race Relations Act) and create a display board (if possible) for the rest of the college to see and be informed by	Materials to create a display board	P4, M1, D1		pp 82–91
2.15	Supporting service users' rights	Weeks 20–24	File	In small groups of two or three, learners research how legislation supports service users' rights		P4, M1, D1		pp 82–91
2.16	The right to confidentiality	Week 25	CD	This PPT introduces the right of every person to have information about them kept confidential. Learner task included		P4, M1, D1	Is there a confidentiality policy in placement? Learners to investigate and record in their reflective journals	pp 82–91

Activity	Title and description	Scheme of work	File/CD	Delivery notes	Additional resources	Links to grading criteria	Activities for placement Links to other units	Links to Student Book 1
Outcome 2.4 Understand how anti-discriminatory practice is promoted in health and social care settings								
Power Point® 4	Introduction to Learning outcome 4	Weeks 26–27	CD	This PPT introduces the concept of the individual's influence on anti-discriminatory practice		**P5, P6, M2, M3, D2**	Learners to record in their reflective journals examples of when they have actively promoted anti-discriminatory practice. What are the strengths and weaknesses of each example and how could they improve? Links to: Unit 6, Learning outcome 3	pp 91–103
2.17	Exploring own attitudes and beliefs	Weeks 28–32	File	In this reflective worksheet/action plan, learners will draw on examples of how they have promoted anti-discriminatory practice, and make plans for improvement		**P5, P6, M2, M3, D2**	Learners to ask themselves if staff in their placement (including themselves) are good role models. They should record their thoughts on this in their reflective journals Links to: Unit 6, Learning outcome 3	pp 91–103
2.18	Review of Unit 2 content	Weeks 33–35	File (Answers on CD)	This crossword is a light-hearted activity to consolidate learners' knowledge and complete the unit		All		pp 91–103

Unit 2 Lesson plan

Aims

- To introduce Unit 2
- To introduce Learning outcome 1

This structure may be spread over a number of lessons as required.

Learning outcomes
- have an understanding of the content of Unit 2
- be able to define some of the relevant terminology.

Timing	Content	Teacher activity	Student activity	Resources	Individualised activity
5 mins	Welcome learners and register				
15 mins	Introduce Unit 2	Tutor to introduce Unit 2 by outlining topics to be covered. Moderate use of language to ensure full understanding of all learners	Learners to answer indirect questions to check understanding		
20 mins	Introduce Learning outcome 1	PPT presentation to be used as reference point/'backdrop' for teaching. Encourage discussion where appropriate. Moderate use of language to ensure full understanding of all learners	Learners to answer indirect questions to check understanding. Contribute to discussion	PowerPoint® 1	
20 mins	Activity 2.1: Understanding terminology	Encourage learners to view this pairing game as a 'fun' activity by offering lots of positive feedback and praise in response to their suggestions	Learners to relate to each other in groups of three or four, and answer indirect and direct questions to check understanding	Activity 2.1	Task to be explained using different levels of language. Circulate around class to check understanding and offer assistance or extension where needed.
10 mins	Return to PowerPoint® 1	Moderate use of language to ensure full understanding of all learners. Check understanding	Learners to answer indirect questions, and contribute to discussion	PowerPoint® 1	
10 mins	Discussion: Inequality and discrimination	Encourage learners to share ideas and views on the terminology in order to discuss issues around inequality and discrimination. Ensure that all learners' contributions receive positive feedback	Learners to answer indirect and direct questions to check understanding. Contribute to discussion		
10 mins	Recap: Quick-fire questions about meaning of terminology	Check Learning outcomes. Ensure that all learners' contributions receive positive feedback	Learners to respond to questions		
5 mins	Thank you. Close				

2.1   Pairing game: Understanding terminology

Student Book 1
pp 50–75

For this activity, your tutor will put you into groups of three or four. Each group will be given a set of cards with meanings written on them. In your groups, place the correct meaning card next to each word on the grid below. You have a time limit of around 5–10 minutes. See if your group can finish first, with all the correct meanings next to the right words.

Words	Correct meanings
Rights	
Covert discrimination	
Abuse	
Empower	
Label	
Stereotype	
Difference	
Overt discrimination	
Values	
Equity	
Independent	
Diversity	
Interdependent	
Opportunity	
Vulnerable	
Equality	
Disadvantage	
Prejudice	
Belief	
Homophobia	
Racism	
Sexism	

2.3 Gapped handout: The benefits of diversity

Student Book 1
pp 50–75

What is diversity?

Diversity is about...

There are many ways in which people are different and these include:

G............................., D............................, R............................,

A............................, C............................, S............................,

A.............................

How else are we all different?

....

....

....

....

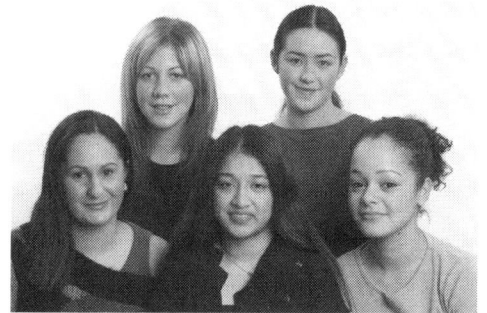

Our society in the UK is made up of people who are different in all these ways. How does this benefit society?

....

....

....

Are there any other benefits you can think of?

....

....

....

2.4   Poster task: Celebrate diversity

Student Book 1
pp 50–75

Britain is a diverse society made up of many different people. Imagine that you work in advertising and you have been asked to advertise 'Diversity' as a new product. How will you sell it?

Create a poster with the title 'Celebrate Diversity'. You might choose to use words or images, or both, to get your message across.

Consider the following ideas:

■ economic benefits

■ social cohesion

■ tolerance

■ different ethnic origins

■ people of different physical abilities

■ different religions

■ different foods/restaurants

■ different fashions

■ and others…

What sort of images would you use to show these ideas?

Make sure that your poster is colourful and eye-catching. After all, no one will buy your product if the advertising isn't good!

       [41]

2.5 Group task: Labelling people

Student Book 1
pp 50–75

For this activity, your tutor will put you into groups of two or three, and give each group a selection of cut-out images of people. In your group, choose one person and stick the image on to a large sheet of paper. Give your person a name and write it at the top. Then consider what type of person they are, based on their appearance.

Your tutor will also give you a set of labels and some glue or sticky tack. Choose the following labels and stick them on to the large sheet of paper with your person:

■ 1 occupation

■ 2 hobbies or leisure activities

■ Married/Unmarried

■ Children/No children

■ A selection of cards to describe the person's character

When the whole class has completed the task, your group can introduce your person and discuss why you chose the labels you did.

2.6 Group task: Individual rights

Student Book 1
pp xx–xx

For this activity, your tutor will put you into groups of three or four. Each group will be given one wall chart or flipchart and two sets of ten cards showing statements of rights.

In your group, draw a vertical line down the middle of the paper and write the headings 'ME' and 'SERVICE USER' at the top. Stick one set of ten cards under the 'ME' heading in order of importance, according to the rights you think you should have.

Then stick the other set of ten cards under the 'SERVICE USER' heading, in order of importance to a service user.

When the whole class has completed the task, you can all look at the differences between the charts. Your group can then explain why you ranked the statements as you did. What are the differences between what you expect for yourselves and what you think is appropriate for service users?

2.8   Gapped handout: Care value base (CVB)

Student Book 1
pp 50–75

What is the care value base?

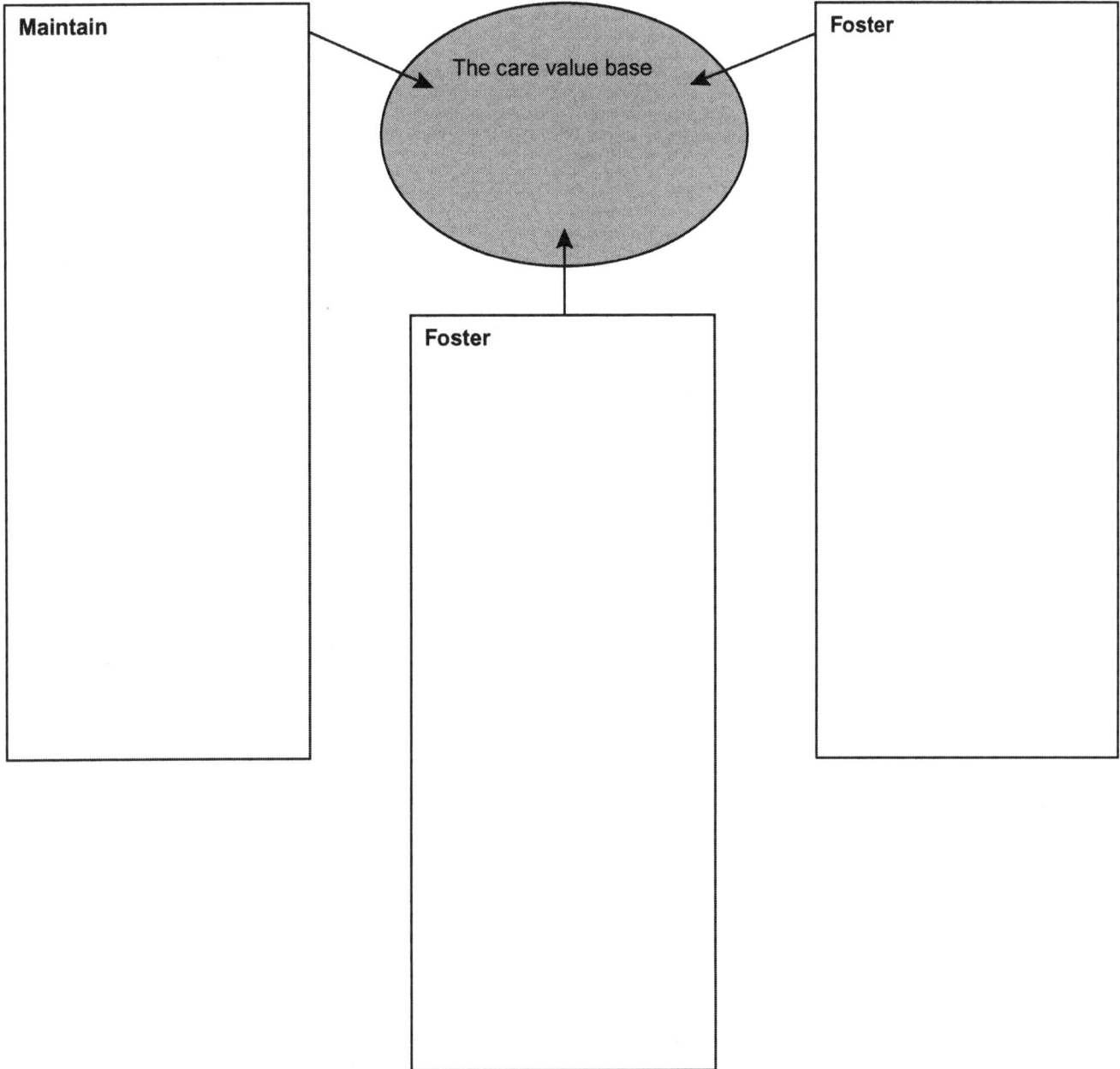

Maintain

The care value base

Foster

Foster

2.10 Complaints case studies

Student Book 1
pp 50–75

Group 1

Lucy, aged 12, says that she is being picked on in the children's home because she is the eldest. She complains that if she doesn't help the younger children with their homework, she either gets grounded, or her pocket money is stopped. Lucy needs your help to be able to make a complaint to the relevant personnel.

You should decide:

- How will you enable Lucy to prepare her complaint (Where is the evidence? How does she feel, etc?)
- How will you empower Lucy to make her complaint? (Will your support be practical, as in writing the complaint? Or will it be personal, as in being there when she complains? Will you be an advocate and voice the complaint on Lucy's behalf?)
- Who will the complaint go to and who will ensure that the complaints procedure is followed?
- How will the complaint and the resulting action be recorded?
- How will you consider confidentiality?

Then consider:

- Did you take sole responsibility for dealing with the complaint?
- Were there potential difficulties for you in supporting the complaint?
- What feelings might Lucy have had when thinking about complaining?
- How would you feel if you were the subject of a complaint?
- What positive and negative effects can complaints have on health and social care services?

Group 2

Joshua, aged 13, is in hospital after an operation. He complains that some of the men on his ward keep talking to him about things he does not want to hear about, especially things about the nurses. He is too embarrassed to talk to his parents and wants to be moved to the children's ward. Joshua needs your help to be able to make a complaint to the relevant personnel.

You should decide:

- How will you help Joshua to prepare his complaint? (Where is the evidence? How does he feel, etc?)
- How will you empower Joshua to make his complaint? (Will your support be practical, as in writing the complaint? Or will it be personal, as in being there when he complains? Will you be an advocate and voice the complaint on Joshua's behalf?)
- Who will the complaint go to and who will ensure that the complaints procedure is followed?
- How will the complaint and the resulting action be recorded?
- How will you consider confidentiality?

Then consider:

- Did you take sole responsibility for dealing with the complaint?
- Were there potential difficulties for you in supporting the complaint?
- What feelings might Joshua have had when thinking about complaining?
- How would you feel if you were the subject of a complaint?
- What positive and negative effects can complaints have on health and social care services?

Continued overleaf

2.10 Complaints case studies (*contd*)

Group 3

John, aged 21, who has a severe speech impediment, says that some of the staff will not wait for him to communicate through his computer; they make their own minds up about what his needs are. This means they insist on making him have a bath, and eating when he does not want to. John needs your help to be able to make a complaint to the relevant personnel.

You should decide:

- How will you help John to prepare his complaint? (Where is the evidence? How does he feel, etc?)
- How will you empower John to make his complaint? (Will your support be practical, as in writing the complaint? Or will it be personal, as in being there when he complains? Will you be an advocate and voice the complaint on John's behalf?)
- Who will the complaint go to and who will ensure that the complaints procedure is followed?
- How will the complaint and the resulting action be recorded?
- How will you consider confidentiality?

Then consider:

- Did you take sole responsibility for dealing with the complaint?
- Were there potential difficulties for you in supporting the complaint?
- What feelings might John have had when thinking about complaining?
- How would you feel if you were the subject of a complaint?
- What positive and negative effects can complaints have on health and social care services?

Group 4

Mabel, aged 87, tells you that the nurse who came to help her to the toilet last night was very rude and rough. Mabel shows you a bruise on her arm. Mabel needs your help to be able to make a complaint to the relevant personnel.

You should decide:

- How will you enable Mabel to prepare her complaint (Where is the evidence? How does she feel, etc?)
- How will you empower Mabel to make her complaint? (Will your support be practical, as in writing the complaint? Or will it be personal, as in being there when she complains? Will you be an advocate and voice the complaint on Mabel's behalf?)
- Who will the complaint go to and who will ensure that the complaints procedure is followed?
- How will the complaint and the resulting action be recorded?
- How will you consider confidentiality?

Then consider:

- Did you take sole responsibility for dealing with the complaint?
- Were there potential difficulties for you in supporting the complaint?
- What feelings might Mabel have had when thinking about complaining?
- How would you feel if you were the subject of a complaint?
- What positive and negative effects can complaints have on health and social care services?

2.11   Gapped handout: The cycle of disadvantage

Student Book 1
pp 75–82

What are the effects of discriminatory practice?

People are discriminated against because of ....,

...., ...

Discriminatory practice is:

S............................., L............................., B.............................,

A............................., I............................., O.............................,

D............................., A............................

Service users and their families who are subjected to discrimination can suffer the following effects:

....

....

....

Fill in the boxes in this cycle.

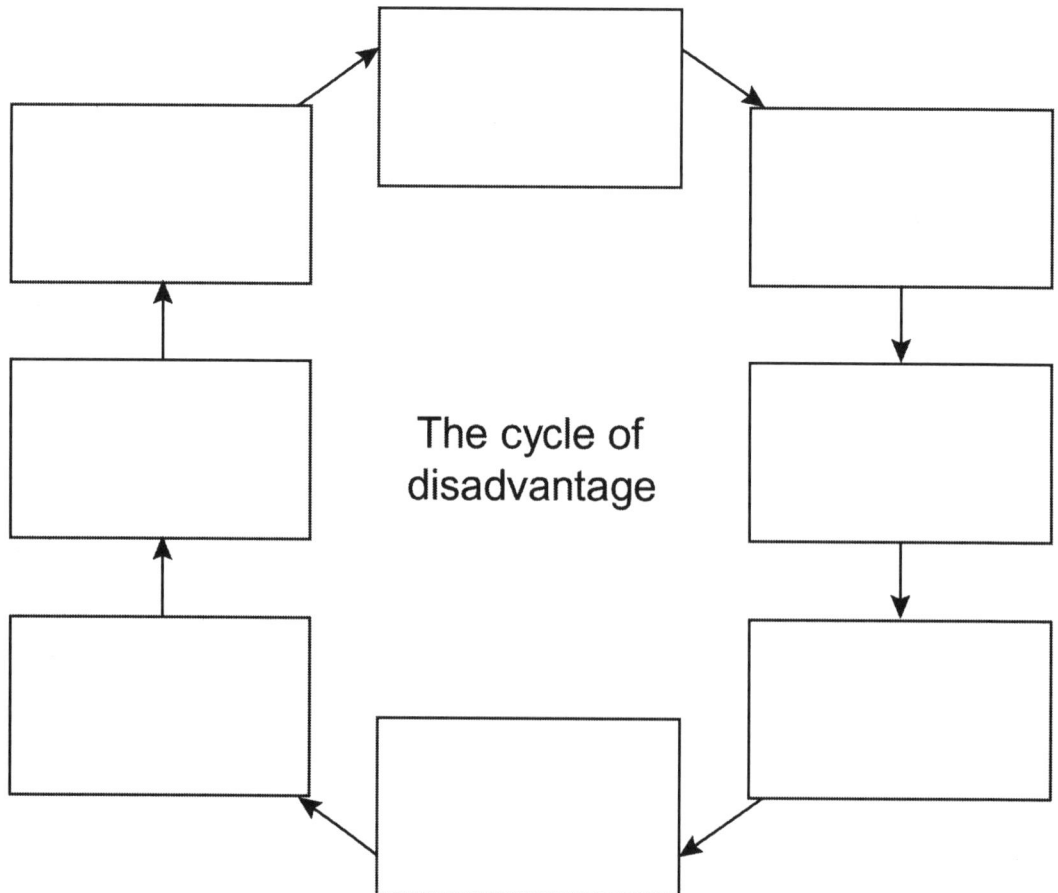

The cycle of disadvantage

2.12   Case studies: The effects of discrimination

Student Book 1
pp 75–82

In groups of three or four, read the following case studies and identify the issues involved. Consider how these issues are related to discrimination.

Group 1
Inquiry into the death of David 'Rocky' Bennett

In the early hours of Saturday 31 October 1998, David 'Rocky' Bennett, a 38-year-old black man, was certified dead. For the past three years he had been a detained patient in a medium-security unit in Norwich.

After an incident in which Bennett was racially abused by a white patient, staff had tried to move him off the ward and Bennett had become angry. Several nurses then held him face down for 25 minutes, and he died of asphyxiation. His family were not told about his death for two days.

In May 2001, an inquest returned a verdict of 'Accidental death aggravated by neglect'. The Coroner made recommendations to improve practices. In particular, he highlighted the need for national standards on restraining patients and for staff to be pro-active in dealing with racist behaviour, both by and against patients.

The campaign group 'Inquest' has been drawing the public's attention to the number of deaths of black people due to the use of force or medical neglect. They stress that there needs to be a system in place to monitor the use and danger of restraint. They campaigned, with Mr Bennett's family, for an extended inquiry looking at national changes, which the government agreed to in April 2003.

Helen Shaw, co-director of 'Inquest', said: 'This is a case that raises significant questions about the treatment of black people in psychiatric custody, institutional racism…and the dangers of restraint… We hope that this inquiry will result in significant and lasting change.' The inquiry will also look into over-diagnosis of black people with mental health problems and the poor treatment of bereaved families.

Group 2
Ministers choose 'business as usual' for mental institutions

In August 2004, a leaked official report showed that most of the findings from the Bennett Inquiry had been ignored, particularly those on restraint procedures and dealing with racism in the mental health system. Campaigners have been protesting for a long time against the health minister's refusal to admit racism in the NHS or embrace the Bennett Inquiry's findings.

Department of Health figures showed that black people are five times more likely to be placed in high security units, six times more likely to be sectioned, and significantly over-medicated compared to white patients.

The leaked report, 'Race Equality In Mental Health: An Action Plan to Engage Communities and Improve Services' ignores the 22 recommendations made by the Bennett Inquiry, and reaction to the report has been highly critical. Professor Sashi Sashidarand said it would allow 'damaging practices of misdiagnosis, over medication and restraint [to] continue in medical wards … without any consequences'. Dr Richard Stone, who sat on the Bennett Inquiry panel, added: 'Two people have already died in psychiatric care after being restrained since the report was published… This move means that black people will remain over-represented within mental health institutions'.

Continued overleaf

2.12 Case studies: The effects of discrimination (*contd*)

Lee Jasper, Chair of the African Caribbean Mental Health Commission, said: 'If the Government refuses to include the bulk of the recommendations included in the Bennett Report then the black community will be outraged. It is beyond comprehension that they would do this. The report seems to have become a victim of the very issue it sought to expose – institutional racism.'

Group 3
'Half a million' elderly people abused, says House of Commons report

A report, issued by the House of Commons, states that of the half a million elderly people who may be being abused, two-thirds of these cases occur in their own homes. Abuse also took place in nursing homes, residential care and sheltered housing.

Abuse could be sexual, physical, financial, or in the form of neglect or over-medication. The committee said: 'Abuse of older people is a hidden, and often ignored, problem in society'. It called for the Department of Health to clarify the full extent of the problem.

The elderly seldom report abuse, due to fear, embarrassment or simply being unable to complain. In addition carers often lack the training needed to recognise the signs of abuse, and the report called for this training to be made 'mandatory'. The report stated that certification of death was a 'particular concern', and called for the Health Care Commission to tackle the problems.

Jonathan Ellis, from Help the Aged, said: 'At present little is known of the prevalence of elder abuse, particularly the abuse of people in their own homes. We urge the government … to act quickly to end elder abuse.'

Group 4
Abuse of disabled children and young people

Some disabled children and young people are mentally or physically more vulnerable than others, which could make it easier for abusers to exploit them. These young people may also find it more difficult to recognise and report abuse, and to be believed. This might be due to:

- limited life experiences leading to undeveloped social skills, or not developing appropriate language skills
- having been encouraged to comply with people's wishes
- being afraid to challenge abusive situations – it is often easier to be compliant or pleasing, rather than angering an authority figure
- being unable to recognise that abuse has taken place
- feeling powerless, as they have to depend on others
- being unable to remove themselves from abusive situations
- having no one to confide in
- feeling guilt or shame at the abuse, or not having a sense of ownership over their own bodies, due to constant medical examination
- having low self-esteem or self-image.

Disabled children may also suffer from two further forms of abuse:

- institutional abuse: when carers override the needs and wishes of a disabled child in favour of the rules and procedures of an organisation
- financial abuse: deliberate misuse and exploitation of a disabled child's money or possessions.

2.13 Handout: Organisational policies and codes of practice

Student Book 1
pp 82–91

Why do health and social care settings have equality and rights policies?

Recruitment and selection of staff	To ensure that staff are recruited fairly and in accordance with legislation such as the Disability Discrimination Act, Sex Discrimination Act and Race Relations Act
Equal opportunities	To form part of all policies to ensure equal treatment and equal chances for both staff and service users and service users' families. This should encourage a 'no blame' culture to cope with change and development of services
Anti-discrimination	To promote opposing and challenging discrimination in every area including language, bullying and covert or unintentional discrimination
Harassment	To give clear guidance on all forms of harassment (e.g. racial or sexual) experienced by staff, service users and their families
Admissions	To provide open and fair admissions systems that can be accessed by all members of the community. Extending knowledge of service to 'hard to reach' sections of community (e.g. translating relevant material into relevant languages)
Relations with families	To state the setting's attitudes and values regarding next of kin and other family members as partners
Staff development and training	To provide on-going training to promote anti-discriminatory practice by raising awareness of discrimination and ensuring that staff understand the issues and support the solutions
Quality standards	To incorporate elements of other policies and ensure that service is of the highest quality across all the setting's work. Also to detail ways of obtaining and using feedback from service users and other agencies. Inspections, codes of practice and the underlying principles of the setting will all contribute to the quality standards
Complaints	To provide details of the complaints procedure in the event of a service user, relative or member of staff making a complaint against the setting. There should be a clear process designed to lead to a resolution of the complaint

2.14 Display task: Understanding legislation

Student Book 1
pp 82–91

Group 1

Design a display board with the title:

Human Rights Act 1998 – Important for health and social care settings…

Research the following:

- Why is this legislation important?
- What does it mean to Britain today?
- Why is it positive?
- Why is it important for health and social care settings?

You need to:

- collect relevant information
- collect images that you can use – you can draw them larger!
- decide on a colour scheme and design your board on paper first
- construct your display.

Ensure that you reference correctly and that you label the display with the following:

- BND Health and Social Care
- Year 1
- Unit 2: Equality, Diversity and Rights in Health and Social Care
- Task: Legislation as a legal framework for health and social care services

Group 2

Design a display board with the title:

Data Protection Act 1998 – Important for health and social care settings…

Research the following:

- Why is this legislation important?
- What does it mean to Britain today?
- Why is it positive?
- Why is it important for health and social care settings?

You need to:

- collect relevant information
- collect images that you can use – you can draw them larger!
- decide on a colour scheme and design your board on paper first
- construct your display.

Ensure that you reference correctly and that you label the display with the following:

- BND Health and Social Care
- Year 1
- Unit 2: Equality, Diversity and Rights in Health and Social Care
- Task: Legislation as a legal framework for health and social care services

2.14 Display task: Understanding legislation (*contd*)

Group 3

Design a display board with the title:

Sex Discrimination Act 1975 – Important for health and social care settings…

Research the following:

- Why is this legislation important?
- What does it mean to Britain today?
- Why is it positive?
- Why is it important for health and social care settings?

You need to:

- collect relevant information
- collect images that you can use – you can draw them larger!
- decide on a colour scheme and design your board on paper first
- construct your display.

Ensure that you reference correctly and that you label the display with the following:

- BND Health and Social Care
- Year 1
- Unit 2: Equality, Diversity and Rights in Health and Social Care
- Task: Legislation as a legal framework for health and social care services

Group 4

Design a display board with the title:

Mental Health Act 1983 – Important for health and social care settings…

Research the following:

- Why is this legislation important?
- What does it mean to Britain today?
- Why is it positive?
- Why is it important for health and social care settings?

You need to:

- collect relevant information
- collect images that you can use – you can draw them larger!
- decide on a colour scheme and design your board on paper first
- construct your display.

Ensure that you reference correctly and that you label the display with the following:

- BND Health and Social Care
- Year 1
- Unit 2: Equality, Diversity and Rights in Health and Social Care
- Task: Legislation as a legal framework for health and social care services

2.15 Group task: How does legislation support service users' rights?

Student Book 1
pp 82–91

How does legislation support service users' rights?

Investigate one of the following:

■ The Sex Discrimination Acts 1975 and 1986

■ The Human Rights Act 1998

■ The Race Relations Act 1976

■ The Disability Discrimination Act 1995

■ The Data Protection Act 1998

■ The Mental Health Act 1983

For your chosen piece of legislation, ask:

1   What does the Act aim to do? What is its purpose?

2   How does the Act define discrimination?

3   What is the relevance of this type of discrimination in a health or social care setting? Who is it relevant to and why?

4   If someone feels they have been discriminated against, under the terms of the Act, what help can they get?

5   Give an example of an act of discrimination in a health or social care setting, which would be illegal under the Act you have researched.

Prepare a short summary of your findings to use in a spoken presentation to the group.

2.17   Worksheet: Reflective practice/Action plan

Student Book 1
pp 91–103

- How well do you think you promote anti-discriminatory practice?

- Have your attitudes towards other people changed?

- Using examples from placement, describe how you have promoted anti-discriminatory practice.

I have promoted anti-discriminatory practice in the following ways:

What do you need to do to improve your own practice?

I could make the following improvements:

How will you achieve these improvements? What will you actually do? For instance, will you actively seek further training in one particular area and/or continually monitor and review your own progress?

Continued overleaf

2.17 Worksheet: Reflective practice/Action plan (*contd*)

Strategies for improvement:

When will you achieve these improvements?

I will aim to achieve these improvements to my own practice by the following date:

Student name……………………………………….…… Date……………………………….

Student signature……………………………………………

Tutor signature………………………………………..…… Date……………………………….

2.18 End-of-unit crossword

Student Book 1
pp 91–103

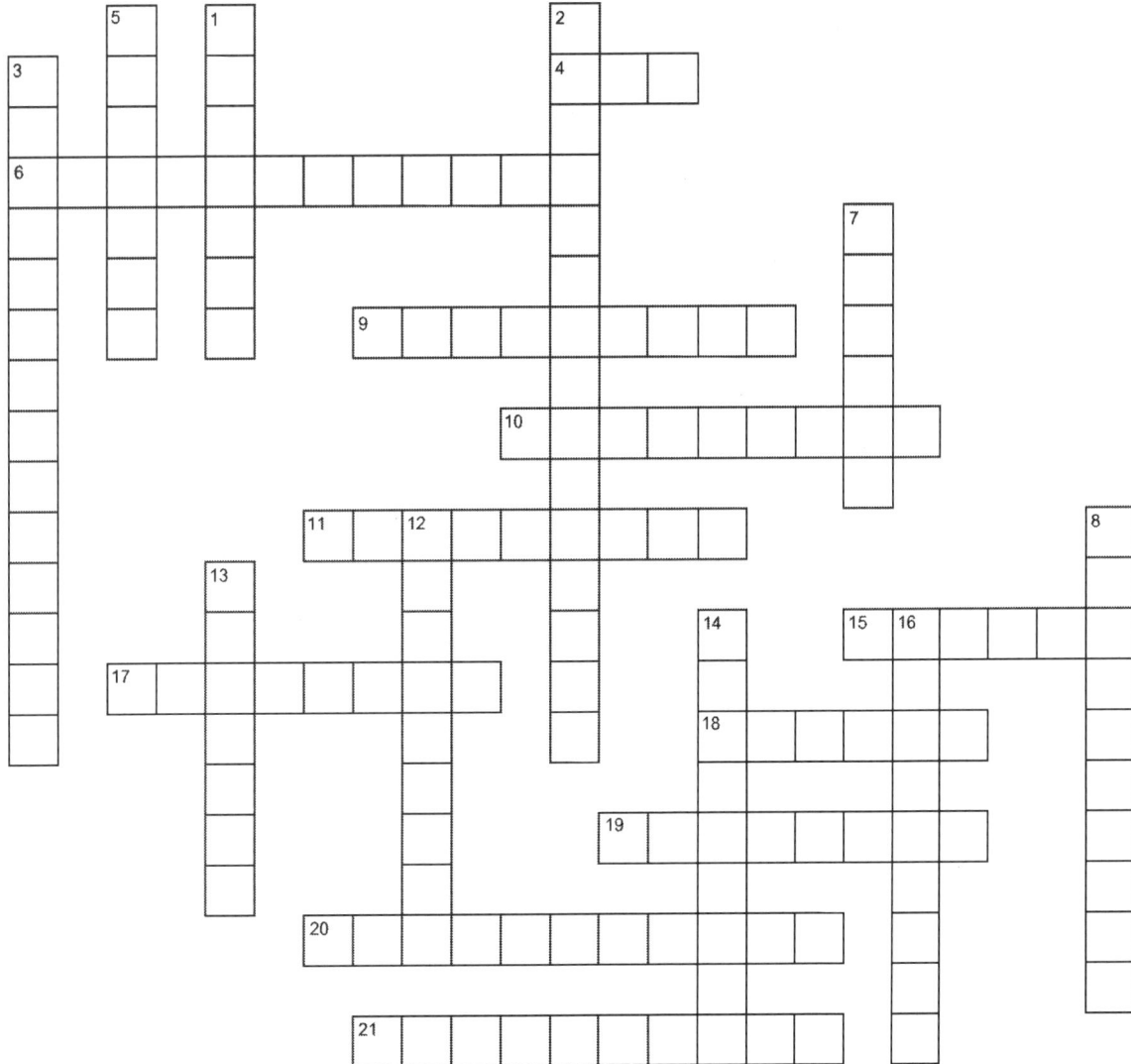

ACROSS

4 New legislation prohibits discrimination on the basis of this
6 A standardised image of a type of person
9 A potential area of discrimination
10 Difference
11 Understanding and accepting differences
15 We all have them; they are our morals and beliefs
17 Created by health and social care settings from conventions, legislation and regulations
18 Fairness, impartiality and reasonableness
19 Treating people according to their individual needs
20 Provides the legal framework for health and social care services
21 A benefit of diversity

DOWN

1 These give us a clue about where someone is from
2 When people are left out
3 Treating one group more or less favourably than another
5 Active promotion of anti-discriminatory practice leads to choice and ....
7 These are set out in legislation
8 To take people's rights away
12 Assigning a name to a type of person
13 This is different in different parts of the UK and other countries
14 An unfavourable view of someone
16 We need to explore our own in order to promote anti-discriminatory practice
17 It is these beliefs and values that can influence the individual's anti-discriminatory practice

3

Health, safety and security in health and social care

unit overview

This unit will give learners an insight into the complex health and safety issues that arise on a daily basis within health and social care settings. Students will learn about the practicalities of providing a safe care environment. They will also develop an understanding of the core principles and legislation underpinning health and social care practice. This unit is split into four Learning outcomes.

Learning outcomes

On completion of this unit learners should:

3.1 understand potential hazards in health and social care

3.2 understand how legislation, guidelines, policies and procedures promote health, safety and security

3.3 understand roles and responsibilities for health, safety and security in health and social care settings

3.4 understand how to deal with hazards in a local environment.

Suggested activities

The At-a-glance activity grid shows how the activities in the Assessment and Delivery Resource (ADR) relate to the content of the unit. The activities include introductory and plenary activities and a variety of case studies, research tasks, discussions and presentations, using written, verbal and presentation skills. The activities may help learners prepare for assessment, and the grid indicates which assessment criteria are relevant for each activity. Copies of activity sheets can be given to learners.

Teaching Unit 3

Unit 3 will assist students with a number of other units in the course, especially Unit 11 (Supporting and protecting adults), as well as with their professional work placements. To meet all the criteria of this unit, learners will need to pass a recognised first aid course. It may also be beneficial for students to undertake a short certificated food hygiene course. However, it is not advisable for learners to undertake a manual handling course, as they may be tempted to carry out activities such as lifting and moving service users, which could put them at risk.

Gaining familiarity with the health and safety legislation related to this unit will provide students with the underpinning knowledge required to meet professional standards. Visiting speakers, such as health and safety officers, care home managers, social workers for the elderly, and nursing staff, can add another dimension to students' learning by giving examples of their experiences of dealing with risks in different health and social care settings. As well as arranging visiting speakers, you should organise visits to different service provision settings.

Students can improve their understanding by investigating current legislation and guidelines and how they are used to produce local polices and procedures. Advise students to use only UK websites when carrying out Internet research, as each country has its own legislation. For instance, they can relate the Control of Substances

Hazardous to Health (COSHH) and Reporting of Injuries, Diseases and Dangerous Occurrences (RIDDOR) regulations to the activities they carry out or observe while on work placement. This will help them see how legislation is put into practice. You will also need to inform students that legislation changes to meet the changing needs of the populace. It is therefore important for them to keep up to date with the latest legislation.

There is a wealth of additional information available on websites including VLE tutor resources, such as short videos introducing heath and safety. It is worth spending time reviewing these sites, as they can add some variety to delivery of these topics. There is also a complete resource file for health and safety in social care available in the Standards Unit Resource Box.

The content of each Learning outcome

Learning outcome 1: Understand potential hazards in health and social care (relevant criteria: P1, P2, P3)

The first Learning outcome begins with a PowerPoint® presentation introducing the importance of health, safety and security and related legislation in health and social care. Activity 3.1 is a worksheet on the safe storage of chemicals. This is followed by Activity 3.2, which requires learners to consider the risks posed by different food allergies.

Learning outcome 2: Understand how legislation, guidelines, policies and procedures promote health, safety and security (relevant criteria: P1, P2, P3, P4, M1, D1)

The second Learning outcome begins with a PowerPoint® presentation introducing the importance of confidentiality in health and social care. In Activity 3.3 learners devise their own emergency evacuation procedure for a nursing home. In Activity 3.4 learners consider how two different hazards can be reduced or avoided. This should help them realise that risks are not always avoidable and that precautions may reduce (but not entirely remove) the risks. This is followed by Activity 3.5, in which students devise a survey questionnaire in order to research the most common types of accident for different age ranges and environments. In Activity 3.6, learners take on the role of a health and safety manager and explain how to carry out risk assessments.

Learning outcome 3: Understand roles and responsibilities for health, safety and security in health and social care settings (relevant criteria: P1, P2, P3, P4, P5, M1, M2, D1, D2)

This Learning outcome is all about understanding the different roles and responsibilities of employers, employees and service users themselves, and it begins with a PowerPoint® presentation explaining the importance of professional logs of tasks carried out. In Activity 3.7, learners consider how to deal with different types of spillages safely. Activity 3.8 focuses on disposing of waste in health and care settings, while protecting service users and staff from cross-contamination. In Activity 3.9 learners consider security of premises and service users, especially in open environments. In Activity 3.10, students look at roles and responsibilities in four different care situations. Activity 3.11 is an individual or group-based task in which learners consider which health and social care workers would benefit from undertaking different training courses.

Learning outcome 4: Understand how to deal with hazards in a local environment (relevant criteria: P1, P3, D1)

The fourth Learning outcome begins with a PowerPoint® presentation explaining the importance of safe employment practices, including the need for anti-discriminatory practice in recruitment. Activity 3.12 is a PowerPoint® presentation that introduces a survey to be completed in work placements. Learners then carry out their surveys and present their results using graphs and/or charts. Activity 3.13 includes three case studies highlighting possible risks for health and social care staff who work on their own in the community.

How this unit will be assessed

To reach Pass level, the evidence must show that the learner is able to:

P1   use work placement experiences to explain a minimum of six potential hazards in a health or social care setting

P2   describe how key legislation, in relation to health, safety and security, influences health and social care delivery

P3   using examples from work experience, describe how policies and procedures promote health, safety and security in the health and social care workplace

P4   examine the roles and responsibilities of key people in the promotion of health, safety and security in a health or social care setting

P5   carry out a health and safety survey of a local environment used by a specific patient/service user group

P6   demonstrate basic first aid skills.

To reach Merit level, the evidence must show that, in addition to the Pass criteria, the learner is able to:

M1   explain how legislation, policies and procedures are used to promote the health, safety and security of individuals in the health and social care workplace

M2   assess the risk associated with the use of the chosen local environment and make recommendations for change

M3   demonstrate first aid skills on a critically injured individual.

To reach Distinction level, the evidence must show that, in addition to the Pass and Merit criteria, the learner is able to:

D1   using examples from work experience, evaluate the effectiveness of policies and procedures for promoting health, safety and security

D2   justify recommendations for minimising the risks, as appropriate, for the setting and service user groups.

The importance of placement experience

It is beneficial for learners to start work on Unit 3 before beginning their first placement, to ensure that they take into account their own safety as well as that of service users and service providers. Students should be told to find out about the evacuation and emergency procedures on their first visit to their allocated work placement. While on their placements, students will benefit a great deal by observing others dealing with hazards. Time should be spent looking at different environments, including service users' homes. Risks covered should include accidents (e.g. falls) resulting in injuries, lack of awareness of danger due to cognitive impairment, caring for people with infectious conditions, improper storage or use of chemicals, and cross-contamination resulting from dealing with waste. If there is a delay in allocating work placements then students can find out about these procedures in their own learning environment instead. While they are on work placements, learners need to follow the individual setting's health and safety policies and procedures. You need to spend some time establishing certain ground rules at the outset, or at the very least before students attend their first placements. For instance, it is vital that learners maintain confidentiality relating to placement staff as well as service users. While on their placements, it is essential for students to keep professional logs. These records will be needed throughout Unit 3.

Assessment tasks

Task 1 (relevant criteria: P2, P4)

* Write a report that clearly explains the roles and responsibilities of key people in the promotion of health, safety and security in a health or social care setting **(P4)** and identify key supportive legislation **(P2)**.

Task 2 (relevant criteria: P5, M2, D2)

* Choose a specific user group and local environment to carry out a health and safety survey **(P5)**.
* Assess the risks associated with this environment and make recommendations to reduce the risks **(M2)**.
* Justify these recommendations **(D2)**.

Task 3 (relevant criteria: P1, P3, M1, D1)

* Complete professional logs covering activities, observations and assessments carried out in placements. **(P1)**
* Write an account reflecting on your individual work placement experiences to describe how policies and procedures promote health, safety and security **(P3)**.
* Explain how legislation, policies and procedures are used to promote health, safety and security **(M1)**.
* Evaluate the effectiveness of these policies and procedures for promoting health, safety and security **(D1)**.

Student logs should be assessed throughout the year so that tutors can make recommendations to ensure that students meet the pass criteria for this unit.

Scheme of work

BTEC National Health and Social Care
Unit 3 Health, safety and security in health and social care

Broad aim: Successful completion of the unit

Teacher(s): ....

Academic year: ....

Number of weeks: 35

Duration of session: 1 hour

Guided learning hours: 35

Week/s	Topic/outcome	Tutor preparation	Student activity	Resources	Links to grading criteria
1–2	Introduction to Unit 3	This PowerPoint® provides an explanation of unit content, ensuring professional logs are in place and understanding the dangers of food allergies. Introduction of the Health and Safety Act, including key points of the Act and policies arising in care settings, undertaking further research of the Act	You may like to give learners hard copies of the PPT presentation with spaces to add notes; these notes can be used as a basis for future discussion	PowerPoint® 1	P1, P2, P3, P4, P5, P6
3–4	Safe storage of chemicals	Specific regulations in relation to control of substances hazardous to health – COSHH and implications for practice. Introduction of key points of RIDDOR. Identifying procedures for reporting injuries, diseases and dangerous occurrences, and risk assessments	Learners can work alone or in small groups before discussing their answers with the rest of the class. As a placement activity, learners can be asked to collect information on specific examples of the safety measures used in the workplace. **Activity for placement: Identify where and how any chemicals are stored in your placement**	Activity 3.1	P2
5	Dealing with food allergies	Introduce specific regulations in relation to the storage and handling of food and implications for practice	Learners can discuss the activity in a whole class session or in small groups. This could also be covered by a 'Food handling' short course. **Activity for placement: Is there anyone in your placement with a food allergy? How is this managed by the staff?**	Activity 3.2	P2
6–7	Investigating the National Standards of Care and the effects and implications for care settings	Investigating the regulations in relation to healthcare providers and the effects and implications for care settings	Learners can carry out their own research to discover how the National Standards work in practice, and measures taken to meet them. **Activity for placement: Ask your placement supervisor how the setting ensures they meet the National Standards for Care**	Access to Internet	P2
8–9	Data Protection Act and confidentiality	This PowerPoint® provides an introduction to the Data Protection Act, right of access and security of records (both paper and electronic)	Ask learners to identify policies and procedures required by health and care settings. You may like to give learners hard copies of the PPT presentation with spaces to add notes	PowerPoint® 2	P2, P4

Unit 3 Health, safety and security in health and social care

Week/s	Topic/outcome	Tutor preparation	Student activity	Resources	Links to grading criteria
10–11	Roles and responsibilities of people in health and care settings	Identifying reasons for evacuating health and care settings. Setting and working on Assessment task 1	Learners can work in small groups to complete the activity, before discussing answers with the class. Ask learners to research other evacuation procedures and compare them to their answers. **Activity for placement: Identify the person who has responsibility for health and safety in your placement. Describe their role and explain their responsibilities**	Activity 3.3	P2, P4
12–13	Responding to hazards and accidents	This introduces learners to hazards in the workplace, especially in relation to poor practice. You need to cover reporting, recording and appropriate responses to accidents	Discussion of case studies in small groups and whole class. Independent research by students (this could be done in pairs or groups) into hazards in the workplace	Activity 3.4, Activity 3.5	P1, P3, M1, D1
14	Risk management	Learners can be asked to carry out some advance preparation before beginning the research and presentation in this activity	Learners take on the role of a health and safety manager for a group of residential care homes for the elderly, and give a presentation on how to undertake a risk assessment. **Activity for placement: Carry out a health and safety audit of your placement, identifying any hazards and potential risks**	Activity 3.6	P1, P3, M1, D1
15	Keeping professional logs	This PowerPoint® provides an introduction to keeping professional logs	You may like to give learners hard copies of the PPT presentation with spaces to add notes	PowerPoint® 3	P1, P3, M1, D1
16–18	Safe disposal of waste and reducing risks of contamination	Learners are introduced to dealing with spillages, recognising possible risks and identifying safe methods of disposal	For both Activities 3.7 and 3.8 learners can work in pairs or groups to discuss the issues. Encourage learners to feed their answers back to the class. Ask learners to carry out research into the differences between policies in specific workplaces and discuss why these differences might exist	Activity 3.7, Activity 3.8	P1, P3, M1, D1
19	Dealing with intruders	Looking at security of premises and service users, especially in open environments	Learners discuss the case studies in small groups. Learners can then carry out research to find specific examples for each policy. **Activity for placement: Identify the precautions your placement takes to stop intruders entering the premises. Do they have a procedure for recording who enters and leaves the building?**	Activity 3.9	P1, P3, M1, D1
20	Roles and responsibilities within health and care settings		Learners consider four different care situations and discuss roles and responsibilities	Activity 3.10	P4

Unit 3 Health, safety and security in health and social care

Week/s	Topic/outcome	Tutor preparation	Student activity	Resources	Links to grading criteria
21–22	Training opportunities	Establishing and maintaining competences and updating professional practice. Setting and working on Assessment task 2	Ask learners to research the training opportunities and gain some understanding of the differences between them. Learners can find out if any career choices need specific qualifications	Activity 3.11	P4, P5, M2, D2
23	Safeguarding vulnerable clients through safe employment practices	This PowerPoint® introduces safe employment practices	You may like to give learners hard copies of the PPT presentation with spaces to add notes	PowerPoint® 4	P2, P3, P4, M1, D1
24–25	Carrying out a survey on accidents	Activity 3.12 is a PowerPoint® that introduces the survey to be completed in work placements	Learners carry out surveys and present their results using graphs and/or charts	Activity 3.12	P5, M2, D2
26	Specialist and adapted equipment that supports independent living	This is an ideal session in which to invite an occupational therapist as a guest speaker	Learners ask guest speaker about specialist and adapted equipment		P1, P2, P4
27	Safe practices for working alone in the community	Encourage learners to discuss their conclusions on the case studies as a whole class	Learners consider three case studies and consider how risks could have been reduced or avoided. This can be done individually or as small group work	Activity 3.13	P1, P2, P4
28	Manual handling	Identify the need for specialist training in manual handling	Learners recognise the dangers of mishandling equipment and service users		P1, P2, P4
29	Policies and procedures in health and social care settings	Evaluating policies and procedures and reflecting on the effects of changes in legislation	Ask learners to research legislative changes. Learners can then produce presentations on the reasons behind specific changes. **Activity for placement: Ask your placement supervisor how health and safety incidents are recorded in the setting**	Access to Internet	P2, P4
30	Assessment of professional logs	Assessment of students' professional logs to ensure recording and students' evaluation of their own practice		Students' professional logs	P1, P3, M1, D1
31–34	First aid course		Learners complete a recognised first aid course		P6
35	Evaluation of professional logs and end-of-unit crossword	Completion of assessment and evaluation of students' logs. You can use the crossword in the final session to review the unit content	Learners complete crossword	Activity 3.14	P5, M2, D2

At-a-glance activity grid
Unit 3 Health, safety and security in health and social care

Activity	Title and description	Scheme of work	File/CD	Delivery notes	Additional resources	Links to grading criteria	Links to Student Book 1
Outcome 3.1 Understand potential hazards in health and social care							
Power Point® 1	Introduction to Health and Safety	Weeks 1–2	CD	Explanation of unit content, ensuring professional logs are in place and understanding the dangers of food allergies. Introduction of the Health and Safety Act, including key points of the Act and policies arising in care settings, undertaking further research of the Act. PPT to work through on a whole class basis	Handouts of PPT	P1, P2, P3, P4, P5, P6	pp 108–117
3.1	Safe storage of chemicals	Weeks 3–4	File (Answers on CD)	Specific regulations in relation to control of substances hazardous to health – COSHH and implications for practice. Introduction of key points of RIDDOR. Identifying procedures for reporting injuries, diseases and dangerous occurrences, and risk assessments		P1, P3	pp 108–117
3.2	Dealing with food allergies	Week 5	File (Answers on CD)	Discuss specific regulations in relation to the storage and handling of food and implications for practice. This could also be covered by a 'Food handling' short course. The worksheet can be used on an individual or group basis	Sample food labels	P1, P3	pp 108–117
	Investigating the National Standards of Care	Weeks 6–7		Investigating the regulations in relation to health care providers and the effects and implications for care settings		P2	pp 108–117
Outcome 3.2 Understand how legislation, guidelines, policies and procedures promote health, safety and security							
Power Point® 2	Security of information	Week 8	CD	PPT relating to the Data Protection Act and the importance of confidentiality	Handouts of PPT	P2, P4	pp 117–129
	Policies and procedures required by health and care settings	Week 9		Identifying policies and procedures required by health and care settings		P2, P4	pp 117–129
3.3	Evacuation procedures	Weeks 10–11	File	Identifying different reasons for evacuation of care settings. Learners write an evacuation procedure for a nursing home for the elderly. May be extended by asking students to evaluate the procedures. This is followed by setting and working on Assessment task 1		P2, P3, P4	pp 117–129
3.4	Hazards in the workplace	Week 12	File	Learners assess hazards in two different situations and reflect on them to find solutions. May be extended by asking students to write their own scenarios		P1, P3	pp 117–129

Activity	Title and description	Scheme of work	File/CD	Delivery notes	Additional resources	Links to grading criteria	Links to Student Book 1
3.5	Responding to accidents	Week 13	File	Individual or group research activity on accidents, followed by presentation of findings	Access to Internet for research	P1, P3, M1, D1	pp 117–129
3.6	Risk assessments	Week 14	File	Learners take on the role of a health and safety manager for residential care homes to plan risk management. May be extended by asking learners to present their findings		P1, P3, M1, D1	pp 117–129
Outcome 3.3 Understand roles and responsibilities for health, safety and security in health and social care settings							
PowerPoint® 3	Professional logs	Week 15	CD	PPT linking the students' professional placement logs to identified criteria for this unit	Students' own professional placement logs	P1, P3, M1, D1	pp 129–136
3.7	Dealing with spillages	Week 16	File (Tutor information and Answers on CD)	This individual matching activity can also be used as a small group activity	Copies of safety symbols, yellow slip warning sign	P1, P3, M1, D1	pp 129–136
3.8	Safe disposal of waste	Week 17	File (Answers on CD)	This activity involves matching appropriate methods to different waste products. It can be extended by changing the setting or service user	Yellow waste bags, sample sharp box (empty)	P1, P3, M1, D1	pp 129–136
	Precautions required to reduce risks of cross-contamination	Week 18		Identifying the risks of cross-contamination and precautions required to reduce the risks		P1, P3, M1, D1	pp 129–136
3.9	Dealing with intruders	Week 19	File (Answers on CD)	Learners match security systems to settings. This activity can be used with small groups or on an individual basis	Invite a safety police officer to give a talk	P1, P3, M1, D1	pp 129–136
3.10	Roles and responsibilities within health and care settings	Week 20	File	This individual task, requiring learners to identify appropriate responses and staff responsibility in four situations, may also be used to lead a discussion		P4	pp 129–136
3.11	Training opportunities	Week 21	File	In this individual or group-based activity, learners identify specific training needs and benefits		P4	pp 129–136
	Assessment task 2	Week 22	File	Setting and working on Assessment task 2		P5, M2, D2	

Outcome 3.4 Understand how to deal with hazards in a local environment

Activity	Title and description	Scheme of work	File/CD	Delivery notes	Additional resources	Links to grading criteria	Links to Student Book 1
Power Point® 4	Safe employment practices	Week 23	CD	PPT that deals with safeguarding vulnerable service users through safe employment practices	Handouts of PPT	P2, P3, P4, M1, D1	pp 137–145
3.12	Planning survey on accidents to be completed in work placements	Week 24	CD	PPT assisting student with identifying their requirements and planning their survey		P5, M2, D2	pp 137–145
	Presenting survey results	Week 25		Learners carry out surveys and present their results using graphs and/or charts		P5, M2, D2	pp 137–145
	Specialist and adapted equipment that supports independent living	Week 26		This is an ideal session in which to have an occupational therapist as a guest speaker		P1, P2, P4	pp 137–145
3.13	Safe practices for working alone in the community	Week 27	File	Learners consider three case studies and consider how risks could have been reduced or avoided. This could lead on to individual learners writing reflective accounts, or the case studies could be used as a basis for group discussions		P1, P2, P4	pp 137–145
	Manual handling	Week 28		Identifying the need for specialist training, and recognising the dangers of mishandling equipment and service users		P1, P2, P4	pp 137–145
	Policies and procedures in health and social care settings	Week 29		Evaluating polices and procedures and reflecting on the effects of changes in legislation		P2, P4	pp 137–145
	Assessment of professional logs	Week 30		Assessment of students' professional logs to ensure recording and students' evaluation of their own practice		P1, P3, M1, D1	pp 137–145
	First aid course	Weeks 31–34		Learners complete a recognised first aid course		P6	pp 137–145
3.14	Evaluation of professional logs and unit review	Week 35	File (Answers on CD)	Completion of assessment and evaluation of students' logs. End-of-unit crossword to review content		P5, M2, D2	pp 137–145

Unit 3 Lesson plan

Aims

- To introduce the unit

This structure may be spread over a number of lessons as required.

Learning outcomes
- recognise topics to be covered
- identify the need for boundaries and confidentiality
- list Learning outcomes for Unit 3
- list information required from placements.

Timing	Content	Teacher activity	Student activity	Resources	Individualised activity
5 mins	Introduction: Lesson aims and objectives written up and explained	Use varied levels of vocabulary to ensure understanding and to extend vocabulary			
15 mins	Explanation of Unit 3 topics and method of delivery	Tutor to ask open questions to confirm understanding		PowerPoint® 1	
15 mins	Explanation of unit assessment strategy, making notes	Note information required for higher grades	Students to respond to questions		
15 mins	The role of work-related placements	Encourage students to identify their areas of concern	Learners to clarify concerns and suggest strategies to overcome them		More able students can offer ideas on how to overcome the concerns raised
20 mins	Confidentiality when discussing instances relating to placements		Learners to work in small groups, considering possible difficulties in relation to confidentiality and suggesting boundaries. Students to give responses in group work	Flipchart	More confident students can make notes on flipchart
10 mins	Group feedback, producing boundaries for the group	Group feedback agreed, boundaries set	More confident students to give feedback for group, offering reasons for the difficulties and asking questions of other groups		
5 mins	Recap, identification of objectives met, information on next lesson to prepare students	Use varied vocabulary and repetition to ensure understanding	Students to respond to questions		

3.1   Safe storage of chemicals

Student Book 1
pp 108–117

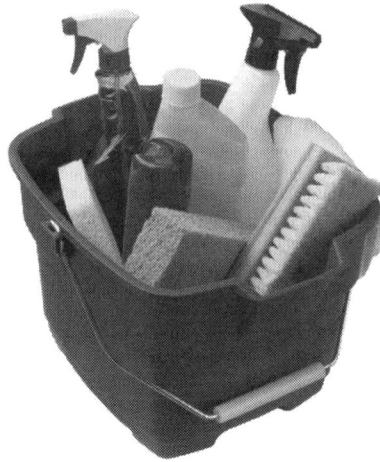

Fill in the following worksheet.

List chemicals that may be used in health or social care settings. Think about those used for cleaning purposes.
Indicate how these chemicals should be stored safely.
Identify safety measures that may need to be taken while using the chemicals.

3.2   Dealing with food allergies

**Student Book 1
pp 108–117**

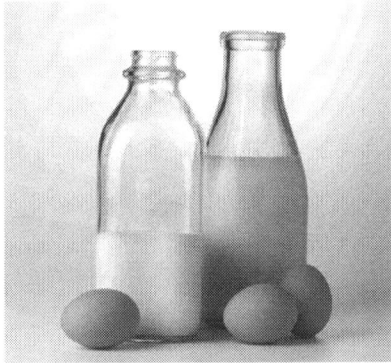

Food allergies can have a wide range of effects on sufferers, from a mild upset stomach to death. Milk is the most common cause of allergic reactions in children, but nuts and fish cause the most severe reactions. People with coeliac disease have an allergy to wheat. It is possible to develop allergies; they are not always evident from childhood. Some types of fish should be avoided because of the risk of choking on bones.

The table below shows six foods that cause around 90 per cent of all food-related allergic reactions. Take some time to consider each food type and then complete the table.

Food type	Describe the type of allergic reaction caused and give it a grade from 1 (mild) to 10 (fatal)	Identify food products that would need to be avoided	Identify precautions needed in care settings	Suggest alternatives to these foods
Eggs				
Fish				
Milk				
Nuts				
Shellfish				
Wheat				

3.3 Evacuation procedures

Student Book 1
pp 117–129

Identify five reasons for evacuating a health or social care setting.

1 ....

2 ....

3 ....

4 ....

5 ....

Now write a procedure for evacuating the nursing home described below in an emergency. Identify any specific roles for staff members and explain how the staff will know their specific roles.

The home provides nursing care for 12 elderly residents, all of whom have different degrees of dementia. Two are also visually impaired, and four are hearing impaired.

There are 17 members of staff in total, some of whom work part time.

Due to shift rotations, the minimum number of staff on site at any time is four and the maximum is eight. There are always eight members of staff on duty between 8 a.m. and 8 p.m. The staff roles are as follows:

- one manager and two deputy managers (one of whom is always on duty)
- a receptionist/administrator who works from 9 a.m. to 5 p.m., Monday to Friday
- three nursing sisters who work on an eight-hour shift rota
- three newly qualified nurses who work on an eight-hour shift rota
- three care workers all of whom have a Level 3 or 2 NVQ in Care who work on an eight-hour shift rota
- two care assistants, one of whom covers for the cook two days a week
- a cook who works five days a week on a rota for six hours a day, from 10.30 a.m. till 4.30 p.m.
- a cleaner who works from 7.30 a.m. till 11.30 p.m.
- two volunteers who provide entertainment for the residents on Mondays, Wednesdays and Fridays from 2 p.m. to 4 p.m.

3.4   Recognising and reducing potential hazards

Student Book 1
pp 117–129

Consider the following information and highlight any potential hazards. Then list them in order, from highest to lowest risk. You can use a grading system of 1 to 5, such as those used when undertaking a risk assessment. Make sure that you explain your grading system. Then discuss how the following hazards could be reduced or avoided.

Situation 1

Someone has walked into a bucket of water, spilling it all over the floor in the waiting area of a very busy hospital accident and emergency unit. The receptionist rings for a cleaner to mop up the water. She is told it will be at least five minutes before they can get anyone there. The receptionist is concerned that someone may slip on the wet floor but there is no warning sign nearby and she is far too busy to go looking for one.

Situation 2

Sam is bedridden and has very bad bedsores. It is Monday morning and his care worker has arrived at his home to help his wife get him washed and turned. Sam and his wife are both in their seventies. His wife is frail and can't manage Sam on her own. When the care worker arrives she finds that Sam's wife is unable to help, as she has flu. It requires two people to lift and turn Sam. The carer did not know Sam's wife was ill. She was fine the last time she visited on Friday, and there are no weekend visits to their home.

Now describe a potential hazard using information from your experiences in placement or the knowledge you have of a health or social care setting. Include your own suggestions for reducing the risks and/or solving the problems. (Remember to preserve anonymity and confidentiality by not giving actual names or identifiable details about settings or individuals.)

Swap your potential hazard situation with one written up by another student, and compare your ideas for reducing the risks and/or solving the problems.

3.5   Research task: Types of accidents

Student Book 1
pp 117–129

Research the most common types of accidents for different age ranges, environments and groups of service users in health and social care settings. Then devise a short questionnaire to collect information on accidents that have occurred within a set time frame within your student group. Extend your time frame until you have sufficient data to identify their most hazardous year for accidents as a group. Present your findings as clearly as possible in a chart or table.

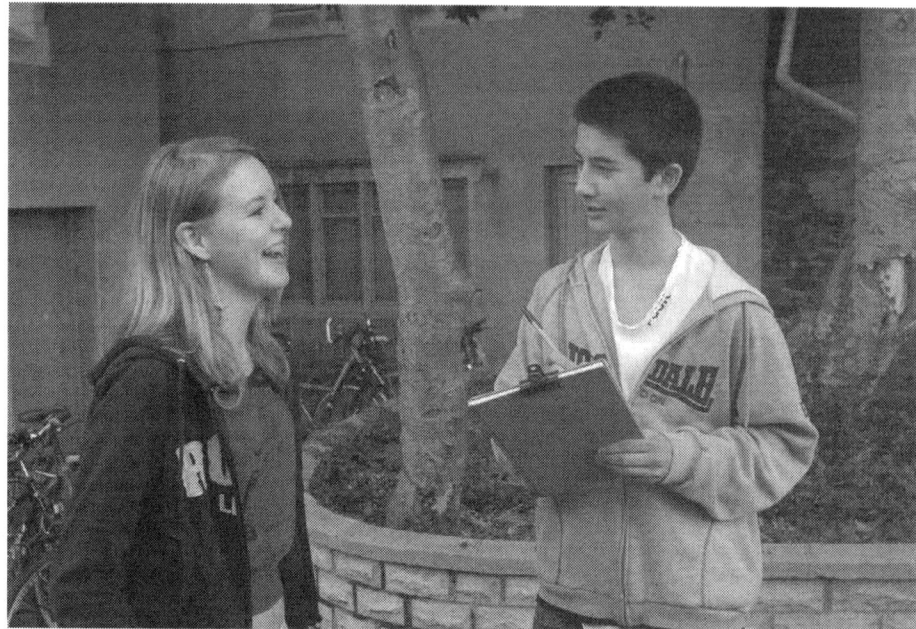

3.6   Risk management

Student Book 1
pp 117–129

For this activity, you will be taking on the role of a health and safety manager for a group of residential care homes for the elderly.

One of your responsibilities is training staff to carry out risk assessments. You should therefore prepare a presentation (in PowerPoint® or any other format) that explains why staff members have to carry out risk assessments and how to undertake one. You will also need to provide a handout to support your presentation. Remember the need:

1   to meet legal requirements

2   to adapt risk assessments to cover different health and care settings (or say if the risk assessment is only relevant to a specific type of setting)

3   to consider levels of risk

4   to consider responsibilities.

3.7 Dealing with spillages

Student Book 1
pp 129–136

Match the following incidents (identified by letters) with the following actions (identified by numbers). Some incidents may require several actions.

Incidents	Actions
(a) A large amount of vomit	1 Call for a cleaner
(b) A spilt bag of transfusion blood	2 Put up a yellow warning sign
(c) A damaged colostomy bag	3 Cover it with sand
(d) A spilt bucket of water that has been used to disinfect an infected area	4 Place paper towels over the area
(e) A spilt canister of slug pellets	5 Remove all service users from the area
(f) A spilt bottle of superglue	6 Inform the manager
(g) A spilt blood sample from a person with HIV	7 Set off the fire alarm to evacuate the building

For incident (a), I would take actions ……………………………..

For incident (b), I would take actions ……………………………..

For incident (c), I would take actions ……………………………..

For incident (d), I would take actions ……………………………..

For incident (e), I would take actions ……………………………..

For incident (f), I would take actions ……………………………..

For incident (g), I would take actions ……………………………..

3.8 Safe disposal of waste

Student Book 1
pp 129–136

Describe in detail the procedure for disposing of the following types of waste materials.

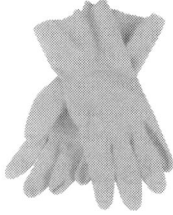

Type of waste	Method of disposal
Tissue used to wipe the mouth of an elderly person with dementia	
Cloth used to clean the highchairs and tables used at mealtimes in a day nursery	
A soiled incontinence pad	
Tissues that have been used by a person with a nose bleed	
A used diabetic syringe	
Gloves and apron used by a member of staff who has cleaned the area and toys where a child has vomited	
Paper towels used by staff and service users to dry their hands	

3.9   Security: Avoiding and dealing with intruders

Student Book 1
pp 129–136

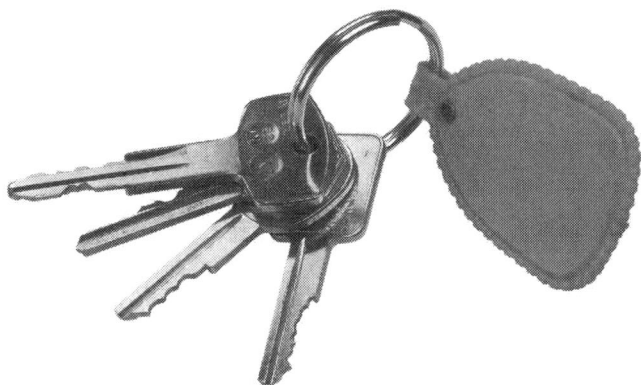

Security of service users and staff has become a major concern over recent years. It is more difficult in some settings to have a secure environment. Take a few minutes to consider the different health and social care environments that you know. How do they ensure the security of their service users and staff, while also allowing freedom of movement and access? Working in pairs or small groups, draw a line matching the best security system to each setting. In each case justify your selection and describe the positive and negative aspects of the system chosen.

Care settings	**Security systems**
Accident and Emergency Department	Standard Yale locks fitted to all doors
Elderly residential care home	Card key lock to main entrance
Community home for adults with learning difficulties	Keypad with a regularly changed code
Children's care home	Security office at front of building staffed from 7 a.m. to 11 p.m.
Day centre for adults with disabilities	Magnetic lock with release control in reception office
Boarding school for children with complex special needs	Intercom with lock release
Elderly residential nursing home	Open entrance with receptionist who has a panic alarm button
Medical centre	Video camera linked to electronic lock

Now write a procedure for dealing with the threat of an intruder for one of the settings.

3.10 Roles and responsibilities

Student Book 1
pp 129–136

Situation 1

The hoist in a service user's home is not working. The care worker used the hoist on Friday. There have been no carer visits since then, as the service user's partner cares for her at weekends. The carer is unable to use the hoist on Monday morning.

■ Who should report the problem with the hoist?

■ Who do you think will cover the cost of the repair?

Explain the reasons for your responses.

Situation 2

A new floor has been laid in the entrance to a care home. The owner came in over the weekend to do the work himself. On Monday morning it started to rain, and the floor became wet and slippery as people entered in wet shoes. The staff were used to walking in onto a tread mat and carpeted area, and some staff members moaned to each other about the lack of a tread mat. Later in the afternoon a visitor arrived. On entering the home, he slipped on the wet floor and hurt his back.

■ How could the manager have warned people of the danger of the wet floor?

■ Was anyone else in a position to deal with the situation?

Explain the reasons for your responses.

Situation 3

While helping the cook in a care home prepare an evening meal, Janice (another staff member) cut her finger. Janice pressed a tea towel on to her finger but the cut would not stop bleeding. The cook got the first aid box down but there were no dressings. The box only contained a pair of scissors, a couple of safety pins, eye wash solution and a sling. The cook used the internal phone to ring reception to ask for a first aider. The receptionist came to the kitchen. On seeing how deep the cut was, she suggested that Janice took herself off to the local hospital accident and emergency unit, which was a few miles away. Janice got her coat and left. However, once outside in the car park, she felt faint. A passer-by stopped and called an ambulance.

■ Should Janice have gone alone?

■ Was an ambulance necessary?

Explain the reasons for your responses.

Situation 4

The previous night was very stormy, and a large tree fell across the garden outside a nursing home. One of the branches broke a window on the ground floor next to the rear entrance. The night staff recorded the information in their shift report. The next day, the area has been swept and a warning sign put up; only staff members use the rear entrance. The duty manager for the day shift reads the report and assumes that the area has been made safe and secure. She rings the maintenance man to inform him. Later that day a staff member notices a stranger in the building. When challenged by the staff member, the man runs out of the back door. The staff member notices that the board covering the broken window has been pushed in, allowing access to the rear door lock.

■ What else could the staff have done to secure the premises?

■ Who was at risk?

Explain the reasons for your responses.

3.11   Training opportunities

Student Book 1
pp 129–136

Consider the following training opportunities and decide which health or social care workers would benefit from taking these courses. Take some time to consider workers in different health and social care settings as well as those working with different groups of service users across a range of ages and abilities. You can use the spare boxes to identify the type of settings that the staff would be employed by.

Manual Handling Operations Certificate	**Control of Substances Hazardous to Health (COSSH)**
First Aider at Work Certificate	**An Introduction to British Sign Language (BSL)**
Food Hygiene	**NVQ Level 3 in Care**
An Introduction to Makaton	**In-House Risk Assessment Training**
Understanding the Data Protection Act 1998	**Reporting of Injuries, Diseases and Dangerous Occurrences Regulations (RIDDOR)**
Counselling Certificate (Level 1 and 2)	**Fire Safety and Evacuation Procedures**

3.13 Case studies: Dangers of working in the community

Student Book 1
pp 137–145

Working alone in the community can be dangerous for a number of reasons. Read the following case studies and write an account that identifies the dangers for the different community workers. Then consider what steps could have been taken beforehand to reduce the risks or avoid the dangerous situations. This may be written as a risk assessment or as a report for each case.

Case study 1

A health visitor is going to visit a mother and her 11-day-old baby. It is her first visit to the family home, as they moved to the area just before the baby was born. The health visitor was due to meet with the midwife who had delivered the baby at the local hospital. However, the midwife had a car accident and was in a coma. The health visitor got the case notes from the hospital but they were hand-written and difficult to read. She gained the following useful information: 'arrived late to hospital, already … dilated, natural birth, no painkillers given, used gas and air, required stitching, … boy, weight 3.7 kg, length (not recorded), admitted for 24 hours.'

The family had registered with a local GP. From the registration documents, the health visitor found out that this was the fourth child born to the mother, and she had had three boys in the previous five years. There were no other records with the same surname recorded as new patients. However, there were four boys of corresponding ages registered, all with different surnames, but the same address. The home was in a rundown part of town, known to have a high crime rate. The health visitor arrives at the house at 4.30 p.m., on a cold, dark December afternoon.

Case study 2

The community occupational therapist (OT) went to the home of a three-year-old child with muscular dystrophy to carry out an assessment. He was met by the family's health visitor outside their home. It was the OT's first visit to the family and he had therefore asked the health visitor (who knew the family well) to introduce him. This was normal practice in the area, designed to put families at ease with professionals visiting them in their homes. Before the visit the OT had done some background reading to help him understand the condition, and make an informed assessment. The boy was the first child of a married couple in their mid-twenties. The father worked full time and the mother had stopped work to care for her child at home. The child had been diagnosed through random blood screening tests when he was ten days old.

The visit went very well and after the introductions the mother was happy for the health visitor to leave. The OT completed his assessment and was explaining to the mother the action plan he proposed to meet the child's needs. The mother went into the kitchen to make tea and the OT followed her to talk through the child's care plan. While the kettle was boiling the mother started drying the dishes that were stacked on the draining board. All was going well until the OT said he would have to contact the physiotherapist and the

Continued overleaf

3.13 Case studies: Dangers of working in the community (*contd*)

wheelchair service. The mother became hysterical. No one had mentioned the word 'wheelchair' to her before. The OT reached out to calm her down, not realizing that she still had a large knife inside the tea towel in her hand. The knife fell and landed tip first on his foot. He felt a piercing pain and collapsed to the floor.

Case study 3

Julie works in the community visiting the elderly and disabled. Her morning duties include helping service users to get out of bed, wash, dress, and prepare breakfast. She returns to the same people in the evening and helps them get undressed and into bed. Julie works for an agency; she has a Level 3 Diploma in Care and enjoys her work. She has a good relationship with all but one service user, who she has been visiting for a couple of weeks. This lady has shouted and sworn at Julie, and complains that Julie is hurting her whenever she moves her limbs while dressing or undressing her.

When Julie arrives one evening the lady's son-in-law is visiting, and the lady looks upset. Julie introduces herself to the relative and goes into the bathroom to ensure that everything is ready for the evening wash routine. When she returns the visitor has left so Julie helps the lady to wash and then undress for bed. As Julie is drying the lady's arms, she notices a large fresh bruise on her upper arm. Julie asks the lady if she has hurt herself. The lady says 'No, but you keep hurting me.'

As Julie walks home she thinks to herself that she needs to write up the information and talk to the agency in the morning. But when Julie arrives home she is met by her son who is really excited and wants to show her what he has made at school.

The next day Julie is met at the lady's home by a social worker. He has received a complaint from the son-in-law. Julie is being accused of abusing the lady. Julie has not recorded any of the information from the previous night; she forgot to write it up.

3.14 End of unit crossword

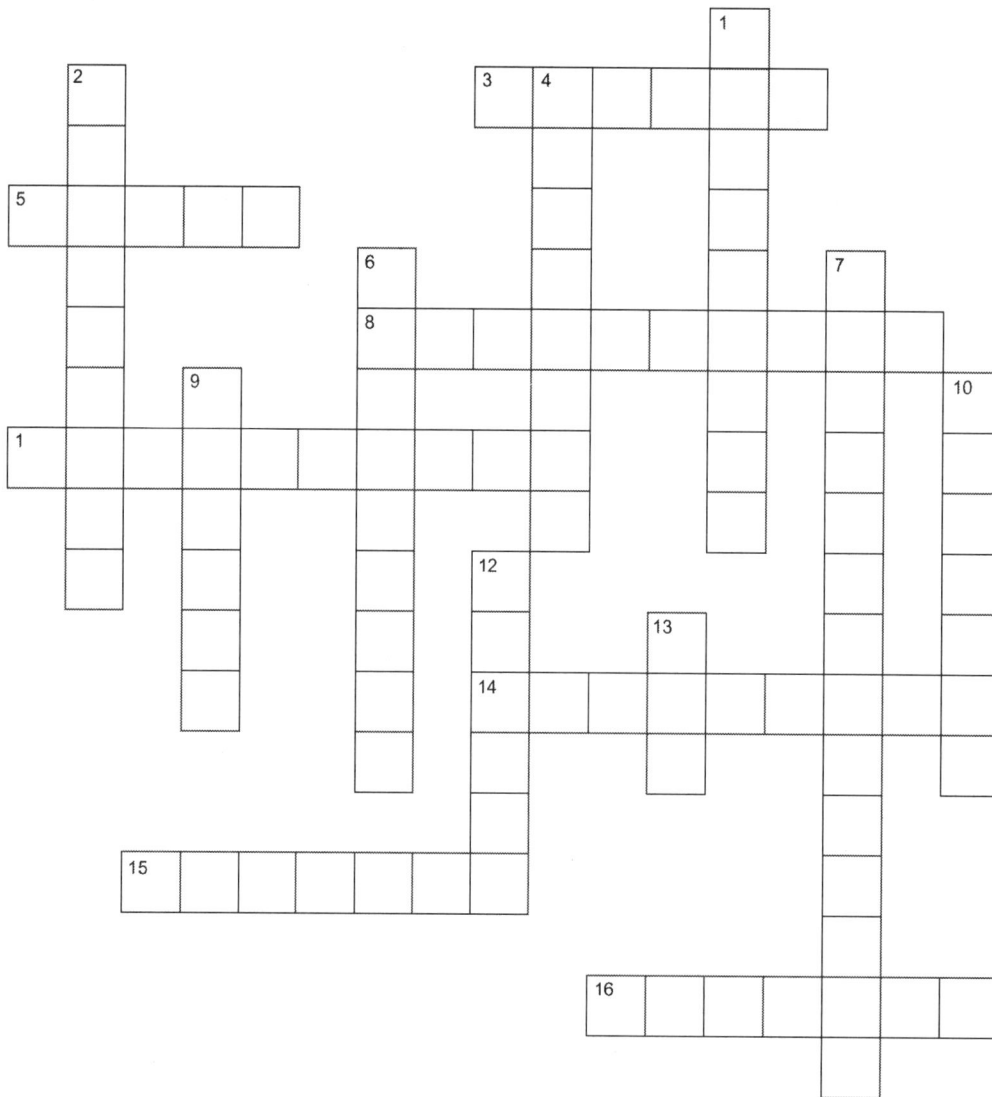

ACROSS

3 Legislation to follow after an accident
5 Legal guidelines that cover the use and storage of chemicals
8 Vehicles called in an emergency
11 To be at risk
14 Watching to learn
15 Dangerous situations
16 Changed to be more suitable

DOWN

1 Collective name used for domestic environments
2 How staff know what to do in a given situation
4 Unwanted visitor
6 They may arrive by ambulance
7 Allocation of duty
9 Possible result of an accident
10 Adverse reaction especially to certain foods
12 You wear them to help prevent cross-contamination
13 An opener

4

Development through the life stages

unit overview

This unit explores the way people develop as life progresses. Learners will gain a valuable insight into the way people's needs and priorities are influenced by their age and stage of development. The unit is split into three distinct Learning outcomes.

Learning outcomes

On completion of this unit learners should:

4.1 understand human growth and development through the life stages

4.2 understand how life factors and events may influence the development of the individual

4.3 understand physical changes and psychological perspectives in relation to ageing.

Suggested activities

The At-a-glance activity grid shows how the activities in the Assessment and Delivery Resource (ADR) relate to the content of the unit. The activities include introductory and plenary activities and a variety of case studies, research tasks, discussions and presentations, using written, verbal and presentation skills. The activities may help learners prepare for assessment, and the grid indicates which assessment criteria are relevant for each activity. Copies of activity sheets can be given to learners.

The content of each Learning outcome

Learning outcome 1: Understand human growth and development through the life stages (relevant criteria: P1, M1, D1)

For this outcome students will learn how human growth and development is categorised and measured. They will become familiar with the language used to describe development, and explore how we respond to people at different stages of development (Activity 4.1). They will see how developmental milestones are created and applied (Activity 4.2), and explore the nature-nurture debate (Activity 4.3). The knowledge gained will be consolidated using a case study approach (Activity 4.4), and finally applied to evidence gained during placement (Activity 4.5).

Learning outcome 2: Understand how life factors and events may influence the development of the individual (relevant criteria: P2, P3, M2)

This Learning outcome begins by focusing on humans as individual organisms, exploring the genetic factors that influence development (Activity 4.6). This view will then widen to include the effect of a person's physical environment, and the impact of interpersonal and social relationships on development (Activity 4.7). This will lead on to a consideration of the way major life events affect personal change and growth (Activity 4.8). Finally learners will explore the impact of these factors on individuals, using experiences from placement combined with case studies (Activity 4.9).

Learning outcome 3: Understand physical changes and psychological perspectives in relation to ageing (relevant criteria: P4, P5, M3, D2)

This last outcome considers the psychology and physiology of maturation and ageing. Learners will research and write about puberty and the menopause (Activities 4.10 and 4.11). They will then focus on the psychological and social effects these changes can bring (Activity 4.12). This will give students an opportunity to review and consolidate points covered in Learning outcome 1, while considering individuals at the end of their lives. Learners will then compare two contrasting theories of ageing (Activity 4.13). They will consider specific medical factors (Activity 4.14) and will be encouraged to gain a balanced view of ageing, in order to promote empathy and respect.

This unit can be taught very effectively using hypothetical and real case studies (Activities 4.15 and 4.16). Learners can compile life histories of two or more individuals, tracking their development from birth to death. These histories should compare and contrast individuals from different backgrounds and circumstances in order to highlight the influence of factors such as gender, poverty and environment. The histories can begin with basic details of life stages and developmental norms. Details such as environmental or social factors can be added, and gradually a more detailed account can be created. Finally, there is a crossword (Activity 4.17), which should demonstrate how much knowledge learners have gained!

How this unit will be assessed

To reach Pass level, the evidence must show that the learner is able to:

P1 describe physical, intellectual, emotional and social development through the life stages
P2 describe the potential influence of five life factors on the development of individuals
P3 describe the influence of two predictable and two unpredictable major life events on the development of the individual
P4 describe two theories of ageing
P5 describe physical and psychological changes caused by the ageing process.

To reach Merit level, the evidence must show that, in addition to the Pass criteria, the learner is able to:

M1 discuss the nature-nurture debate in relation to individual development
M2 explain how major life events can influence the development of the individual
M3 use examples to compare the influence of two major theories of ageing on health and social care provision.

To reach Distinction level, the evidence must show that, in addition to the Pass and Merit criteria, the learner is able to:

D1 evaluate the nature-nurture debate in relation to the development of the individual
D2 evaluate the influence of two major theories of ageing on health and social care provision.

The importance of case studies and placement experience

Four of the activities are case studies. Three of the case studies are provided in full, with questions that enable learners to consider all the relevant issues (Activities 4.4, 4.9 and 4.15). The fourth case study (Activity 4.16) is created by students themselves. These four case studies are included in addition to the developmental timeline (Activity 4.2), which tracks an individual's whole lifespan. Where possible, learners can incorporate the experiences of older people they have met on placements in their case studies. However, it is very important that students respect the confidentiality and vulnerability of such individuals, and only use material that is kept anonymous, and has been gathered sensitively.

The case studies can be utilised effectively for assessments, supplemented where necessary with alternative pieces. The P1 criteria can be met with a written piece, outlining expected development through the life stages. This could be presented as separate strands for physical, intellectual, emotional and social development. The P2 and M2 criteria are directly addressed by Activity 4.2. This could simply be written up and assessed accordingly.

The P3 and M3 criteria can use the case studies, combined with a discussion of psychology and sociology research evidence. Care should be taken to ensure that students understand the difference between predictable and unpredictable life events, as these two types of events can have very different effects on individual development.

The P4, P5, M3 and D2 criteria should draw heavily on out-of-classroom experience, through placements, visits or community engagements. Learners should, wherever possible, base their answers on the testimony of the elderly people they have met, while taking care to respect their dignity and privacy. The case study approach can also be applied to presentations or videos, allowing students to share with the class their experiences of working with the elderly.

Assessment tasks

Task 1 (relevant criteria: P1, P2, M1, D1)

Create a timeline, which follows an individual from conception to death. Include:

- A clear identification of each life stage
- The major milestones associated with each stage
- At least five factors that could influence your individual's development (e.g. genetic, environmental, etc)
- For each of the five factors, explain their influence on development in terms of the nature-nurture debate.
(P1, P2, M1)

Using your timeline, write a brief (500 words maximum) account that explains how useful the nature-nurture debate is in explaining human development. Include consideration of the following questions:

- Is it possible to decide which factors are nature and which are nurture?
- Does this distinction really help us understand how people grow and change?
- How does this debate relate to personal beliefs?
- Is each side of the argument based on a different view of people? **(D1)**

Task 2 (relevant criteria: P3, M3)

Select two major unpredictable life events, and two major predictable life events. For each one, write an advice leaflet that will explain:

- Whether they are predictable or unpredictable
- What short-term effects they will have on an individual's development
- What long-term effects they will have on an individual's development
- Whether those effects are positive or negative

You may want to describe events that have happened to yourself or to someone you know. If so, please remember to keep your answers anonymous by making sure that no one can identify the people you write about. **(P3)**

Continue your discussion, including other major life events. Consider how the individual's development might have been different if those events had not happened, and explain the specific ways in which those events caused a **change**. **(M3)**

Task 3

Consider the **disengagement theory** and the **activity theory** of ageing.

Create two care plans for two individuals: one who is typical of disengagement theory, and another who is typical of activity theory. Your plans should help someone who has just begun working with these two people to understand and meet their needs with respect and dignity. Include:

- The major physical changes the two individuals experience as they age
- The major psychological changes they experience as they age

*NB: These should include both positive **and** negative changes.* **(P5)**

- How they interact with others
- The changes they have made to their daily routines **(P4)**
- How they are similar, and how they differ **(M3)**
- What care and health services they will require
- How those services should be provided
- How their individual life choices affect the types of care they require. **(D2)**

Scheme of work

BTEC National Health and Social Care
Unit 4 Development through the life stages
Broad aim: Successful completion of the unit
Teacher(s): ....

Academic year: ....
Number of weeks: 30
Duration of session: 2 hours
Guided learning hours: 60

Week/s	Topic/outcome	Tutor preparation	Student activity	Resources	Links to grading criteria
1–2	Introduction to Unit 4: Define and describe different life stages	You may like to give learners hard copies of the PowerPoint® presentation with spaces to add notes	Learners can carry out Activities 4.1 and 4.1a using other writing, photographs, paintings or video clips	PowerPoint® 1, Activity 4.1, Activity 4.1a	P1, P2, M1, D1
3–4	Describe the expected phases of normal physical development	This piece of work would be very effective if prominently displayed in the classroom	Learners work in groups to create a timeline of the average lifespan. Learners can add to and adapt as the unit progresses, either in the form of a display or as a folder or file for each student.	Activity 4.2	P1, P2
5–6	Describe the expected phases of normal intellectual and language development to explore the nature-nurture debate	You should emphasise that there are no right or wrong answers, and encourage learners to discuss the issues raised	Learners to look at a list of statements and decide which best apply to them, and then discuss further in a whole class setting. Ask learners to create a few questions of their own	Activity 4.3	P1, M1, D1
7–8	Describe the expected phases of normal emotional and social development	You can use the case studies as ongoing examples, to illustrate unit themes	Learners discuss the themes raised in the case studies, and complete written answers to the questions either in pairs or individually	Activity 4.4 (Case study one)	P1, P2, P3 M1, M2, D1
9–10	Explore the potential problems of delayed development, and how development can be supported	This task should be set before learners go out into placement	Learners to prepare a short presentation on their placements, which they then present to the rest of the class. Encourage learners to field questions on their presentations	Activity 4.5	P2, P3, M2
11–12	List the genetic and biological factors that impact on development	You may like to give learners hard copies of the PowerPoint® presentation with spaces to add notes. Activity 4.6 should be divided over two sessions	Learners work in groups to create a presentation. You should select groups to allow differentiation across ability and learning style. Learners can record their own impressions and understandings from each presentation. These can be used as a basis for whole class discussion	PowerPoint® 2, Activity 4.6	P2, P3, M2

Unit 4 Development through the life stages

Week/s	Topic/outcome	Tutor preparation	Student activity	Resources	Links to grading criteria
13–14	Investigate the environmental and socio-economic factors that impact on development	This activity is particularly suitable for visual learners	Learners work individually to produce mind maps® around themes of their choice. You should encourage students to produce a mind map® in whichever way suits them best	Activity 4.7	P2
15–16	List and describe major life events and evaluate their influence on development	In Activity 4.8 you should emphasise the contents of the list, and ask students to evaluate these events	Learners individually complete a stress test, then discuss the issues raised either in small groups or as a whole class. Ask learners to suggest ways in which stress can be reduced	Activity 4.8	P1, P2, P3, M1, M2, D1
17–18	Explore and discuss the interrelationships between factors that influence development	In Activity 4.9 you can use the case studies as ongoing examples, to illustrate unit themes		Activity 4.9 (Case study two)	P1, P2, P3, M1, M2, D1
19	Define and describe the physical and psychological changes in ageing	You may like to give learners hard copies of the PowerPoint® presentation with spaces to add notes		PowerPoint® 3	P4, P5, M3, D2
20–21	Outline the role of hormones in puberty and menopause	Activities 4.10 and 4.11 will need to be focused on the way these stages affect psychological as well as physical development	Learners work in groups to prepare a poster, and have a whole class discussion of the themes covered. Learners then individually prepare a pamphlet for Activity 4.11	Activity 4.10, Activity 4.11	P1, P5
22–23	Assess the effects of life factors	For Activity 4.12, learners will need to be fully briefed before going into placement, and will need to show sensitivity to service users	Learners use experience gained from placement to complete a table showing the effects of life factors	Activity 4.12	P2, P3, M2
24–25	Describe and compare theories of ageing	This activity should draw on placement experience	Learners to apply theories to practice. Learners could expand this activity with role play	Activity 4.13	P4, P5, M3, D2
26–27	Assess the impact of the major physical effects of ageing	This activity should be handled sensitively	Learners to discuss their own feelings about the physical deterioration associated with ageing. Learners carry out research in groups	Activity 4.14	P5
28	Assess the impact of the major psychological effects of ageing	You can use the case studies as ongoing examples, to illustrate unit themes		Activity 4.15 (Case study three)	P1, P2, P3, P4, P5, M2, M3, D2

Unit 4 Development through the life stages

Week/s	Topic/outcome	Tutor preparation	Student activity	Resources	Links to grading criteria
29	Assess the impact of major life events on people at different life stages	You can use the case studies as ongoing examples, to illustrate unit themes	Learners discuss the themes raised in the case studies, and complete written answers to the questions either in pairs or individually	Activity 4.16 (Case study four)	All
30	Unit review and evaluation	You can use this crossword in the final session as a recap	Learners complete crossword	Activity 4.17	All

At-a-glance activity grid
Unit 4 Development through the life stages

Activity	Title and description	Scheme of work	File/CD	Delivery notes	Additional resources	Links to grading criteria	Links to Student Book 1
Outcome 4.1 Understand human growth and development through the life stages							
PowerPoint 1	Define and describe the different life stages	Week 1	CD	This PPT presentation introduces the key concepts and activities for the first Learning outcome. You may like to give learners hard copies of the PPT presentation with spaces to add notes	Copies of PPT presentation	P1, P2, M1, D1	pp 152–164
4.1	Life stages	Week 1	File	This activity uses a passage by Shakespeare to stimulate reflection on the different stages in a human life. You may wish to adapt this activity using other articles, video clips, etc	Articles, video clips, etc	P1	pp 152–164
4.1a	Life stages	Week 2	File	Discussion based on photograph of multi-generational family. You may wish to adapt this activity using other photographs or paintings	Photographs, paintings, etc	P1	pp 152–164
4.2	Developmental timeline	Weeks 3–4	File	This is an ongoing activity, which can be used to produce a holistic documentary record of all aspects of the unit. This piece of work would be very effective if prominently displayed in the classroom. It can be added to and adapted as the unit progresses, in the form of a display or as a folder or file for each student	Long piece of paper (e.g. fax roll) and sticky notes or paper and sticky tack	P1, P2	pp 152–164
4.3	The nature-nurture debate	Weeks 5–6	File	This is a self-assessment activity that explores the nature-nurture debate. You should emphasise that there are no right or wrong answers, and encourage students to discuss the issues raised		P1, M1, D1	pp 152–164
4.4	Case study one	Weeks 7–8	File	This is a short case study with progressively more difficult discussion/individual work questions. You can use the case studies as ongoing examples, to illustrate unit themes		P1, P2, P3, M1, M2, D1	pp 152–164
4.5	Services at your placement	Weeks 9–10	File	This task should be set before students go out into placement. They need to give presentations on how placements meet the developmental needs of service users	Placement journals	P2, P3, M2	pp 152–164
Outcome 4.2 Understand how life factors and events may influence the development of the individual							
PowerPoint 2	Life factors and events	Week 11	CD	This PPT presentation introduces the key concepts and activities for the second Learning outcome. You may like to give learners hard copies of the PPT presentation with spaces to add notes	Copies of PPT presentation	P2, P3, M2	pp 165–184
4.6	Genetic factors in development	Weeks 11–12	File	This research and presentation activity for small groups should be divided over one or two sessions. You should select groups to allow differentiation across ability and learning style		P2	pp 165–184

Activity	Title and description	Scheme of work	File/CD	Delivery notes	Additional resources	Links to grading criteria	Links to Student Book 1
4.7	Impact of socio-economic factors on development	Weeks 13–14	File	This mind mapping® activity is particularly suitable for visual learners. You should encourage students to produce a mind map® in whichever way suits them best	Materials needed for mind mapping® (e.g. coloured pens, sticky notes, etc)	P2	pp 165–184
4.8	Major life events	Weeks 15–16	File	This activity uses Holmes and Rahe's list of major life events to measure stress levels. You should emphasise the contents of the list, and ask students to evaluate these events		P1, P2, P3, M1, M2	pp 165–184
4.9	Case study two	Weeks 17–18	File	This is a short case study with progressively more difficult discussion/individual work questions. You can use the case studies as ongoing examples, to illustrate unit themes	Placement journals	P1, P2, P3, M1, M2, D1	pp 165–184
Outcome 4.3 Understand physical changes and psychological perspectives in relation to ageing							
Power Point® 3	Define and describe the physical and psychological changes in ageing	Week 19	CD	This PPT presentation introduces the key concepts and activities for the third Learning outcome. You may like to give learners hard copies of the PPT presentation with spaces to add notes	Copies of PPT presentation	P4, P5, M3, D2	pp 185–197
4.10	Puberty	Week 20	File	This group activity defines and describes puberty. Learners will need to be encouraged to act professionally when dealing with sensitive issues of sexual development. Tutors may like to encourage this by asking males to research and describe females, and vice versa	Poster paper, sticky notes, coloured pens	P1, P5	pp 185–197
4.11	Menopause	Week 21	File	This individual or pair work explores the effects of menopause. You may like to open this session with a discussion about how menopause has affected learners' own families		P1, P5	pp 185–197
4.12	The effects of life factors	Weeks 22–23	File	This placement-based activity uses real examples to illustrate the ideas in this unit. Learners will need to be fully briefed before going into placement, and will need to show sensitivity to clients	Placement journals	P2, P3, M2	pp 185–197
4.13	Theories of ageing	Weeks 24–25	File	This task compares activity and disengagement theory. It should draw on placement experience, and enable learners to apply theories to practice	Placement journals	P4, P5, M3, D2	pp 185–197
4.14	Physical changes of ageing	Weeks 26–27	File	This worksheet focuses on the physical effects of growing older, and then explores the major medical conditions that affect the elderly. This activity gives an opportunity for learners to discuss their own feelings about the physical deterioration associated with ageing, and should be handled sensitively		P5	pp 185–197

Activity	Title and description	Scheme of work	File/CD	Delivery notes	Additional resources	Links to grading criteria	Links to Student Book 1
4.15	Case study three	Week 28	File	This is a short case study with progressively more difficult discussion/individual work questions You can use the case studies as ongoing examples, to illustrate unit themes	Placement journals	P1, P2, P3, P4, P5, M2, M3, D2	pp 185–197
4.16	Case study four	Week 29	File	This is an opportunity for learners to consolidate their knowledge by constructing a case study that explores all the course themes. You can use the case studies as ongoing examples, to illustrate unit themes	Placement journals	All	pp 185–197
4.17	End-of-unit crossword	Week 30	File (Answers on CD)	This activity could also be used at the beginning of the unit. Comparing learners' answers will demonstrate and reinforce learning		All	pp 185–197

Unit 4 Lesson plan

Aims

- To introduce the unit

This structure may be spread over a number of lessons as required.

Learning outcomes

- list the learning outcomes for this unit
- describe different stages of life development
- discuss life stage development issues.

Timing	Content	Teacher activity	Student activity	Resources	Individualised activity
5 mins	Introduction	Introduce unit: tutor to display lesson aims and objectives on flipchart		Flipchart	
20 mins	PowerPoint® presentation	Define, facilitate discussion	Question and answer; discussion	PowerPoint® 1	Copies of PPT with note spaces to be made available for those who require them
30 mins	Small group work		Each learner group is given a copy of the extract, or photograph to discuss. Learners will answer worksheet questions for the piece, and produce a flipchart poster about it	A small range of pieces of writing and images of different life stages	Groups can be allocated according to ability. Different pieces of writing, images or other media could be selected according to complexity to match group ability. Group roles (e.g. scribe, spokesperson, artist) can reflect individual learning styles
20 mins	Presentation of posters		Each group to describe their piece to the whole class	Flipchart paper and pens	Visual learners can be encouraged to make flipchart posters. More confident learner can act as spokesperson for group
10 mins	Plenary session	Tutor can guide learners to add any key points that have been missed, and reinforce lesson themes	Whole group to discuss themes and issues raised	Worksheets	Worksheets can be handed in for assessment at the end of the session
5 mins	Recap: whole class teaching to highlight where lesson objectives have been achieved		Contribute to discussion		Directed questioning

4.1   Introductory activity: Life stages

Student Book 1
pp 152–164

Read the passage below. (You may recognise it from English lessons at school!) Then, in small groups, discuss the questions that follow. Make notes on your answers so that you can share them with the class later.

The Seven Ages of Man
All the world's a stage,
And all the men and women merely players:
They have their exits and their entrances;
And one man in his time plays many parts,
His acts being seven ages. As, first the infant,
Mewling and puking in the nurse's arms.
And then the whining schoolboy, with his satchel
And shining morning face, creeping like snail
Unwillingly to school. And then the lover,
Sighing like furnace, with a woeful ballad
Made to his mistress' eyebrow. Then a soldier,
Full of strange oaths, and bearded like the pard,
Jealous in honour, sudden and quick in quarrel,
Seeking the bubble reputation
Even in the cannon's mouth. And then the justice,
In fair round belly with good capon lined,
With eyes severe and beard of formal cut,
Full of wise saws and modern instances;
And so he plays his part. The sixth age shifts
Into the lean and slipper'd pantaloon,
With spectacles on nose and pouch on side;
His youthful hose, well sav'd, a world too wide
For his shrunk shank; and his big manly voice,
Turning again toward childish treble, pipes
And whistles in his sound. Last scene of all,
That ends this strange eventful history,
Is second childishness and mere oblivion;
Sans teeth, sans eyes, sans taste, sans every thing.

From *As You Like It*, Act II, Scene VII
By William Shakespeare (1554–1616)

1   Can you identify the seven stages Shakespeare mentions here?

2   Can you say what age group each stage represents?

3   Do you think Shakespeare's descriptions still apply today? Can you suggest modern equivalents?

4   Does this description of a man's life tell us about a rich man or a poor man?

5   Shakespeare describes old age as 'second childishness and mere oblivion'. Is this a fair way to describe the elderly people you know?

6   Can you describe the seven stages of a woman's life?

4.1a Life stages

Student Book 1
pp 152–164

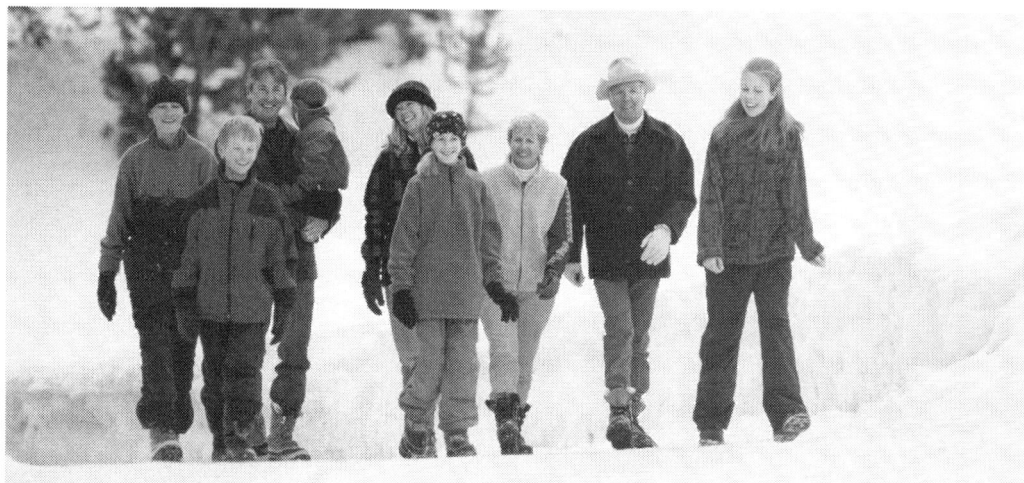

▲ **Figure 4.1: This family includes three generations: grandparents, parents and children.**

Look at the photograph above. Then answer the questions below, and make notes on your answers so that you can share them with the class later.

1   Can you identify the different life stages each person represents?

....

....

....

2   What do you think are the typical characteristics for each stage?

....

....

....

3   Are the people in the photograph typical of the people you know at that stage?

....

....

....

4   Does each age group experience the same problems?

....

....

....

[90]

4.2   Activity: Developmental timeline

Student Book 1
pp 152–164

Work in groups of four or five. You will need a long piece of paper for this activity and some sticky notes, or paper and sticky tack.

The aims of this exercise are:

■ to define the major life stages

■ to consider the impact of major life changes on life expectancy

■ to list some potential effects of major life changes.

Begin by deciding on the average lifespan of a person born in Britain today. Then mark your paper from <u>conception</u> to that age, and divide it into five-year segments. Next, use your sticky notes to show the beginning and end of each of the following stages:

■ conception

■ pregnancy

■ birth

■ infancy

■ childhood

■ adolescence

■ adulthood

■ older adulthood

■ final stages of life

■ death.

Now use another set of sticky notes to add at least five of the following major life changes. You may also like to add some of your own.

Becoming homeless	Becoming a parent	Getting married
Getting divorced	Parent dying	Moving house
Retiring	Partner dying	Being seriously injured
Getting arthritis	Having a heart attack	Losing a job
Being unable to pay bills	Taking up smoking	Leaving education
Getting asthma	Being abused by partner	Being bullied at work

Now look at your first set of sticky notes. Are they still in the right place? Which ones should you move? Why? Finally, compare your timeline to those of the other groups in your class. What differences have you found? Are your timelines similar?

[91]

4.3 The nature-nurture debate

Student Book 1
pp 152–164

This activity will:

- enable you to define the nature-nurture debate
- give you an insight into your own feelings on this issue
- help you debate nature-nurture issues
- think about your understanding of these issues.

First, look at the statements below and tick the boxes that apply to you.

	Statement	Strongly agree	Agree	Agree slightly	Disagree slightly	Disagree	Strongly disagree
1	Some children are born evil.						
2	With the right education and support, anyone could be prime minister.						
3	People cannot get out of poverty just by working harder.						
4	Overweight parents will always have overweight children.						
5	There is a link between nutrition and crime.						
6	I believe in fate: what will happen in your life is out of your control.						
7	All children should reach developmental milestones at the same age.						
8	Some people are born lazy.						
9	If your father died of a heart attack, you probably will too.						
10	People who think positively are generally healthier.						
11	Most crime could be prevented by better parenting.						
12	I believe that someone can be born with an 'addictive personality'.						
13	People with Down's syndrome need to be in special schools.						
14	I believe it is up to me whether I am a success or a failure.						

Now score each of your answers as follows.

For questions 1, 4, 6, 7, 8, 9, 12, 13:

Strongly agree	= 6
Agree	= 5
Agree slightly	= 4
Disagree slightly	= 3
Disagree	= 2
Strongly disagree	= 1

For questions 2, 3, 5, 10, 11, 14:

Strongly agree	= 1
Agree	= 2
Agree slightly	= 3
Disagree slightly	= 4
Disagree	= 5
Strongly disagree	= 6

You should now have a score between 14 and 84.

Continued overleaf

4.3 The nature-nuture debate (*contd*)

If your score is 14–28

You seem to believe strongly in nurture. You think people are the way they are because of the way they are brought up, the way society treats them, and the decisions they make for themselves. You believe your fate lies in your own hands. (And you probably never play the lottery!)

If your score is 29–42

You believe most things in life are decided before we are born. However, you do realise that there are some things that are within our own power to change.

If your score is 43–56

You are in the middle of the debate. Although you believe certain characteristics or events are inevitable, you also realise that the way other people treat us can change our lives for good or bad.

If your score is 57–70

Although you believe we are in charge of our own fate most of the time, you believe that some things in our lives are influenced by factors that occur before we are born.

If your score is 71–84

You seem to feel that our lives are decided before we are born, and that our personalities and the events in our lives are determined by fate or luck. (You probably play the lottery quite often!)

　　　　　　　　　　　　　　[93]

4.4   Jonathon: Case study one

Student Book 1
pp 152–164

Jonathon is 12. He has Down's syndrome. When he was born, his mother gave up her well-paid job as a corporate banker to care for him. The family hired specialist nurses and portage workers to help with Jonathon's care, and Jonathon has regular appointments with private doctors to monitor his progress. He lives with his mother and his sister Charlotte, who is 15. Jonathon's mother and father were divorced five years ago, but his father sees him and his sister every weekend, and pays a very large amount of maintenance. Jonathon attends the local secondary school in the wealthy area he lives in. He is also a member of the local scout group, and a performing arts project for people with special needs. Because of his Down's syndrome, Jonathon must take regular medication for his heart condition.

1   What are the main symptoms of Down's syndrome?

2   What is portage?

3   Jonathon is about to experience a major developmental stage. Can you name it and explain what will happen?

4   How do you think Jonathon's life would be different if his parents were not wealthy?

5   What difficulties might Jonathon experience at school? How could he be helped to deal with these?

6   How will Jonathon's time at scouts and the performing arts project help his development?

7   What do you think Jonathon's life will be like in 10, 20, and 30 years' time?

8   What does the nature/nurture argument tell us about Jonathon's development? (Look back at question 4.)

4.5   Services at your placement

Student Book 1
pp 152–164

For this activity you need to prepare a short PowerPoint® presentation to give to your class. Your presentation should describe how your placement offers different services to individuals at different times in their lives. For example, your placement may have:

■ special equipment such as ramps or adapted toilets for people with mobility problems

■ organised trips for individuals who want to keep active

■ doctor or nurse visits for those who are experiencing the effects of ageing

■ special diets available for individuals who need to control their weight, or have a particular cultural need

■ counsellors or pastors available to help with psychological or spiritual issues

■ user groups to involve residents in the day-to-day running of the facility.

Explain what the facilities are, how they are used, which life factors or changes they support, and how they might be improved or adapted. Your presentation should be 8–10 minutes long, with about five or six slides.

4.6　Genetic factors and development

Student Book 1
pp 165–184

For this activity you will need to split into four groups, with one for each of the following conditions:

■ Phenylketonuria

■ Cystic fibrosis

■ Down's syndrome

■ Sickle cell anaemia/trait/disorders.

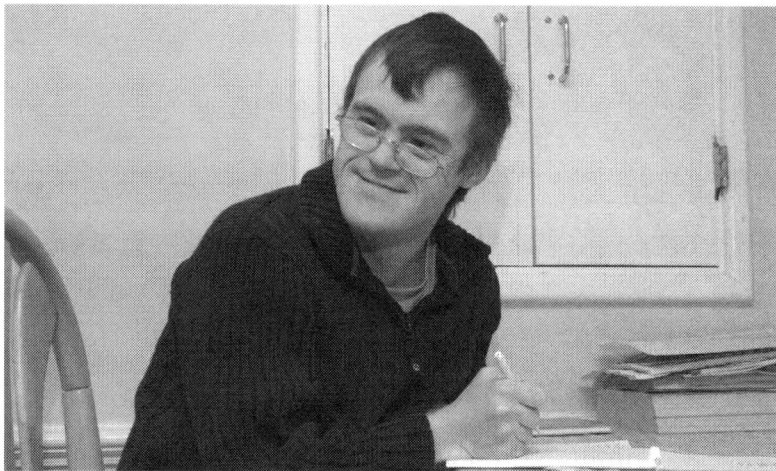

▲ **Figure 4.2:　This student has Down's syndrome.**

Using your library or resource centre, research the condition, and prepare an 8- to 10-minute PowerPoint® or poster presentation to share with the class.

Your presentation should include:

■ the link between genetics and the condition

■ the main signs and symptoms

■ the incidence (i.e. how many people are affected?)

■ treatments and interventions

■ long-term outcomes

■ effects on 'normal development'

■ illustrations.

Overleaf is a grid, which will allow you to record each group's findings as they make their presentations. You can add your own too! Once you have all the information, you may wish to include one or more conditions in your case study.

4.6 Genetic factors and development (*contd*)

Condition	Genetics	Signs and symptoms	Incidence	Treatments and Interventions	Long-term outcomes	Effects on development
Phenylketonuria						
Cystic fibrosis						
Down's syndrome						
Sickle cell anaemia/ trait/disorders						

4.7 The impact of socio-economic factors on development

Student Book 1
pp 165–184

Think about two people. They could be characters from fiction. For instance, they might come from your favourite soap opera or TV show, or they could be characters from a novel or film. Alternatively, you could use real people – either celebrities or people you know.

Using the diagram below as an example, draw a mind map® of all the possible social or economic factors that have had an influence on that person's development.

Add the effects that these could have. In the example below, the Queen has excellent housing. This puts her at far less risk of stress-related disorders, or environmentally influenced illnesses such as asthma.

Draw your mind map® however you want to. You could use sticky notes or scraps of paper at first, then draw a final version by hand or using a computer. Use colours, capital letters and underlining, drawings or whatever methods help you to understand the concepts. Remember this is a diagram for *you* to use, so it does not have to make sense to anyone else!

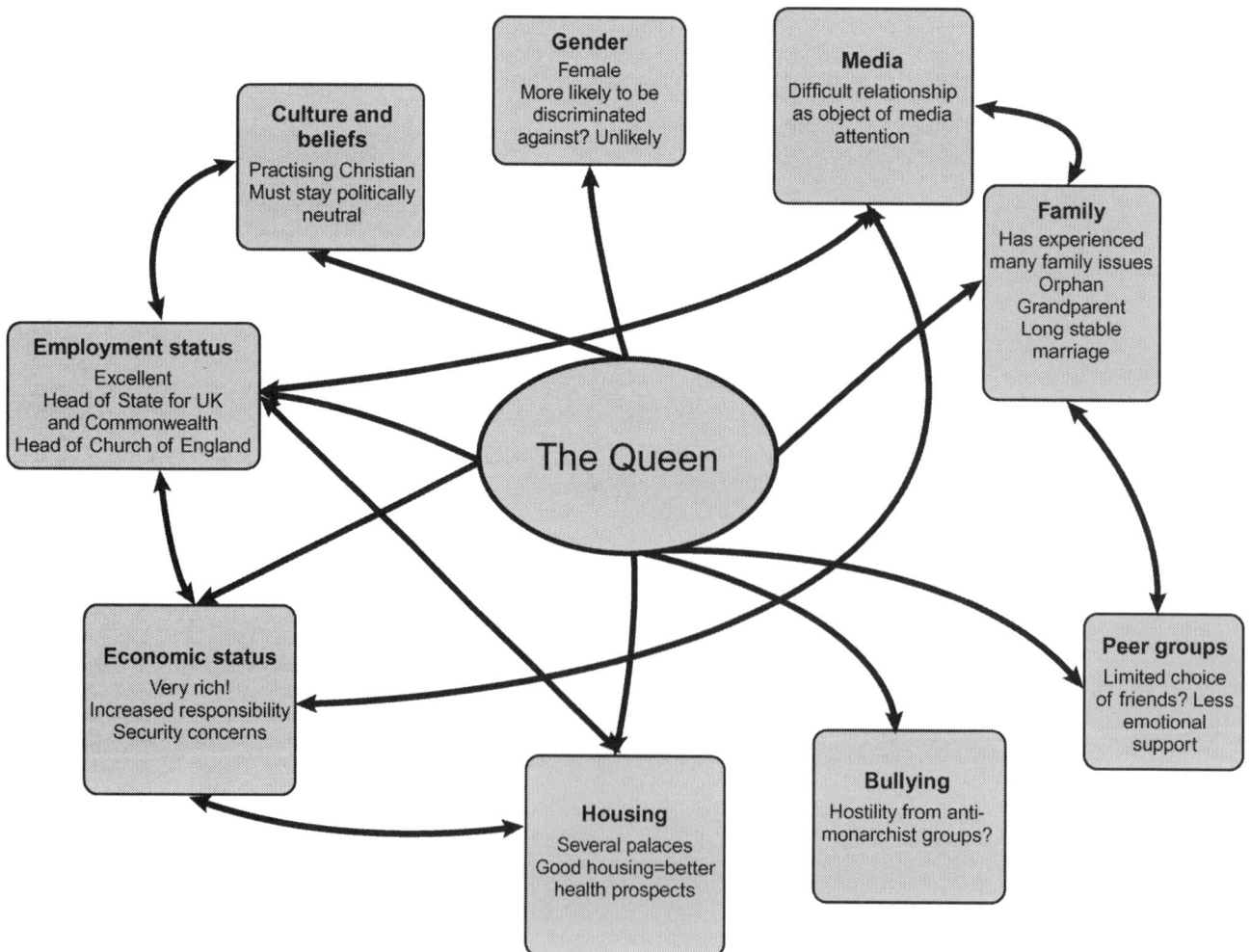

▲ Figure 4.3: Mind map® showing the impact of socio-economic factors on the Queen

4.8   Major life events

Student Book 1
pp 165–184

In 1967 two doctors, Thomas Holmes and Richard Rahe, developed a rating scale to measure how much stress a person was experiencing. To do this, they compiled a list of major life events, and gave each one a score for how stressful it was. They called it 'The social readjustment rating scale' (SRRS).

Calculate your level of stress by looking at the list below*, and ticking every event that has happened to you in the past six months. Then add up your scores to get your total.

1.	Death of a spouse	100 -------
2.	Divorce	73 -------
3.	Marital separation	65 -------
4.	Jail term	63 -------
5.	Death of a close family member	63 -------
6.	Personal injury or illness	53 -------
7.	Marriage	50 -------
8.	Fired at work	47 -------
9.	Marital reconciliation	45 -------
10.	Retirement	45 -------
11.	Change in health of family member	44 -------
12.	Pregnancy	40 -------
13.	Sex difficulties	39 -------
14.	Gain of a new family member	39 -------
15.	Business readjustments	39 -------
16.	Change in financial state	38 -------
17.	Death of a close friend	37 -------
18.	Change to different line of work	36 -------
19.	Change in number of arguments with spouse	35 -------
20.	Taking on a mortgage	31 -------
21.	Foreclosure of mortgage	30 -------
22.	Change in responsibilities at work	29 -------
23.	Son or daughter leaving home	29 -------
24.	Trouble with in-laws	29 -------
25.	Outstanding personal achievements	28 -------

Continued overleaf

4.8 Major life events (*contd*)

26.	Wife begins or stops work	26 -------
27.	Begin or end school	26 -------
28.	Change in living conditions	25 -------
29.	Revision of personal habits	24 -------
30.	Trouble with boss	23 -------
31.	Change in work hours or conditions	20 -------
32.	Change in residence	20 -------
33.	Change in school	20 -------
34.	Change in recreation	19 -------
35.	Change in religious activities	19 -------
36.	Change in social activities	18 -------
37.	Taking out a loan	17 -------
38.	Change in sleeping habits	16 -------
39.	Change in number of family get-togethers	15 -------
40.	Change in eating habits	15 -------
41.	Going on holiday	13 -------
42.	Christmas holidays	12 -------
43.	Minor violation of laws (speeding, parking tickets, etc)	11 -------

Your stress score:

less than 149	=	Low
150-200	=	Mild
200-299	=	Moderate
more than 300	=	Major

Think about this study for a moment, and discuss the following questions.

■ Can you think of any difficulties it raises?

■ Look at the dates the research was carried out. Is it relevant to current British life?

■ What about the life events it considers. How many affect your own life?

■ Are all the events negative, or do they change according to personal circumstances (e.g. numbers 12 or 32)?

■ Which of these life events do you think are predictable, and which are unpredictable?

■ Do you think this study proves that stress causes illness?

*Reprinted from the *Journal of Psychosomatic Research*, Vol. 11, T.H. Holmes & R.H. Rahe, 'The social readjustment rating scale', pp 213–218, 1967, with permission from Elsevier Inc.

4.9   Steffi: Case study two

Student Book 1
pp 165–184

Steffi is 17. She lives in a squat in a run-down part of the city. Steffi left home two years ago to get away from her stepfather who regularly beat her. She hated school, where she found reading and writing very difficult, and where she was often bullied and called 'thick'. Since then she has spent time living on the streets, making money by begging and occasionally picking pockets. Since she started drinking more regularly, Steffi has also made money through prostitution. She often drinks a whole bottle of vodka in a day. Steffi hates her life, and has tried to kill herself several times. Her diet is mainly fast food, or soup and sandwiches from the local homeless project. Steffi avoids contact with social services, as she does not trust them. Steffi has missed three periods now, and she is sure she is pregnant.

1   Which developmental stage is Steffi at?

2   What has affected Steffi's emotional development?

3   What illnesses and infections is Steffi vulnerable to?

4   What could happen to Steffi's baby?

5   Steffi may have a learning difficulty. Can you suggest what it might be?

6   Which professional services can help Steffi and her baby?

7   Do you think Steffi's baby could have a good life with Steffi?

8   Would it be better to take Steffi's baby away from her?

4.10 Puberty

Student Book 1
pp 185–197

In this activity you will learn about the major changes that take place during puberty, and how and when they happen. You will also discuss some of the difficulties that people may experience during puberty.

Split into two groups. One group will look at girls, and the other group will look at boys. In your group, sketch an outline of an adolescent boy or girl on a large piece of poster paper. Using information from your textbooks, add details and labels to your drawing to indicate the physical changes that take place during puberty. For every change, include:

■ the **typical age** at which it happens

■ **why** it happens (e.g. testicles grow in order to produce sperm, pelvis widens to allow for childbirth, etc)

■ what **emotional and social** effects these changes can have

■ the role of **hormones**, including oestrogen and testosterone, in puberty.

You should also give each change a number to show the **order** in which the changes occur.

When you have finished your poster, present it to the rest of the group. Then compare the experience of puberty for boys and girls.

Finally, as a whole class, discuss the issues surrounding puberty. Here are some suggested questions to get you started:

■ Is it easier for either sex?

■ How does society treat people who are going through puberty?

■ Puberty seems to be happening earlier. Can you suggest any reasons for this?

■ What factors might affect an individual's normal development during puberty?

■ How can we make puberty easier for adolescents?

4.11   The menopause

Student Book 1
pp 185–197

During this activity you will find out about the major physical changes that occur during menopause, as well as the emotional and medical effects it can have. For many women, menopause can be a distressing or difficult experience. Their families may not always be able to understand what is happening.

Write an information leaflet for the partner and family of a woman who is experiencing menopause. The leaflet should explain:

■ what menopause is

■ what physical changes take place

■ what physical symptoms a woman may experience

■ what psychological symptoms a woman may experience

■ which treatments and therapies can help

■ which aspects of menopause are positive

■ how partners, families and friends can help.

4.12 The effects of life factors

Student Book 1
pp 185–197

This activity should be completed using evidence from your placement. Think about the life factors that the people you met have experienced. Write a list of all the life factors that you think have changed or influenced their development. You should set your list out like the example table below. Keep your finished list to use when you are completing your case studies and timeline.

Placement one: St Saviour's nursing home
Life factors affecting residents

Resident	Event	Effects on individual	Type of factor? *(genetic, biological, environmental, socio-economic, lifestyle)*	Predictable or unpredictable?
Mr C.	Fought in France during World War Two	Still has nightmares and disturbing memories, made long-lasting friendships	Socio-economic, lifestyle, environmental	Unpredictable
Mrs F.	Losing sight due to Glaucoma	Reduced mobility, more dependent on others, depression	Biological	Predictable

Placement two: Rose Street drop-in centre
Life factors affecting clients

Resident	Event	Effects on individual	Type of factor? *(genetic, biological, environmental, socio-economic, lifestyle)*	Predictable or unpredictable?
Miss L.	Has been forced to leave home after an argument with her mother	Sleeping on friends' floors, increased drug and alcohol use, stress and depression	Socio-economic, lifestyle	Unpredictable
Mr W.	Offered a secure job at end of training course	Steady income, able to move out of hostel accommodation, happier	Environmental, socio-economic	Predictable

4.13 Theories of ageing

Student Book 1
pp 185–197

Your task is to create a weekly schedule for a retired person. Your schedule should include whatever activities you think are appropriate for a reasonably healthy 75-year-old. For each day, list activities for morning, afternoon and evening. Hint: Think about the retired people you know, and include some of the things they usually do.

When you have completed your schedule, answer the following questions:

1   How much physical exercise have you included?

2   How many social opportunities have you included?

3   How much time will be spent alone?

4   Have you included any type of paid or voluntary work?

5   Do any activities rely on help from other people?

6   How does this schedule compare to your typical week?

Now consider the two theories of ageing below:

> **Activity theory:** This is the idea that older people benefit from being as active as possible. By taking part in social events or employment, or actively pursuing hobbies and interests, older adults seem healthier and happier. This is true even for those who have disabilities or other impairments that make going out more difficult or painful.

> **Disengagement theory**: This theory states that it is normal for older people to withdraw from social activities, and separate themselves from other people. Their lives 'shrink', so they have fewer roles and relationships, and they are not expected to follow the normal rules of social life (for example, they can be late, or rude, or leave early). Disengagement theory also says that it is normal for older people to accept these changes and reduce their interactions with other people.

Which theory do you think best describes the schedule you have drawn up? Compare your ideas to those of the rest of the class, and discuss the two theories. Is either theory a better explanation of normal ageing? Which one best describes the older people you know?

4.14   Physical changes of ageing

Student Book 1
pp 185–197

Look at the pictures below. There is an obvious difference in the powers of sight, but what other physical differences would the elderly and the younger men have?

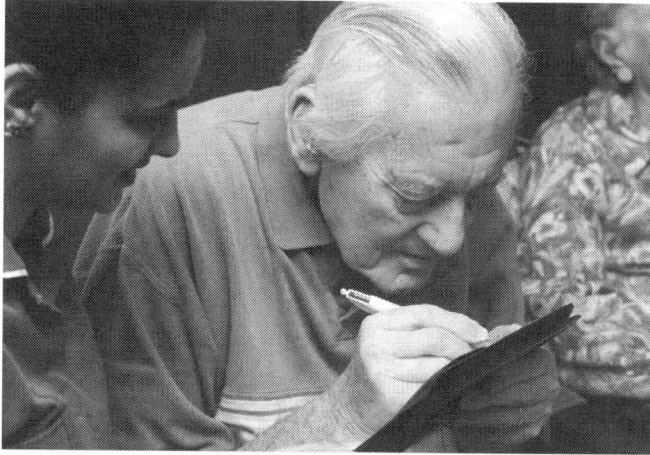

▲ Figure 4.4: An elderly man fills in a form.

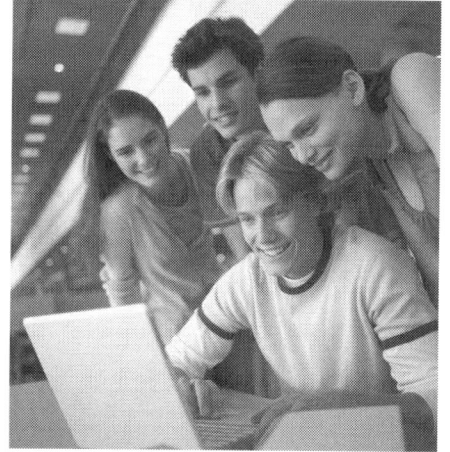

▲ Figure 4.5: Young people look at a laptop computer screen.

In pairs, write down all the physical systems that change or deteriorate with age, and how they are affected. (For example, skin loses elasticity, becomes more translucent, fragile and lined.)

Finally, working in groups of four or five, use your Student Books and library resources to complete the table below. This table lists some typical medical conditions that are associated with ageing.

Name	Symptoms	Treatments
Atherosclerosis		
Coronary heart disease		
Asthma		
Emphysema		
Chronic obstructive pulmonary disease		
Motor neurone disease		
Athritis		
Alzheimer's disease		
Hearing loss		

4.15 Priya: Case study three

Student Book 1
pp 185–197

Priya is 67. She was born in the Punjab, and moved to England with her husband when she was 22. She lives with her son and his young family in a house next door to the shop she ran with her husband for 40 years. Priya's eldest son died after he was hit by a car when he was seven years old. Her husband died of a heart condition three years ago, and Priya misses him very much. Now that her younger son and his wife run the shop, Priya spends much of her time at home. Her grandchildren are teenagers now, and she does not need to spend as much time caring for them. Priya is feeling old and useless. She has put on some weight recently, and is finding it hard to walk very far. She would love to go back to the Punjab to visit her relatives, but there is not enough money to do that at the moment. A friend from temple has invited Priya to join the women's group there, and her GP has suggested she goes to the keep-fit class at the local community centre. Her grand-daughter has offered to take her to the cinema several times. Priya says she does not want to be a burden, and would rather just stay at home.

1 Which life stage is Priya facing?

2 Which recent, or less recent, events have affected her?

3 What factors may be affecting her health?

4 Can you suggest reasons why Priya and her husband may have moved to England?

5 Which theory of ageing best fits Priya's behaviour?

6 What physical changes may be affecting Priya?

7 Should care services encourage Priya to be more active?

8 What are the psychological effects that Priya is likely to be experiencing?

4.16   Create your own case study: Case study four

Student Book 1
pp 185–197

You have read the three case studies of Jonathon, Priya and Steffi.

Now you need to create a case study of your own. Your individual should:

■ be at a recognisable life stage

■ have been influenced by several life factors (genetic, biological, environmental, socio-economic, lifestyle)

■ have experienced some major life events (e.g. bereavement, divorce, parenthood, etc).

You may want to use case studies of people you know or have encountered in placement. Remember, nothing in your case study should enable readers to identify the individual. Don't use the name of your placement, or any specific details. For example, if your individual was once your school's lollipop man then putting that fact in will mean that everyone will know who he is! Change names, and only give relevant details.

Remember to include the theories and definitions that best describe your individual's development.

4.17　End-of-unit crossword

Student Book 1
pp 185–197

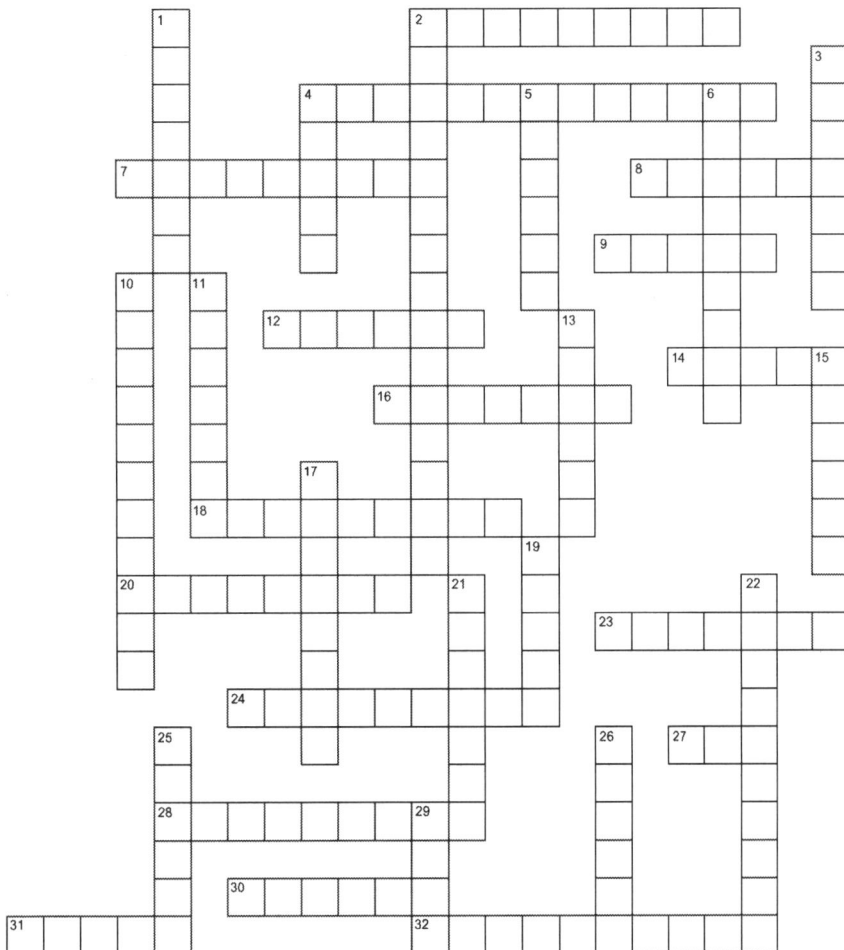

ACROSS

2　Unwanted environmental factors that can cause problems with development

4　A theory of ageing

7　Also known as gestation period

8　The idea that our personality is formed before birth

9　Type of partnership

12　How an organism changes and develops over time

14　A type of chromosomal syndrome

16　Period of a child's life before it can use language

18　Time spent in school, college, etc

20　This is essential for good health

23　Chemical that influences physical development

24　Disease that affects the joints

27　This can be chronological or intellectual

28　The end of fertility

30　Our sexual identity

31　An individual who intimidates or attacks others

32　Provision of clean water and sewerage

DOWN

1　Stage when body becomes sexually mature

2　Disorder diagnosed by heel prick test

3　To do with inherited traits

4　End of life

5　Discrimination against seniors

6　This must be adequate to provide the correct vitamins and minerals

10　Our everyday surroundings

11　The end of a marriage

13　Unusual blood cell shape

15　This can contribute to many diseases

17　A theory of ageing

19　Acronym for different types of development; another name for haemorrhoids

21　The idea that our personalities develop as a result of our experiences

22　When sperm meets egg

25　The people closest to us

26　Respiratory tract disorder

29　Holmes and Rahe's scale of stressful events

5

Fundamentals of anatomy and physiology for health and social care

unit overview

This unit explores both the anatomy and physiology of the human body. More specifically, it describes the gross structures and related functions of the main body systems. It also explains the importance of energy metabolism, of homeostatic mechanisms, and of taking measurements (such as breathing rate) in order to maintain healthy functioning of these systems. This unit is split into four Learning outcomes.

Learning outcomes

On completion of this unit learners should:

5.1 understand the organisation of the human body
5.2 understand the functioning of body systems associated with energy metabolism
5.3 understand how homeostatic mechanisms operate in the maintenance of an internal environment
5.4 be able to interpret data obtained from monitoring routine variations in the functioning of healthy body systems.

Suggested activities

The At-a-glance activity grid shows how the activities in the Assessment and Delivery Resource (ADR) relate to the content of the unit. The activities include introductory and plenary activities and a variety of case studies, research tasks, discussions and presentations, using written, verbal and presentation skills. The activities may help learners prepare for assessment, and the grid indicates which assessment criteria are relevant for each activity. Copies of activity sheets can be given to learners.

The content of each Learning outcome

Learning outcome 1: Understand the organisation of the human body (relevant criteria: P1, P2, P3, D1)

For this outcome, learners study the structure and function of an animal cell, the four types of tissues found in the human body, and the structure and function of the six body systems. This outcome is closely related to the first Learning outcome of Unit 13 (Physiology of fluid balance), which provides more in-depth information on the structure of a cell. Activity 5.1 is a game in which learners have to match a function with a body system. In Activity 5.2 learners label a diagram of a cell and learn more about the structures within a cell. Activity 5.3 begins with learners matching types of tissue with their functions. In Activity 5.4 groups of learners complete a drawing and writing task describing the main functions of the six body systems. Most students enjoy drawing activities, and such tasks can reinforce their learning very effectively. The writing task, in which learners briefly describe the relationship between the structure and the function of an organ, will enable you to measure their communication key skill level 3. Whenever possible, encourage learners to keep in mind a whole picture of the main functions of body systems.

Learning outcome 2: Understand the functioning of body systems associated with energy metabolism (relevant criteria: P4, P5, M1, D2)

In this outcome, learners focus on how food, blood and air circulate in the human body and how energy is supplied to maintain the healthy functioning of the respiratory, cardiovascular and digestive systems. Interactive activities and video clips provide useful resources to deliver this part of the unit. By understanding the normal functioning of some body systems, students will gain an insight into the physiology of a disorder such as Crohn's disease. This outcome has links with Unit 14 (Physiological disorders). In Activity 5.5, groups of learners produce annotated charts showing the roles of the three main body systems in relation to energy metabolism. This is a good exercise to improve their motivation, confidence and communication skills. Activity 5.6 is a writing task in which students write about energy generation and the physiology of the digestive system.

Learning outcome 3: Understand how homeostatic mechanisms operate in the maintenance of an internal environment (relevant criteria: P5, D2)

Homeostasis is another way of maintaining healthy functioning of the body systems and therefore of the human body. In this outcome, students learn how the stability of the body's internal environment (including blood glucose level, body temperature, breathing and heart rate) is maintained. Again, this part of the unit is closely related to Unit 14. Activity 5.7 is a gapped handout that helps learners understand the meaning of homeostasis. This is followed by Activity 5.8, which requires students to label diagrams and write their own explanation of a homeostatic mechanism.

Learning outcome 4: Be able to interpret data obtained from monitoring routine variations in the functioning of healthy body systems (relevant criteria: M2, P6)

This outcome is about monitoring variations such as breathing rate and pulse. Activity 5.9 gives students practice in using three types of measuring equipment, and in Activity 5.10 they use their understanding of homeostasis and the physiology of the respiratory system to complete a writing task.

How this unit will be assessed

To reach Pass level, the evidence must show that the learner is able to:

P1   describe the functions of the main cell components
P2   describe the structure of the main tissues of the body and their role in the functioning of two named body organs
P3   describe the gross structure and main functions of all major body systems
P4   describe the role of energy in the body and the physiology of three named body systems in relation to body metabolism
P5   describe the concept of homeostasis and the homeostatic mechanisms that regulate heart rate, breathing rate, body temperature and blood glucose levels
P6   measure body temperature, heart rate and breathing rate before and after a standard period of exercise, interpret the data and comment on its validity.

To reach Merit level, the evidence must show that, in addition to the Pass criteria, the learner is able to:

M1   explain the physiology of three named body systems in relation to energy metabolism
M2   explain the probable homeostatic responses to changes in the internal environment during exercise
M3   analyse data obtained to show how homeostatic mechanisms control the internal environment during exercise.

To reach Distinction level, the evidence must show that, in addition to the Pass and Merit criteria, the learner is able to:

D1   use examples to explain how body systems interrelate with each other
D2   explain the importance of homeostasis in maintaining healthy functioning of the body.

To assess students, you need to consider the practical activities carried out in the classroom, such as the measurement of breathing rate. During practical work, you will be able to measure your students' achievement of two key skills: level 3 in application of numbers and ICT (Information and Communication Technology). As future nurses and carers, students need to get some practice in taking measurements, and presenting and interpreting data, and these subjects are covered in Learning outcome 4. Learners will need to be guided in the use of measurement techniques, and they will gain useful experience of these aspects in their work placements. However, they should be assessed on the interpretation of obtained data and not on the methodology and techniques of using equipment. You will monitor how students use formulae to work out a measurement (e.g. breathing rate), how they comment on the validity of data, and how they present and interpret the result of their calculations (such as the inspiratory reserve volume). Learners also need to submit three Assessment tasks (see below) covering the four Learning outcomes of this unit.

Assessment tasks

These three tasks can each have their own submission date. Each task will contain a number of assessment criteria to achieve Pass, Merit or Distinction grades. According to the different learning capacities of your students, some of them may aim for Pass grade, others for Merit.

Task 1 (relevant criteria: P1, P2, P3, D1)

Describe:

- the functions of the main cell components **(P1)**
- the structure of the main tissues of the body and their role in the functioning of two named body organs **(P2)**
- the gross structure and main functions of all major body systems **(P3)**.

Finally, use examples to explain how all the body systems interrelate with each other **(D1)**.

Task 2 (relevant criteria: P4, P5, M1, D2)

Describe:

- the role of energy in the body and the physiology of three named body systems in relation to energy metabolism **(P4)**
- the concept of homeostasis and the homeostatic mechanisms that regulate heart rate, breathing rate, body temperature and blood glucose levels **(P5)**.

Explain:

- three named body systems in relation to energy metabolism **(M1)**
- the importance of homeostasis in maintaining the healthy functioning of the body **(D2)**

Task 3 (relevant criteria: P6, M2, M3)

Using Activity 5.9 (Measurement of breathing rate), measure body temperature, heart rate and breathing before and after a standard period of exercise.

- After completing Activity 5.9, interpret the data and comment on its validity **(P6)**.
- Then explain the probable homeostatic responses to changes in the internal environment during exercise **(M2)**.
- Finally, analyse the data obtained to show how homeostatic mechanisms control the internal environment during exercise **(M3)**.

Scheme of work

BTEC National Health and Social Care
Unit 5 Fundamentals of anatomy and physiology for health and social care

Academic year: ....
Broad aim: Successful completion of the unit
Teacher(s): ....

Number of weeks: 35
Duration of session: 100 mins
Guided learning hours: 60

Week/s	Topic/outcome	Tutor preparation	Student activity	Resources	Links to grading criteria
1–3	Introduction to Unit 5: Understand the structure and function of parts of the human body	Introduce unit; monitor students' participation; practical work (e.g. pig's heart dissection)	Learners work in pairs to complete tables and diagrams, before taking the theory into practical work and discussions	PowerPoint® 1, Activity 5.1, Activity 5.2, interactive whiteboard (e.g. for location of organs in the body), video clips from BBC Education Internet, anatomical models, bioviewers to show cell structures	P1, P3
4–5	Understand the main tissues of the body	You can create similar activities with the main tissues of the heart and their corresponding functions to complete the P2 grading criteria	Learners define and draw diagrams of muscle, epithelial, nervous and connective tissues	Activity 5.3	P2
6–10	Understand the main functions of body systems	This drawing and writing activity can be split between two groups of learners, each group working on three body systems	Both groups of learners can collaborate on a chart where they interrelate body systems with each other	Activity 5.4	P3, D1
11–14	Understand body systems and energy metabolism	Monitor learners' participation; practical work (e.g. an enzyme reaction)	Learners carry out group work to produce annotated chart with pictures of three body systems and related energy metabolism activities	PowerPoint® 2, Activity 5.5, interactive whiteboard, BBC Education Internet resources	P4, M1
16–18	Understand the digestive system and energy metabolism	You can create similar activities for the cardiovascular and respiratory systems	Learners write a few lines on the relationship between energy generation and the physiology of the digestive system	Activity 5.6	P4, M1

Unit 5 Fundamentals of anatomy and physiology for health and social care

Week/s	Topic/outcome	Tutor preparation	Student activity	Resources	Links to grading criteria
20–24	Understand homeostasis	Introduce the concept of homeostasis with the PowerPoint® and video clips from BBC Education Internet	The gapped handout reinforces learners understanding. Learners to discuss the contents of the video clips and Internet research	PowerPoint® 3, video clips from BBC Education Internet, interactive whiteboard, Activity 5.7	P5
25–27	Understand the homeostatic mechanism of gluco-regulation	You can create similar activities to explain thermo-regulation (using the structure and functions of the skin) and osmo-regulation	Learners fill in the gaps in the diagram labels to gain a more in-depth understanding of the importance of homeostasis	Activity 5.8	P5, D2
28–31	Understand how to interpret data obtained from monitoring healthy body systems	Monitor students' participation; practical work (e.g. Harvard step test, or breathing rate when walking up and down stairs)	Learners should generate data to use in writing Assessment task 3. Learners carry out practical tasks individually and record their findings, before a group discussion	PowerPoint® 4, Activity 5.9	M2, P6
32–34	Understand how breathing rate is adapted to an activity	You can create an activity where homeostatic mechanisms do not work efficiently	Learners fill in the gaps in the diagram to analyse how breathing rate is adapted to an activity to maintain a stable internal environment	Activity 5.10	M3
35	End-of-unit crossword	You can use this crossword in the final session to recap the unit content	Learners to complete crossword	Activity 5.11	All

At-a-glance activity grid
Unit 5 Fundamentals of anatomy and physiology for health and social care

Activity	Title and description	Scheme of work	File/CD	Delivery notes	Additional resources	Links to grading criteria	Links to Student Book 1
Outcome 5.1 Understand the organisation of the human body							
Power Point® 1	Introduction to Unit 5 and Learning outcome 1	Week 1	CD	This PPT gives an overview of the unit. Encourage learners to discuss their previous knowledge of the subject so that you can implement appropriate differentiation	Video clips from BBC Education Internet resources	P1, P2, P3	pp 202–222
5.1	Understand the structure and function of parts of the human body	Week 1	File (Answers on CD)	In this activity, learners have to match a function to a body system, as well as finding out which tissues and organs each system is made of	Interactive whiteboard (e.g. for location of organs in the body), anatomical models, practical work (e.g. pig's heart dissection)	P3	pp 202–222
5.2	Understand the structure of a cell	Week 2	File (Answers on CD)	You need to explain that organelles work separately and together to maintain cell function. Learners label a diagram as well as matching definitions with particular cell organelles	Use bioviewers to show cell structures	P1	pp 202–222
5.3	Understand the main tissues of the body	Week 4	File (Answers on CD)	In part A of this activity, learners match a specific function to a specific tissue. In part B they look at four types of epithelial tissue and draw two others. Finally, in part C, they write about the role of the tissues in the small intestine. You can create a similar activity with the main tissues of the heart and their corresponding functions to complete the P2 grading criteria	Use bioviewers to show tissue structures	P2	pp 202–222
5.4	Understand the main functions of body systems	Week 6	File (Answers on CD)	This drawing and writing activity can be split between two groups of learners, with each group working on three body systems. Both groups can then collaborate to produce a chart that interrelates body systems with each other (e.g. to explain the respective roles of the cardiovascular and respiratory systems, or how the endocrine system operates with the nervous system)		P3, D1	pp 202–222
Outcome 5.2 Understand the functioning of body systems associated with energy metabolism							
Power Point® 1	Introduction to Learning outcome 2	Week 11	CD	This PPT introduces the role of energy in the body		P4	pp 222–243

Activity	Title and description	Scheme of work	File/CD	Delivery notes	Additional resources	Links to grading criteria	Links to Student Book 1
5.5	Understand body systems and energy metabolism	Week 11	File (Answers on CD)	This activity can be used before or after the lecture. If you use the activity after lecturing, you can still start with a brainstorming session that students will use at the end of the lesson to complete the activity. You can use it to help learners with a few key words. Follow this with group work to produce an annotated chart with pictures of the three body systems and related activities that involve energy metabolism (e.g. anabolism and catabolism)	Interactive whiteboard, BBC Education Internet resources	P4, M1	pp 222–243
5.6	Understand the digestive system and energy metabolism	Week 16	File (Answers on CD)	This is an analysis activity, in which learners write about the relationship between the generation and use of energy and the physiology of the digestive system. You can use it to help learners with a few key words. You can also create a similar activity for the cardiovascular and respiratory systems	Practical work (e.g. an enzyme reaction)	P4, M1	pp 222–243
Outcome 5.3 Understand how homeostatic mechanisms operate in the maintenance of an internal environment							
PowerPoint® 3	Introduction to Learning outcome 3	Week 20	CD	Introduce the concept of homeostasis with the PPT		P5	pp 244–254
5.7	Understand homeostasis	Week 20	File (Answers on CD)	This is a fill-the-gaps activity, which introduces learners to homeostatic mechanisms	Video clips from BBC Education Internet	P5	pp 244–254
5.8	Understand the homeostatic mechanism of gluco-regulation	Week 25	File (Answers on CD)	In this activity, students need to fill in the gaps in two diagrams with the given key words, and then write a few lines on this mechanism. This will encourage students to write in more depth about the importance of homeostasis in maintaining the healthy functioning of the body. You can create similar activities to explain thermo-regulation (using the structure and functions of the skin) and osmo-regulation		P5, D2	pp 244–254
Outcome 5.4 Be able to interpret data obtained from monitoring routine variations in the functioning of healthy body systems							
PowerPoint® 4	Introduction to Learning outcome 4	Week 28	CD	Introduce the concept of monitoring healthy body systems with the PPT		M2	pp 255–265
5.9	Measuring breathing rate	Week 28	File (Answers on CD)	This is a practical activity. Before starting the experiment, you need to demonstrate the use of the three instruments, and then go through any health and safety requirements. Learners should generate data to use in writing Assessment task 3	Practical work (e.g. Harvard step test, or breathing rate when walking up and down stairs)	M2, P6	pp 255–265

Activity	Title and description	Scheme of work	File/CD	Delivery notes	Additional resources	Links to grading criteria	Links to Student Book 1
5.10	Breathing rate and exercise, homeostatic mechanism	Week 32	File (Answers on CD)	This is a fill-the-gaps activity. Students should be able to analyse how breathing rate is adapted to an activity to maintain a stable internal environment. You can also create an activity in which homeostatic mechanisms do not work efficiently.		M3	pp 255–265
5.11	End-of-unit crossword	Week 35	File (Answers on CD)	You can use this crossword in the final session to recap the unit content		All	pp 255–265

Unit 5 Lesson plan

Aims

- To introduce the structure and function of the heart

Learning outcomes
- recognise the main structure of the heart
- explain the cardiac cycle
- link the tissue structure with the functioning of the heart.

Timing	Content	Teacher activity	Student activity	Resources	Individualised activity
10 mins	Introduction	Explain the objectives and get ready for the experiment. Organise group work			Mix students in groups according to their learning capabilities
40 mins	Dissection of a pig's heart and recognition of the major chambers, valves and vessels	Monitor students' work	Carry out dissection		Give advice and guidance when needed
20 mins	Label a heart diagram	Discuss the circulation of the blood through the heart. Discuss the relationship between the cardiac tissue and its function		Lesson plan worksheets (see overleaf, labelled diagram in Activity answers on CD)	Monitor the group work
30 mins	PowerPoint® presentation	Give a PPT presentation to explain the cardiac cycle as part of the cardiovascular system. Ensure that the objectives of the lesson have been covered. Ask questions to reinforce the learning. Relate to previous and coming topics. End the session	Learners to respond to questions		

Lesson plan worksheet

Add labels to this diagram of a human heart.

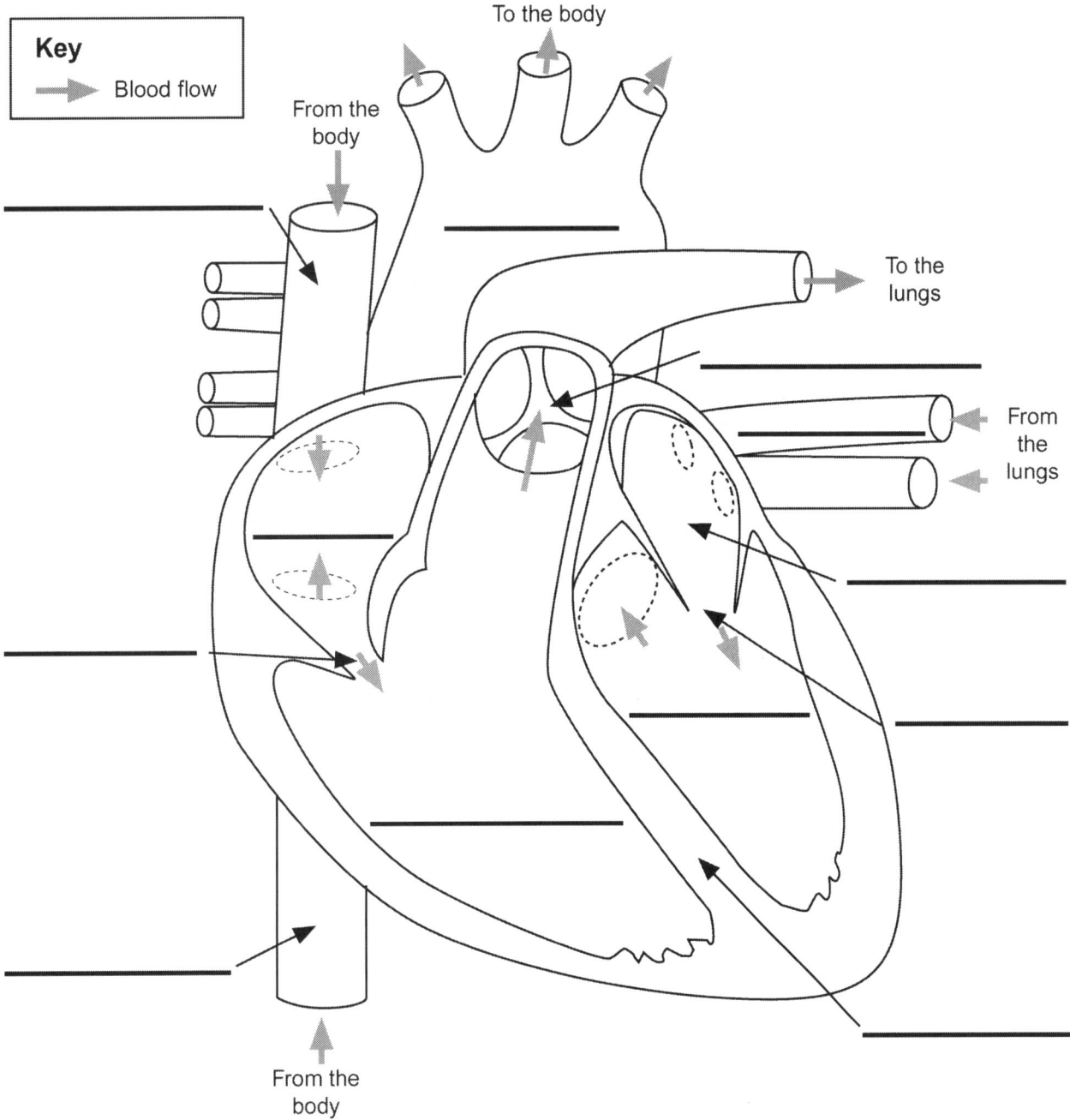

Key

⮕ Blood flow

To the body

From the body

To the lungs

From the lungs

From the body

5.1   Introductory activity: Understand the structure and function of parts of the human body

Student Book 1
pp 202–222

In this unit you will study the anatomy (structure of different parts) and the physiology (function of different parts) of the human body. The table below gives a list of body systems, organs, functions of body systems or organs, and tissues. Choose one of the ten body systems and try to match it with its main function, and with the corresponding organs and tissues. For example: the <u>nervous system</u> has a <u>co-ordination function</u>. It is made of <u>nervous tissue</u> that makes <u>the brain</u> and <u>spinal cord</u>.

Body systems	Functions	Tissues	Organs
Respiratory system	Digestion	Epithelial	Heart
Cardiovascular system	Co-ordination	Connective	Liver
Nervous system	Reproduction	Muscle	Lung
Digestive system	Respiration	Nervous	Intestines
Endocrine system	Energy metabolism		Bladder
Muscular-skeletal system	Maintenance of blood pressure		Brain
Immune system	Maintenance of heart rate		Spinal cord
Lymphatic system	Maintenance of breathing rate		Pancreas
Reproductive system	Thermo-regulation		Larynx
Urinary system	Osmo-regulation		Stomach
	Gluco-regulation		Uterus
	Defence against infections and diseases		Kidney
	Elimination of excess fluids from tissues		Testis
	Movement		Aorta
	Production of immune cells		Trachea
	Protection of internal organs		Gall bladder
			Ovaries
			Penis
			Endocrine glands
			Lymph capillaries
			Colon
			Skeletal muscles
			Lymph nodes

5.2   Understand the structure of a cell

Student Book 1
pp 202–222

First, label the following diagram of a eukaryotic cell (a cell with a visible nucleus), using words taken from the first column (organelles of the cell) in the table below. Then, using the same table, try to find the right definition for each organelle of the cell.

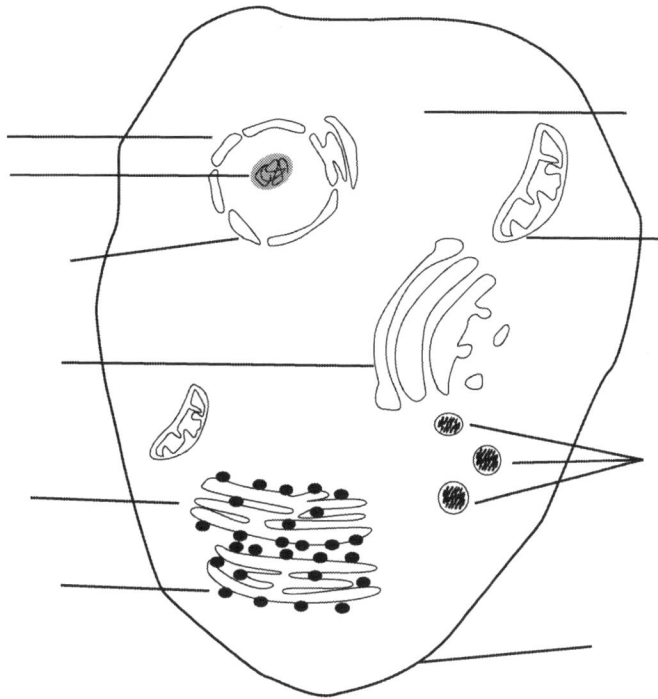

Organelles of the cell	Definition
Mitochondria	Contains various organelles such as mitochondria and lysosomes. Defined by a cell membrane
Lysosome	Composed of three distinct smooth-membrane-limited compartments. Plays a role in glycosylation, sulfation, phosphorylation, and proteolysis of proteins. It initiates concentration and storage of secretory products
Nucleus	Small electron-dense particles composed of ribosomal RNA
Cell membrane	Has a spherical structure and is rich in rRNA and protein
Endoplasmic reticulum	Contains DNA, synthesises RNA, contains a double-layered membrane
Nucleolus	Allows the transport of water-soluble molecules across the nucleus
Cytoplasm	A network of membranes in the cytoplasm. This is where proteins and complex lipids are synthesised
Golgi complex	Organelle within the cytoplasm and contains some DNA. A source of energy in the form of adenosine triphosphate
Ribosome	Made of double-layered phospholipids. Separates the inside of the cell from the external environment. Has proteins embedded in its surface that act as receptors
Nuclear pores	Membrane-bound vesicle that contains hydrolytic enzymes. Plays a role in cellular digestive system

5.3 Understand the main tissues of the body

Student Book 1
pp 202–222

A The table below shows the four main tissues of the body (first column), and the structure and function of each tissue (second column) in random order. Try to match the right structure and function to each tissue.

Tissue name	Structure and function of a tissue
Muscle	Composed of a layer of cells that are tightly packed, this tissue lines the outside and inside cavities of the body. It has various functions such as secretion, transcellular transport, sensation detection, absorption, protection and selective permeability
Epithelial	Composed of cells spaced by an extra-cellular matrix, this tissue provides structure and support in the body
Nervous	This is a contractile tissue composed of differentiated cells containing myofibrils
Connective	Composed of glial cells and neurones, this tissue controls and co-ordinates the activities of the body

B The epithelial tissue is made up of cells with varied forms and dimensions. Can you differentiate below between squamous epithelium (simple or stratified) and cuboidal epithelium (simple or stratified)? Now draw a simple ciliated columnar epithelium and a transitional epithelium.

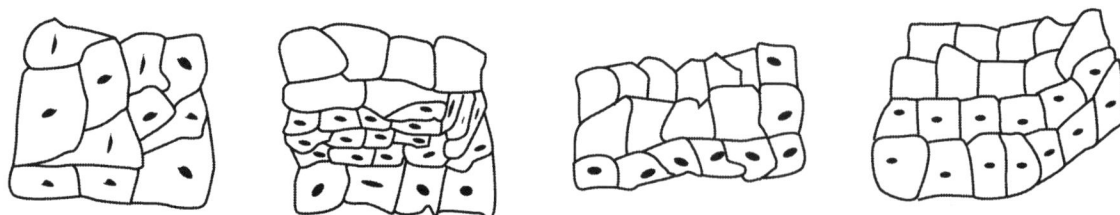

C The diagram below shows a dissection through the small intestine, revealing the different types of tissues the small intestine is made of. Can you write a few lines about the role of these tissues in the functioning of the small intestine as part of the digestive system?

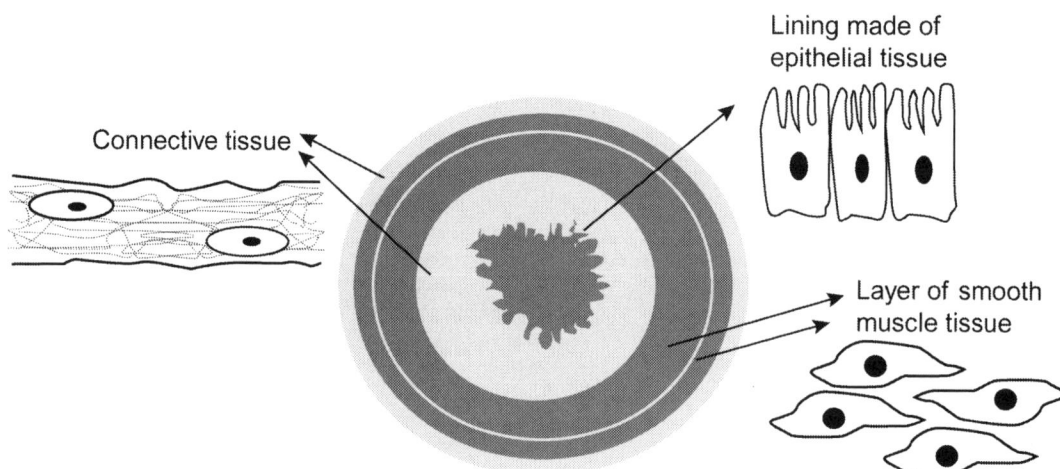

Connective tissue

Lining made of epithelial tissue

Layer of smooth muscle tissue

5.4   Understand the main functions of body systems

Student Book 1
pp 202–222

The table below shows the names of body systems with the organs, which they are composed of. These organs work together to keep each body system functioning. Draw the gross structure of each body system, then write a few lines explaining its main function.

Cardiovascular system (composed of: inferior and superior vena cava, pulmonary arteries and veins, heart and aorta) **Function**	**Diagram**
Respiratory system (composed of: nasal cavity, larynx, trachea, lungs, pharynx, bronchus and diaphragm) **Function**	**Diagram**
Endocrine system (composed of: pituitary, pineal, adrenal and thyroid glands as well as pancreas, testis and ovaries) **Function**	**Diagram**

Continued overleaf

5.4 Understand the main functions of body systems (*contd*)

Urinary system (composed of: kidneys, ureter, bladder, urethra, and renal veins and arteries) **Function**	**Diagram**
Digestive system (composed of: salivary gland, oesophagus, stomach, liver, pancreas, appendix, small intestine, rectum and anus) **Function**	**Diagram**
Reproductive system (composed of: bladder, urethra, penis, epididymis, testis, seminal vesicle, and prostate gland for the male; fallopian tubes, ovaries, uterus, endometrium, cervix, and vagina for the female) **Function**	**Diagram**

5.5   Understand the role of energy in the body

Student Book 1
pp 222–243

There are many links between energy metabolism and the functioning of the cardiovascular, respiratory and digestive systems. Use the brainstorming activities summarised below, and what you know about the structure and function of the above body systems, to write 20–40 lines describing the role of energy in the body.

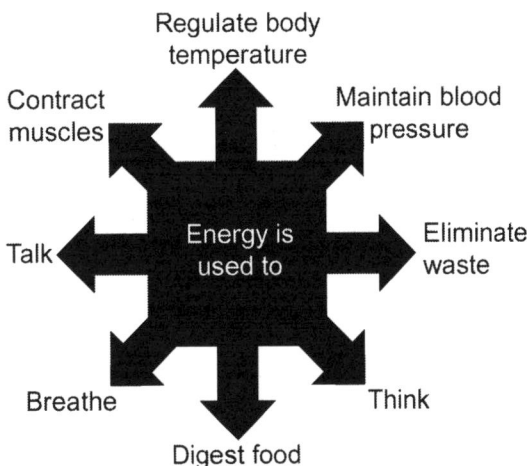

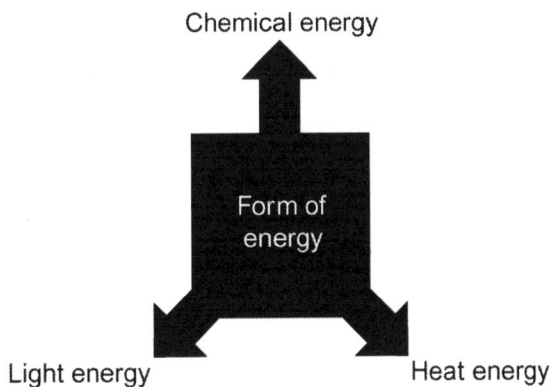

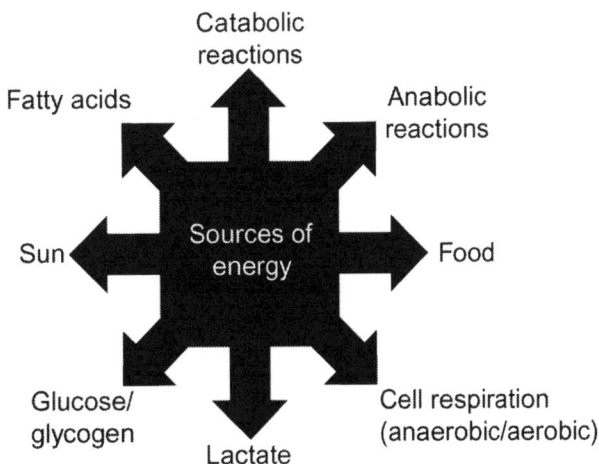

Regulate body
temperature

Contract
muscles

Maintain blood
pressure

Talk

Energy is
used to

Eliminate
waste

Breathe

Think

Digest food

Chemical energy

Form of
energy

Light energy

Heat energy

Catabolic
reactions

Fatty acids

Anabolic
reactions

Sun

Sources of
energy

Food

Glucose/
glycogen

Lactate

Cell respiration
(anaerobic/aerobic)

5.6   Understand the digestive system and energy metabolism

Student Book 1
pp 222–243

Using the information below, write a few lines to explain how the physiology of the digestive system is related to energy metabolism. In other words, how does each organ alone, or with another organ as part of the digestive system, contribute to energy generation?

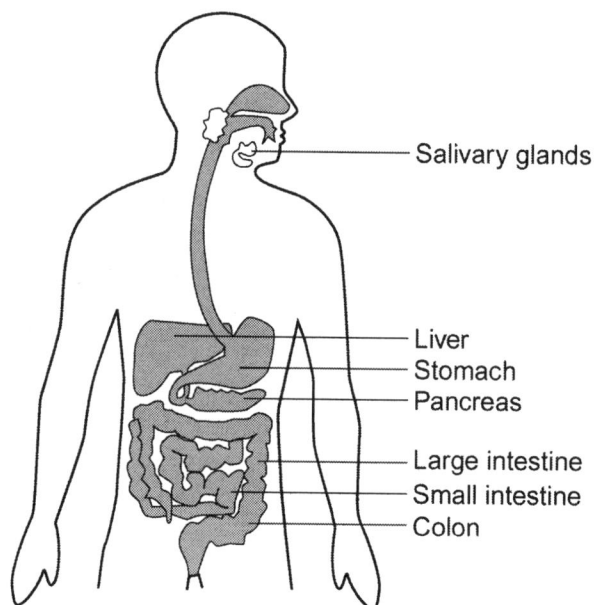

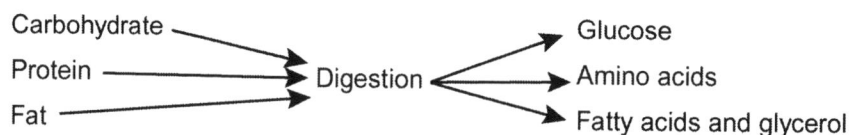

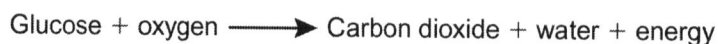

5.7   The concept of homeostasis

Student Book 1
pp 244–254

Use the words in the box to fill in the gaps in the passage below. Then answer the questions.

| homeostasis   thermo-regulation   glucose   glucagon   anti-diuretic hormone |
| negative feedback   hypothalamus   insulin   osmo-regulation   brain |

The main source of energy in our body is .... This blood sugar is maintained at an approximate level of 0.8–1 g/l by two hormones called ....

and .... The control of blood sugar is part of .... Any rise or fall in the normal blood sugar level will trigger a specific corrective mechanism to bring this level back to normal. That is called a .... mechanism. Water balance of the blood, which we call ...., and body temperature regulation, which we call ...., are two other aspects of homeostasis (a mechanism that maintains a constant internal environment). Osmo-regulation is a process that controls both water and salt content in the blood. Any increase or decrease in salt and water content in the blood will be detected by the .... In this case, a hormone called ....….. will be produced at a higher or lower concentration. Again, this negative feedback mechanism will bring the salt and water concentration in the blood back to normal. The skin, with its varied functions, plays a major role in controlling our body temperature. Skin receptors will sense any external temperature changes and inform the .... This will alter the person's behaviour (e.g. they might close the window when they feel cold).

1   Give a short definition of homeostasis.

2   What is an internal environment?

3   What is a negative feedback mechanism?

4   How do we keep our body's internal environment stable?

5.8 Understand the homeostatic mechanism of gluco-regulation

Student Book 1
pp 244–254

Using the key words in the box, complete diagrams **A** and **B**.

insulin	glucose	liver	glucogen	Islets of Langerhans	glucagon

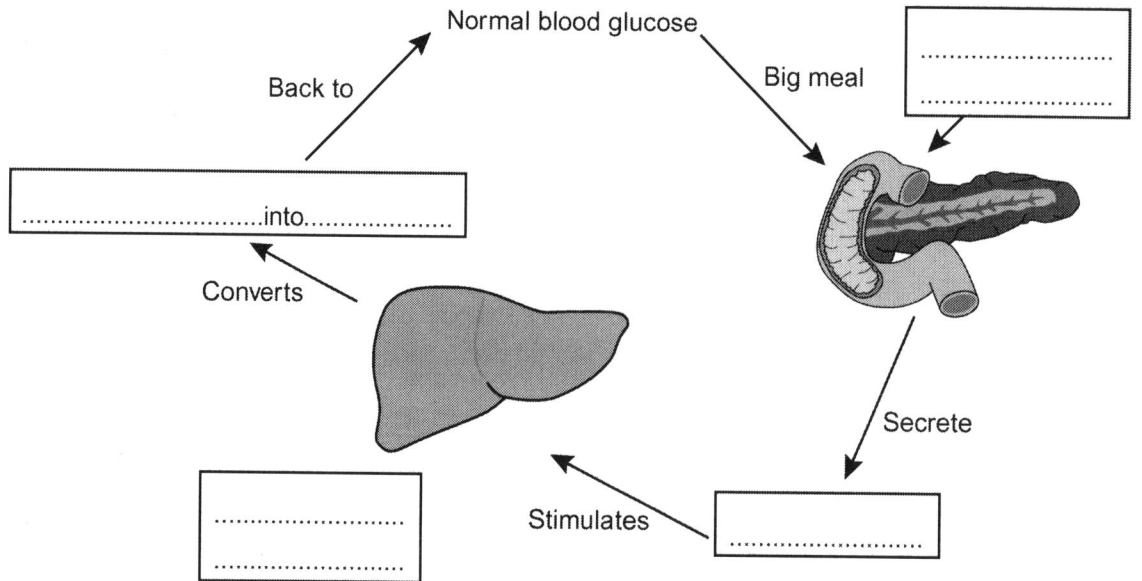

DIAGRAM A

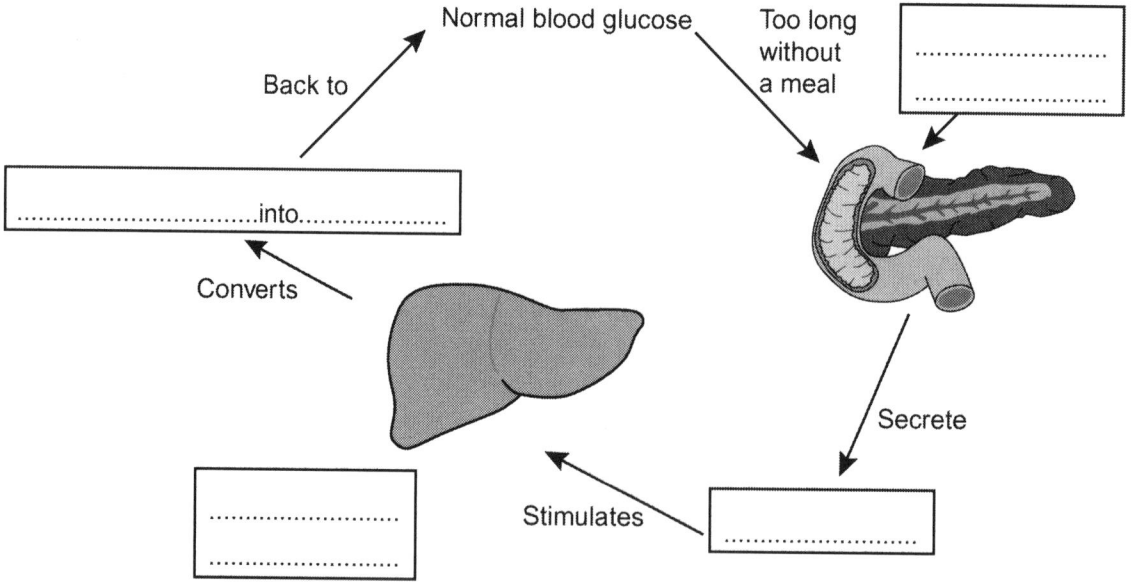

DIAGRAM B

Now write a few lines to explain what happens when:

1   glucose concentration in the blood is above the norm after a big meal

2   glucose concentration in the blood is below the norm after a long time without food.

Finally, can you explain the importance of homeostasis in maintaining a normal blood glucose concentration?

5.9   Measuring breathing rate

Student Book 1
pp 255–265

Part A

During this practical activity, you will use three instruments to measure five parameters:

1   the spirometer to measure the tidal volume, the breathing rate, and the inspiratory reserve volume at rest and during exercise (the breathing rate is the number of inspirations and expirations in a given time)

2   the pulse watch to measure the pulse rate at rest and during exercise

3   the strip thermometer to measure body temperature at rest and during exercise.

You will gather your data by filling in the given table (see page 132). Then answer the questions below.

Part B

Before starting the experiment, let's get familiar with lung volumes. You need to match six definitions to six terms you can read on the spirometer trace (see page 131). For example, the letter A on the spirometer trace corresponds to the tidal volume that we define as the volume breathed in and out in one cycle. You have one box with the terms, a second box with the corresponding definitions, and a spirometer trace labelled with the letters A to F.

> total lung capacity / residual volume / expiratory reserve volume / tidal volume / vital capacity / inspiratory reserve volume

> maximum volume of air forced out after the deepest inspiration / maximum volume of air in your lungs / volume breathed in and out in one cycle / extra volume of air you can inspire above the tidal volume / extra volume of air you can expire above the tidal volume / volume of air in the lungs after forced expiration

A:

B:

C:

D:

E:

F:

Continued overleaf

5.9 Measuring breathing rate (*contd*)

Equipment needed:

- spirometer

- pulse watch

- strip thermometer

- skipping rope.

Method

Take four measurements, as explained, using the spirometer, the pulse watch, and the strip thermometer. The measurements should be taken at rest and then again after using the skipping rope for 1, 2 and 3 minutes.

Collect your spirometer trace, and then transfer the data to the given table (see page 132). Each measurement should be carried out for 12 seconds.

To work out the breathing rate, you need to calculate the number of peaks (breathing in and out) per minute. That gives the breathing rate per minute. For example, at rest when you breathe in and out five times (5 peaks on the spirometer trace) during a period of 12 seconds, your breathing rate will be equal to 25 per minute (5 peaks × 60 secs/12 secs).

Questions

1   How do the breathing cycle patterns differ from each other, when you are at rest and when you are exercising?

2   What happens to the volume of air you breathe in or out when you are exercising?

3   How does your breathing rate change in order to adapt to the effort of exercise?

4   What happens to the inspiratory reserve volume during exercise?

5   What happens to your body temperature during exercise, and does it have any effect on your breathing rate?

6   What happens to your pulse rate during exercise?

7   Why does the residual volume of air stay the same?

Share your results with another student and see how valid your data are. Then try to interpret the changes in breathing rate during exercise.

Continued overleaf

5.9 Measuring breathing rate (*contd*)

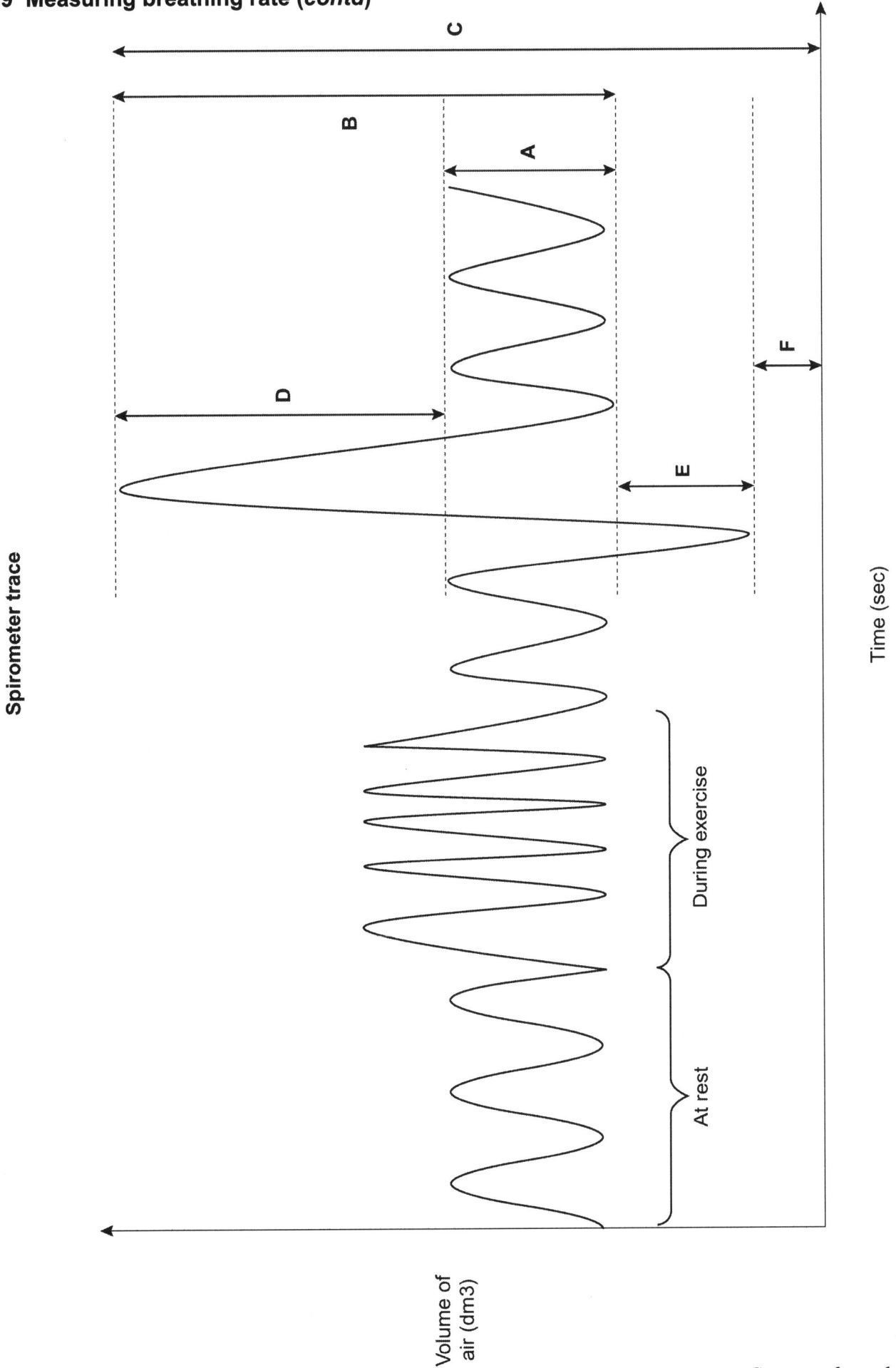

Spirometer trace

Volume of air (dm3)

Time (sec)

At rest

During exercise

Continued overleaf

5.9 Measuring breathing rate (*contd*)

Table to record your results

Time	Spirometer trace for a 12-second period	Breathing rate per min	Tidal volume (litre)	Inspiratory reserve volume (litre)	Body temperature (°C)	Pulse rate (beats per min)
At rest						
1 min						
2 mins						
3 mins						

5.10   Understand breathing rate and exercise (the homeostatic mechanism)

**Student Book 1
pp 255–265**

Use your answers from Activity 5.9 to explain the homeostatic mechanism involved in adapting the breathing rate to exercise. You will also need to use your knowledge of the physiology of the respiratory system to explain this mechanism.

The box below lists a number of key actions, which involve both the nervous and respiratory systems, to adapt your breathing rate to the activity you are doing. Use these key actions to fill in the diagram below.

Contraction of intercostal muscles and diaphragm / increase of carbon dioxide in the blood / increase of breathing rate / nerve impulses from receptors in the blood vessels to the brain / nerve impulses from the brain to the intercostal muscles and diaphragm

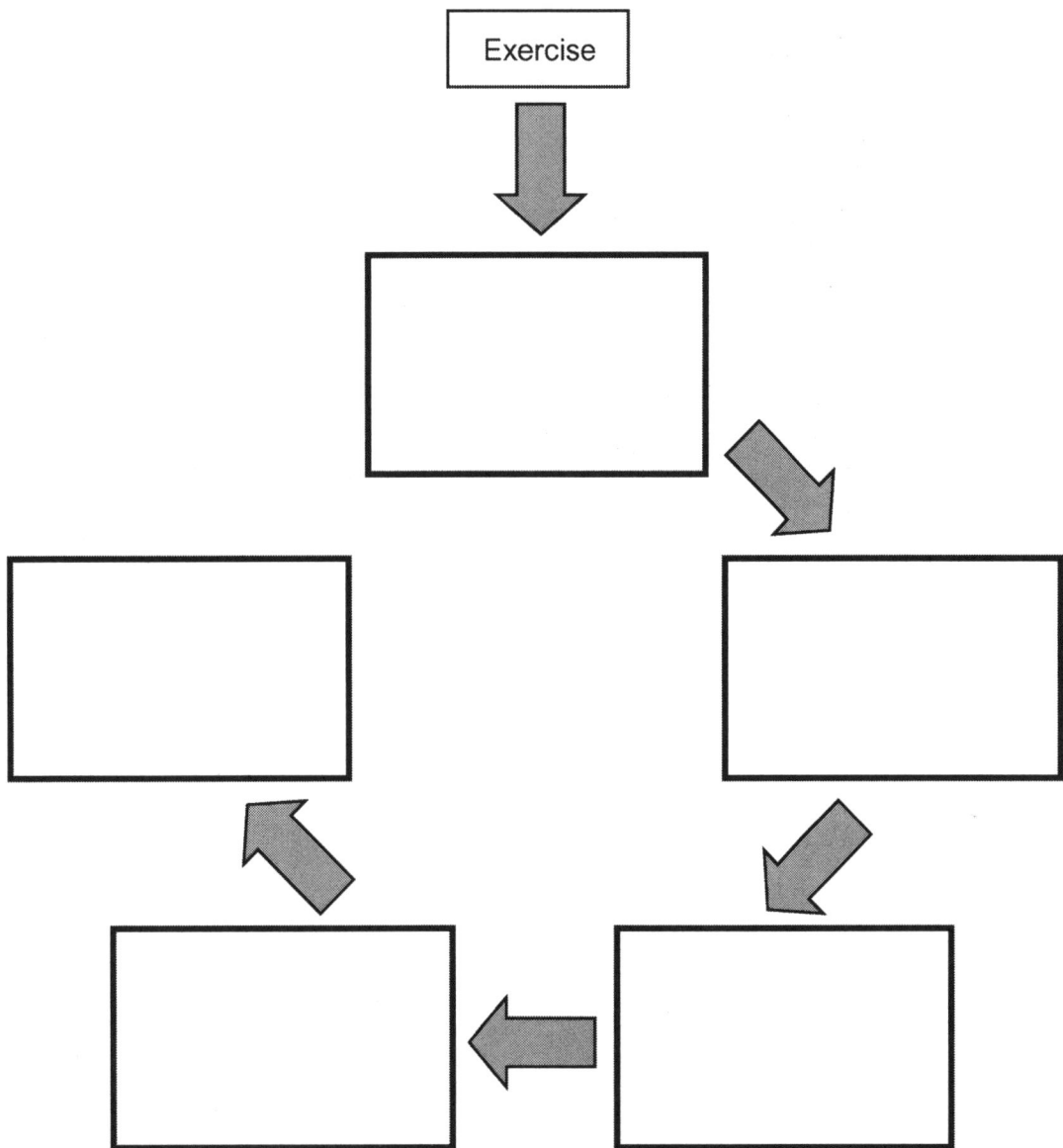

Exercise

Now write a few lines to explain how the brain controls your breathing at rest and when you are exercising to maintain a stable internal environment.

5.11 End-of-unit crossword

Student Book 1
pp 255–265

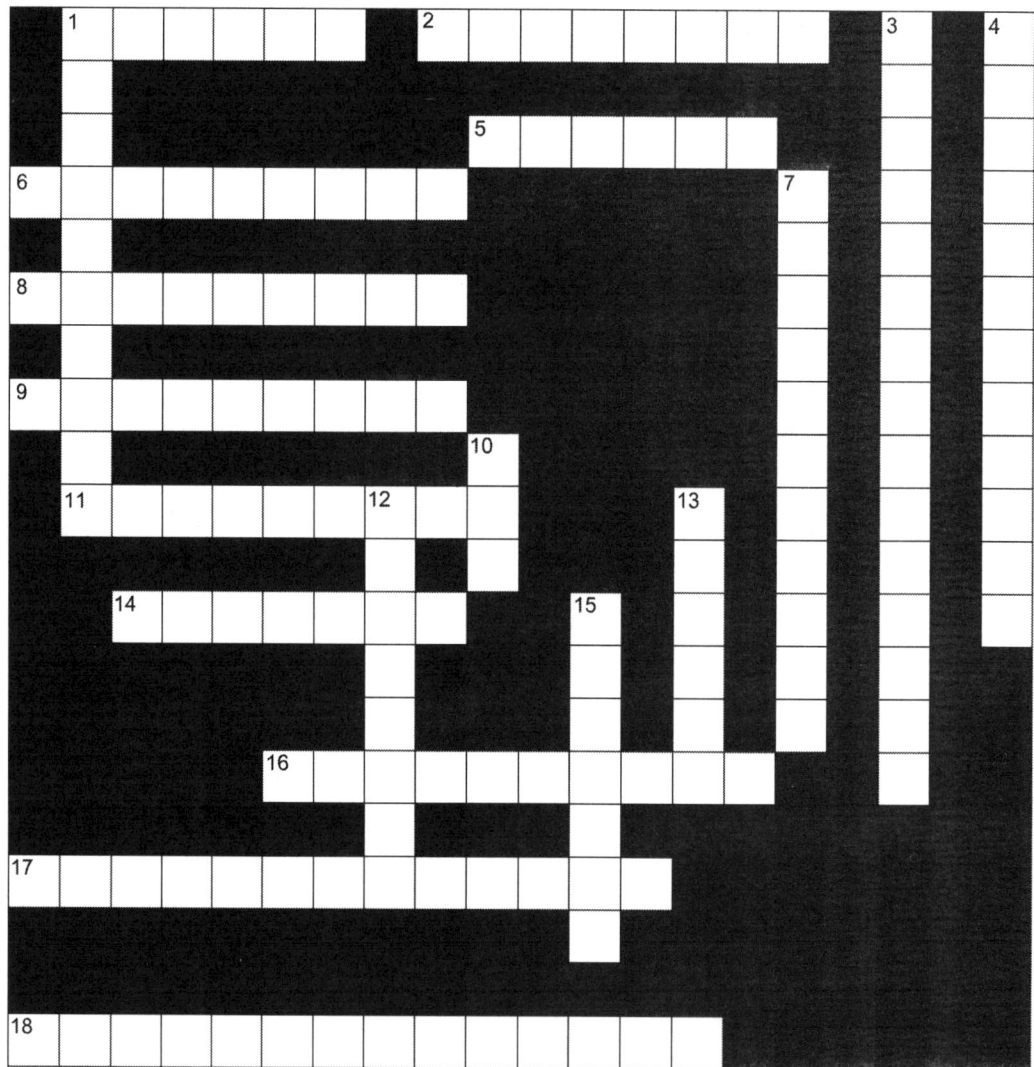

ACROSS

1. An upper chamber of the heart
2. A hormone that changes glycogen into glucose
5. Tube that carries urine from the kidney to the bladder
6. One way to measure breathing rate
8. A graphic representation of discrete data
9. Graph to show frequency distribution of data
11. Elimination of waste products
14. Gap between neurons
16. Used for measuring lung volumes
17. One beat of the heart
18. The force of blood on blood vessels

DOWN

1. Hormone produced by adrenal gland
3. Part of endocrine system that produces hormones
4. Part of the brain responsible for water regulation
7. Maintains the internal environment
10. Central nervous system
12. Hormone produced by the pancreas to lower blood sugar
13. Helps to break down food in digestion
15. Lung tissue

Note: In this crossword, you need to leave one blank square between the words in two-word answers.

The content of each Learning outcome

Learning outcome 1: Understand sociological approaches to study (relevant criteria: P1, M1)

The first outcome begins with a PowerPoint® presentation introducing the learner to the key terminology used in sociology. Understanding of these terms will be checked through the gapped handout (Activity 7.1), the worksheet (Activity 7.2) and the definition matching activity (Activity 7.3), before being applied to diversity issues in a health and social care context (Activity 7.4). Learners will then be introduced to the principal sociological perspectives. The case study (Activity 7.5) provides a care context in which to apply these theories. The mix and match activity (Activity 7.6) will check basic understanding and the group activity (Activity 7.7) provides an opportunity to describe the theories more fully. Three more PowerPoint® presentations introduce other sociology terms that learners will use and explore in this unit.

Learning outcome 2: Be able to apply sociological approaches to health and social care (relevant criteria: P2, P3, P4, P5, M2, M3, D1, D2)

This outcome begins by introducing learners to the different concepts of health (PowerPoint® 5). Activity 7.8 then requires them to explain these concepts and share their learning with the rest of the class. Learners will then apply these concepts within a case study (Activity 7.9). Using PowerPoint® 6, learners can be introduced to the models of health and ill health, before debating and discussing these models in Activity 7.10. This debate activity and the case study (Activity 7.11) will enable learners to develop the skills needed to achieve the merit and distinction grades (M2 and D1).

Learners will be introduced to concepts of ill health using PowerPoint® 7, and directed questioning can generate examples to illustrate the terms. The worksheet (Activity 7.12) provides a mental health context in which to apply and use these terms, and the mix and match activity (Activity 7.13) will test knowledge of the vocabulary. The group activity (Activity 7.14) provides an opportunity to describe and compare different patterns of health and illness in different social groups. This knowledge will be consolidated and further developed by using sociological explanations to account for patterns of health and illness in different groups (Activity 7.15). This activity allows learners aiming for distinction grades to evaluate the four sociological explanations for health inequalities (D2). Finally, the Activity 7.16 group presentation task will help learners review the content of the whole unit.

How this unit will be assessed

This is an internally assessed unit.

To reach Pass level, the evidence must show that the learner is able to:

P1   use sociological terminology to describe the principal sociological perspectives
P2   describe different concepts of health
P3   describe the bio-medical and socio-medical models of health
P4   explain different concepts of ill health
P5   compare patterns of health and illness in three different social groups.

To reach Merit level, the evidence must show that, in addition to the Pass criteria, the learner is able to:

M1   use two sociological perspectives to explain different concepts of health
M2   explain the bio-medical and socio-medical models of health
M3   use sociological explanations for health inequalities to explain the patterns and trends of health and illness in three different social groups.

To reach Distinction level, the evidence must show that, in addition to the Pass and Merit criteria, the learner is able to:

D1   evaluate the bio-medical and socio-medical models of health
D2   evaluate four sociological explanations for health inequalities in terms of explaining the patterns and trends of health and illness in three different social groups.

Assessment tasks

Learners can gather and record evidence for the Assessment tasks at their work placements. They can also read recommended texts and carry out research on the Internet, either through appropriate search engines or specific websites.

Task 1 (relevant criteria: P1)

Using sociological terms introduced within this unit, produce seven handouts, each briefly describing one of the following seven sociological perspectives (write no more than 150 words for each perspective):

1   functionalism
2   Marxism
3   feminism
4   interactionism
5   postmodernism
6   collectivism
7   New Right.

Task 2 (relevant criteria: P2)

Briefly describe the following concepts of health:

- negative
- positive
- holistic
- the World Health Organisation definition.

Task 3 (relevant criteria: M1)

Choose two of the sociological perspectives described in Task 1 and use them to explain more fully the different concepts of health described in Task 2.

Task 4 (relevant criteria: P3, M2, D1)

Describe and explain, using examples, the bio-medical and socio-medical models of health. **(P3, M2)**

Statistics show that around 25 per cent of the world's children live in absolute poverty. These children usually have a shorter life expectancy due to malnutrition, disease and poor housing conditions. They lack access to healthcare and education, and they are often socially excluded.

Evaluate the usefulness of the bio-medical and the socio-medical models of health in this situation. **(D1)**

Task 5 (relevant criteria: P4)

Define and describe the following terms in the context of ill health:

- disability
- illness and disease
- iatrogenisis
- the sick role
- the clinical iceberg.

Task 6 (relevant criteria P5, M1)

Drawing on the statistical information generated from your group activities and other research tasks:

- Compare and explain the patterns of health and illness in three different social groups. **(P5)**
- Evaluate the four sociological explanations for health inequalities as they apply to these groups. **(M1)**

Scheme of work

BTEC National Health and Social Care
Unit 7 Sociological perspectives in health and social care

Academic year: ....
Broad aim: Successful completion of the unit
Teacher(s): ....

Number of weeks: 17
Duration of session: 2 hours
Guided learning hours: 70

Week/s	Topic/outcome	Tutor preparation	Student activity	Resources	Links to grading criteria
1	Introduction to Unit 7: What is sociology?	Introduce key terms using PowerPoint® 1 and present a brief outline of the unit. Provide examples, and encourage learners to provide examples, to illustrate the meanings of the terms.	Allow a maximum of 5 minutes for learners to discuss 'What is sociology?' prior to feedback. Encourage them to write a definition, then discuss and display an agreed definition. All learners to complete Activity 7.1 gapped handout	PowerPoint® 1, Activity 7.1	All
2–3	Applying sociology to learners' life experience	Introduce further key terms using PowerPoint® 2. Learners to complete the Activity 7.3 (definition) matching task in pairs	In pairs or small groups, learners should discuss their responses to the tasks set in Activity 7.2.	Activity 7.2, PowerPoint® 2, Activity 7.3	P1
4–5	Applying sociology to health and care – social diversity	Introduce the Activity 7.4 research tasks. Ensure that all learners make a record of the key points raised.	Task 1 should be a group activity. Task 2 should be completed individually to check understanding across the group. Task 3 learners should share ideas in small groups and give feedback to a full class plenary session.	Activity 7.4	P1
6–7	Introduction to sociological perspectives (functionalism, Marxism, feminism)	Introduce the key sociological perspectives using PowerPoint® 3. Provide examples, and encourage learners to provide examples, to illustrate the key points.	In groups, learners discuss which perspective they think best describes our society. In pairs, learners should complete Assessment task 1 before feeding back to the whole class. Then, in pairs, they can discuss and make notes for Assessment task 2, before full class discussion and completing the written work	PowerPoint® 3, Activity 7.5, Assessment tasks 1 and 2 (see Introduction)	P1
8–9	Introduction to sociological perspectives (collectivism, the New Right, interactionism, postmodernism)	Introduce collectivism and the New Right, using PowerPoint® 4, providing social care examples and generating others from the learners to illustrate these approaches. Introduce interactionism and postmodernism using PowerPoint® 4.	Learners complete Activity 7.5 and Assessment task 3 either individually or in pairs. Learners complete the definition matching task in Activity 7.6, working in pairs or small groups. Learners can be encouraged to discuss their answers with the rest of the class.	PowerPoint® 4, Activity 7.5, Assessment task 3 (see unit introduction), Activity 7.6	P1
10	The sociological perspectives	Consolidate learning of the sociological perspectives.	In groups, to confirm learning and understanding, learners should complete the Activity 7.7 poster task	Activity 7.7	P1

[177]

Unit 7 Sociological perspectives in health and social care

Week/s	Topic/outcome	Tutor preparation	Student activity	Resources	Links to grading criteria
11–12	Concepts of health	Introduce concepts of health using PowerPoint® 5. Describe and discuss with learners how two sociological perspectives explain different concepts of health. Set Task 3 for homework	Ask learners to discuss in pairs what they mean by 'being healthy' and to describe somebody who they regard as being particularly healthy. Activity 7.8 is a group activity that will check understanding of the concepts of health introduced. Learners could be encouraged to share the information as an electronic document. In four groups, learners should complete the three tasks in Activity 7.9 (Cathy's story). Tasks 1 and 2 apply learning to a care context	PowerPoint® 5, Activity 7.8, Activity 7.9	P2, M1
13–14	The bio-medical and socio-medical models of health	Use PowerPoint® 6 to introduce the models of health. Then use the debate in Activity 7.10 to confirm learning and understanding and apply knowledge to health and care policy and practice	Learners should work in teams preparing and then taking part in a debate, using both research and presentation skills. Learners should work in pairs to complete the Activity 7.11 case study before feeding back to the full class. Task 3 will be helpful to those aiming for a Distinction grade	PowerPoint® 6, Activity 7.10, Activity 7.11	P3, M2, D1
15–16	Concepts of ill health	Using PowerPoint® 7, introduce concepts and measures of ill health	Using the PowerPoint® slides and the textbook, learners should complete the Activity 7.12 worksheet. In groups, learners to complete the Activity 7.13 definition matching task	PowerPoint® 7, Activity 7.12, Activity 7.13	P4
17	Patterns of health and illness in different social groups	Following the group presentations, support learners in completing the Activity 7.15 research task	Divide the class into six small groups and ask learners to complete the Activity 7.14 diagram and presentation task. Learners then to work individually preparing written answers to Activity 7.15.	Activity 7.14, Activity 7.15	P5, M3, D2
17	Sociology and working in health and social care	This group presentation task will help learners review the content of the whole unit	Learners to work in small groups to prepare a presentation covering the themes of the whole unit	Activity 7.16	All

At-a-glance activity grid
Unit 7 Sociological perspectives in health and social care

Outcome 7.1 Understand sociological approaches to study

Activity	Title and description	Scheme of work	File/CD	Delivery notes	Additional resources	Links to grading criteria	Activities for placement Links to other units	Links to Student Book 1
Power Point® 1	Introduce key sociological terms	Week 1	CD	Use PowerPoint® 1 to introduce the sociological terms used in this unit. Provide clear examples. Learners, working in small groups or in pairs, should generate examples of their own		All		pp 336–350
7.1	Gapped handout: Key sociological terms	Week 1	File (Answers on CD)	Use the gapped handout in conjunction with PowerPoint® 1 to confirm individual understanding of the key terms		All		pp 336–350
7.2	Applying sociology to everyday life	Week 2	File	In pairs or small groups, learners should discuss their response to the tasks set in the Activity 7.2 worksheet		All	Learners may draw from placement experience to illustrate the concepts introduced. Activity 7.2, Task 3 specifically requires learners to draw on their placement experience to illustrate understanding	pp 336–350
Power Point® 2	Further key sociological terms	Week 3	CD	Introduce further key terms relating to social structure		All		pp 336–350
7.3	Mix and match: Understanding the key terms	Week 3	File (Tutor information and Answers on CD)	Use this definition matching activity to check understanding of the key terms	Thin card cut into sets (see Tutor information on CD)	All		pp 336–350

Activity	Title and description	Scheme of work	File/CD	Delivery notes	Additional resources	Links to grading criteria	Activities for placement Links to other units	Links to Student Book 1
7.4	Research activity: Cultural diversity	Weeks 4–5	File	In Activity 7.4, Task 1 should be a group activity. Task 2 should be completed individually to check understanding across the group. For Task 3, learners should share ideas in small groups and then feed back to a full class plenary session. Ensure that all learners make a record of the key points raised	Library and Internet access. Learners may use ideas and resources from home and/or from their work placements	P1	Learners may be able to provide specific examples from their work placements to illustrate how the needs of people from minority groups are met	pp 336–350
Power Point® 3	Sociological perspectives	Weeks 6–7	CD	Use PPT 3 to introduce feminism, Marxism and functionalism, and give examples of these perspectives		P1		pp 336–350
7.5	Case study: The impact of poverty	Weeks 6–7	File	Through the Activity 7.5 case study, learners apply the sociological perspectives to a health and care context. This could be an individual or group activity		P1		pp 336–350
Power Point® 4, 7.5	Case study: The impact of poverty	Week 8	CD, File	Introduce other perspectives (e.g. collectivism, interactionism and postmodernism) using PPT 4. Learners complete the Activity 7.5 case study to apply and check understanding of the collectivist and New Right approaches		P1		pp 336–350
7.6	Mix and match: Sociological perspectives	Week 9	File (Tutor information and Answers on CD)	This definition matching activity is an opportunity to check understanding in groups	Thin card cut into sets (see Tutor information on CD)	P1		pp 336–350
7.7	Group activity: Sociological perspectives poster	Week 10	File	This is a group activity, in which learners describe the sociological perspectives required for P1	Library and Internet access, materials for creating posters	P1		pp 336–350

Outcome 7.2 Be able to apply the sociological approaches to health and social care

Activity	Title and description	Scheme of work	File/CD	Delivery notes	Additional resources	Links to grading criteria	Activities for placement Links to other units	Links to Student Book 1
Power Point® 5, 7.8	Group activity: Concepts of health	Week 11	CD, File	Use PPT 5 to introduce concepts of health. In groups, learners prepare and circulate handouts on the concepts of health	Access to computers	P2		pp 350–367
7.9	Case study: Cathy's story	Week 12	File	This case study provides a care context in which to apply the concepts of health. It also provides opportunities for learners who are working towards the merit grade		P2, M1	Learners should consider whether the positive or negative concepts of health are applied in their placement settings	pp 350–367
Power Point® 6	Models of health	Week 13	CD	Use PPT 6 to introduce the bio-medical and socio-medical models of health		P3		pp 350–367
7.10	A debate: Bio-medical versus socio-medical models of health	Week 13	File	This debate enables learners to develop an understanding that will lead to pass, merit and distinction grades	Access to computers	P3, M2, D1	Learners should consider whether the bio-medical model or the socio-medical model of health guides the policy and practice at their placement settings	pp 350–367
7.11	Case study: Mrs McPatrick	Week 14	CD	The Activity 7.11 case study provides an opportunity to apply the models of health to a health and care context		P3, M2, D1		pp 350–367
Power Point® 7	Concepts of ill health	Week 15	CD	Use PPT 7 to introduce concepts and measurements of ill health		P4		pp 350–367
7.12	Concepts of ill health	Week 15	File	This activity uses material from the Mind website to check understanding of the concepts of ill health		P4		pp 350–367
7.13	Mix and match: Concepts of ill health	Week 16	File (Tutor information and Answers on CD)	This definition matching activity is an opportunity to check understanding in groups	Thin card cut into sets (see Tutor information on CD)	P4		pp 350–367

Activity	Title and description	Scheme of work	File/CD	Delivery notes	Additional resources	Links to grading criteria	Activities for placement Links to other units	Links to Student Book 1
7.14	Diagram activity: Patterns of health and illness in different social groups	Week 16	File	A group activity to summarise patterns of health and illness in different social groups. The diagrams could be displayed when they are finished	Library and Internet access, materials for creating diagrams	**P5, M3**		pp 350–367
7.15	Research activity: Inequalities in heath and well-being	Week 17	File	This research activity supports learners in working towards pass, merit and distinction grades	Library and Internet access	**P5, M3, D2**		pp 350–367
7.16	Sociology and working in health and social care	Week 17	File	This group presentation task will help learners review the content of the whole unit		**All**		pp 350–367

Unit 7 Lesson plan

Aims

- To introduce learners to the structure and main content of Unit 7
- To introduce key sociological terms used in this unit
- To use learners' knowledge and experiences to illustrate the key sociological terms.

This structure may be spread over a number of lessons as required.

Learning outcomes
• be able to define the terms sociology and society
• be able to identify the main sources of information about our society
• be able to define the following terms used by sociologists in their study of society: culture, value, norms, social role, social status, socialisation, primary socialisation, secondary socialisation
• be able to provide simple illustrations of these terms using appropriate examples from own experiences or from placement settings.

Timing	Content	Teacher activity	Student activity	Resources	Individualised activity
5 mins	Welcome	Welcome learners and register			
15 mins	Introduce the unit content and display the Learning outcomes	Prepare a clear, well-spaced and attractive handout, summarising the key learning points for this unit. Ensure that the language and vocabulary used are appropriate for all learners. Remember that most will have not studied sociology before		Copies of handout	
15 mins	What do we mean by sociology?	Ask learners to work in pairs to discuss the meaning of sociology, then feed back their ideas to the rest of the class. Explain that different sociologists will have slightly different definitions. If necessary, introduce your own definition at the end of the feedback (e.g. 'Sociology is the study of society and how society influences our behaviour.') Make sure you respond positively to all contributions. By the end of the discussion, all learners should have recorded a clear 'working definition' of sociology. Display the definition in the classroom	In pairs, learners try to agree a definition of sociology, then feed back their ideas and contribute to discussion		

Timing	Content	Teacher activity	Student activity	Resources	Individualised activity
15 mins	What do we mean by society?	Introduce the concept of society as a spidergram with 'Society' in the centre and the main institutions as the 'legs': the family, the education system, the health and care services, and the economy. Introduce a definition of society (e.g. 'A society is made up of key institutions or building blocks, including the family, the education system, work and the economic systems, the political system, religious groups and the mass media. Sociologists are concerned with the way these institutions relate to each other and influence our behaviour.'). Display the definition and diagram in the classroom. Explain that the term 'society' can be used slightly differently by different writers.	Learners answer direct questions, and record the diagram and definition	Flipchart or whiteboard	Ensure that all learners have individual records of the definition and diagram. Ensure that the language and vocabulary used are appropriate for all learners. Check understanding through questioning. Direct your questions to students by name to elicit contributions from across the group
20 mins	How can we find out about our society?	Put learners in small groups to discuss the following questions: 1 How or where can we find reliable information about our society? 2 Where might we find the strongest and most reliable evidence? Follow group work with full-class feedback	For question 1, learners should present the information as a spidergram or a list. For question 2, learners should present their key sources in order of reliability, from most reliable to least reliable	Spare paper for groups to draw their diagrams and write their lists	You may choose to organise 'mixed ability' groups to progress discussion. Following feedback, ensure that all learners have individual records of the key learning points
20 mins	Introduce key sociology terms	Use PPT 1 to introduce key sociology terms. Ensure that the language and vocabulary used are appropriate for all learners, and select examples, to which all will relate, to illustrate the points. Check understanding through questioning	Learners answer questions and provide examples from their own experience	PowerPoint® 1	Learners will generate examples according to their understanding and ability

Timing	Content	Teacher activity	Student activity	Resources	Individualised activity
20 mins	Check understanding of the key sociology terms	Ask learners to complete the gapped handout (either individually or in pairs) to check their understanding of the key terms. Ask direct questions to check understanding	Learners to complete the gapped handout and answer questions	Activity 7.1 (Answers on CD)	
10 mins		Revisit the learning objectives, summarising the key learning points and explaining how a knowledge of sociology will help the students in health and care practice. Direct them to the relevant section in their textbook to consolidate their learning. Introduce the topic to be covered next week: How can we apply sociology to everyday life?			

7.1 Gapped handout: Key sociological terms

Student Book 1
pp 336–350

Use the words in the box below to fill the gaps in the text. Be careful – some terms may be used more than once!

culture	primary socialisation	secondary socialisation
social status	norms	values	socialisation

The term used in sociology to describe the values, beliefs, language, rituals, customs and rules that are associated with a particular society or social group is the .... of that society or group. The .... of the society are the beliefs and principles that underpin what is important and seen as worthwhile in a society, what is good or bad, what we are proud of and what should be discarded.

Children and other new members of a society will learn the usual ways of behaving in a society through the process of .... The .... that takes place within the family is called .... The .... that takes place through nursery, school friendship groups and in the wider community is called ....

Children will become familiar with the expected ways of behaving of key people in their lives. These are people who hold the social position or .... of carers, brothers and sisters, playgroup leaders or childminders, for example. Through the process of .... children will begin to understand the .... or usual ways of behaving in their society.

7.2   Applying sociology to everyday life

Student Book 1
   pp 336–350

In all societies there are key values that every person is aware of. These key values dictate most of our behaviour when we interact with other people.

For the following activity you will need to work in pairs.

1   Identify four key values that you think underpin life in our society.

2   Identify and describe three key aspects of the culture of our society.

3   Identify and describe the norms associated with the social status (or social position) of one person that you work with at your placement.

Compare your answers to the questions with others in the class. What differences have you come up with and why?

If you have time, answer the following:

4   Describe situations that you have observed where people may have the challenge of role conflict.

5   Can you think of occasions when you have to address problems that arise from role conflict?

7.3   Mix and match: Understanding the key terms

Student Book 1
   pp 336–350

For this activity, your tutor will put you in pairs and give you a set of cards (showing sociological terms and their definitions), in random order. You need to match each term with its correct definition.

[187]

7.4 Research activity: Diversity

Student Book 1
pp 336–350

Imagine that you are working in a day centre for older people based in a multicultural area in a large industrial city. The users of the centre come from a wide range of ethnic groups and different religious backgrounds. There are some Muslim men and women (many of whom moved to this country from Pakistan), Jews (many of whom have lived in England all their lives) and Hindus (who moved to this country from the Indian subcontinent). The staff at the centre are committed to providing quality care for all.

1   Carry out research in small groups. Write a brief report describing the specific cultural needs of the three religious groups identified. You may consider issues of diet, gender, religious practice and the celebration of religious festivals.

2   Use the following terms to explain the challenges that face the users and staff at the centre. This explanation should be presented in one paragraph of no more than 100 words: culture, values, socialisation, primary socialisation, secondary socialisation, norms, social role.

3   How might the study of sociology help staff to understand and meet the health and care needs of all users of the centre?

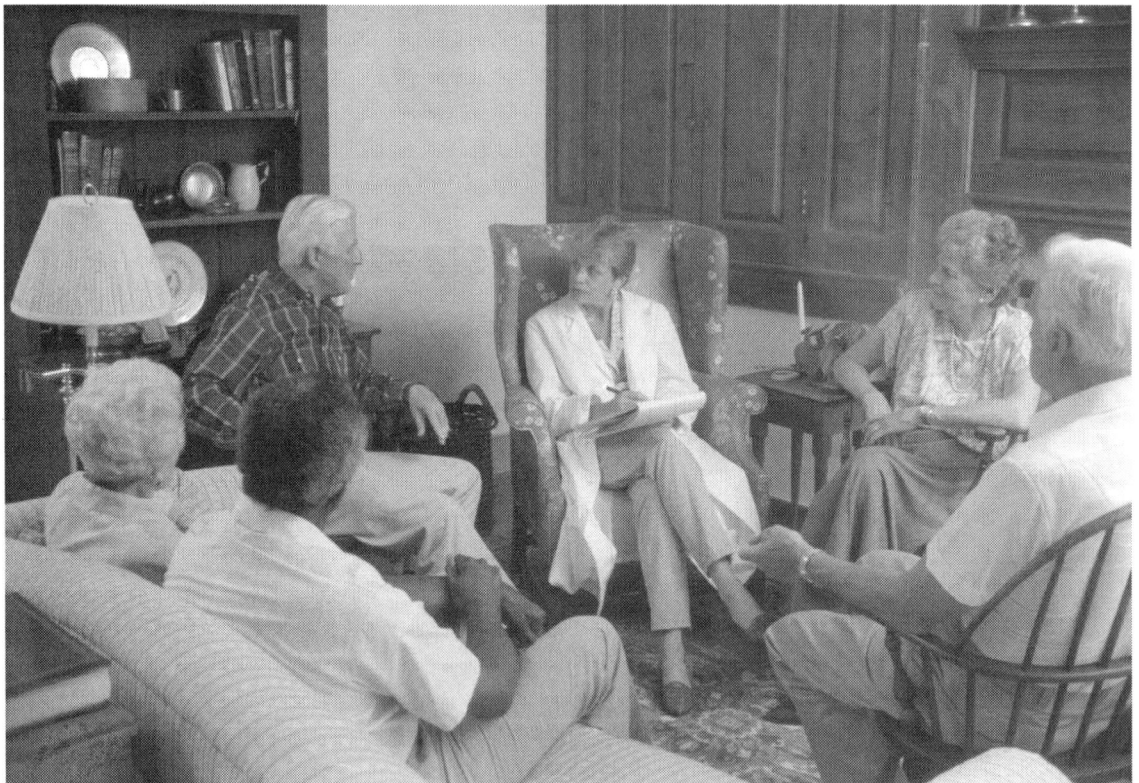

7.5   Case study: The impact of poverty

Student Book 1
pp 336–350

Sadie is a lone parent. She has two children, Sarah aged seven and Tom who is three years old. Sadie's only source of income is her state benefits. Their two-bedroom flat is in a very poor part of a large industrial city, near a motorway and a chemical works. The accommodation is damp. Even in cold weather Sadie does not always put on the heating because she is frightened that she will not be able to pay the electricity bill.

1   Briefly describe the likely impact of poverty on the health and well-being of the two children.

2   Briefly explain how a Marxist, a feminist and a functionalist sociologist would probably respond to these circumstances.

3   Compare and contrast the collectivist and New Right approaches to meeting these needs.

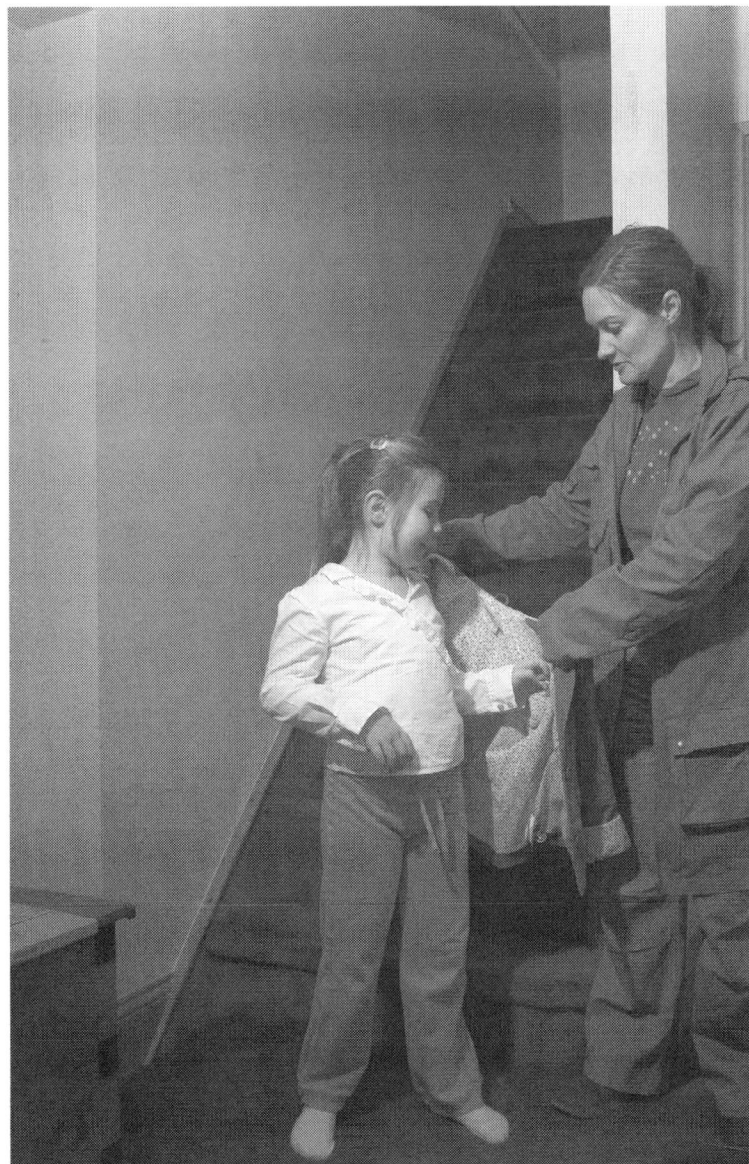

7.6 Mix and match: Understanding sociological perspectives

Student Book 1
pp 336–350

For this activity, your tutor will put you in pairs and give you a set of cards (showing sociological perspectives and their definitions), in random order. You need to match each term with its correct definition.

7.7 Group activity: Sociological perspectives poster

Student Book 1
pp 336–350

Divide into a maximum of seven groups. Each group has to design a poster presenting information about one of the sociological perspectives introduced in this unit. The poster is for a government information campaign, looking to teach people about society. It should be visually interesting and convey lots of information – you will have to choose the information you put on carefully!

1 Design a poster identifying the key features of the sociological perspective your group has chosen.

2 Using the poster, prepare a five-minute presentation to the rest of the class about the sociological perspective.

3 Using a computer, your group should also produce a brief written summary of the perspective (approximately 150 words) that can be copied to all other learners.

7.8 Concepts of health

Student Book 1
pp 350–367

Much of the work done in health and social care requires an understanding of the sociological concepts of health. The four main concepts of health are:

- negative

- positive

- holistic

- the World Health Organisation definition.

Divide into four groups. On a computer, each group can prepare a handout (no longer than one side of A4 paper), explaining the four concepts of health and how they are used in the study of health and social care. The handouts can be handed out to the rest of the class either as printouts or in electronic form.

7.9 Case study: Cathy's story

Student Book 1
pp 350–367

Cathy is 38, a mother of two, and homeless. The two small rooms she is staying in are cramped and filthy, and smell of beer and cigarette smoke from the pub below. Cathy has to share a bed with her eleven-year-old daughter, while her nine-year-old son sleeps on the sofa. The noise of the pub keeps them awake at night and both children have started to do badly at school. There is no kitchen and their only source of water is a shower.

Working individually or in pairs, complete the following tasks:

1 Identify the factors in Cathy's situation that may lead to ill health for herself and her family.

2 Describe how Cathy's needs and her children's health needs would be addressed using:

   a   a negative concept of health

   b   a positive concept of health.

3 Use two sociological perspectives to explain different concepts of health.

7.10 Debate: The socio-medical model versus the bio-medical model

Student Book 1
pp 350–367

There are two main models for the causes of health and ill health in the population. The PowerPoint® 6 presentation will introduce you to the basics of each model. However, you will need to know more. Do some research, using the Internet and books from the library, in order to describe and explain the two models of health. Then prepare a short report on the information you find. The report can either be written or presented to other learners. If writing a report, write no more than 100 words for each model.

Using the information you have collected, split into two teams and prepare to debate the material, with one learner acting as chairperson. Each team will have to debate in favour of one of the following arguments:

■ Argument A – We believe that the bio-medical model of health and illness should guide policy and practice in health and social care.

■ Argument B – We believe that the socio-medical model of health and illness should guide policy and practice in health and social care.

Use your research notes to prepare your team's case. Each team must appoint one person to present their case to the group. The debate will then be opened for all to contribute. This activity will be chaired by the chosen learner.

After the debate, all students need to summarise the key points made in order to evaluate the bio-medical and socio-medical models of health.

Finally, hold a secret ballot to see which team has won.

7.11   Case study: Mrs McPatrick

Student Book 1
pp 350–367

'Mrs McPatrick is only 26 but looks 46, worn out by giving birth every year since she was 16. Three of her babies died, but she still has seven, all of them crammed into two rooms and sleeping end to end in what looked like a big wooden box. They share a privy with four other families [...] there is no bath, just a tin tub brought out from under the kitchen table once a week – though I suspect that does not happen very often... The father is out of work of course and Mrs McPatrick supports the family by cleaning offices at night. But now she is pregnant again and too sick to work, and so they have no income at all and have applied for relief. They are Irish Catholics and get some contribution from the Church – but not nearly enough to provide for even their basic needs.'

From *Diary of an Ordinary Woman*, by Margaret Forster (Chatto & Windus, 2004), a fictional account of a social worker's home visit in 1931, when social workers were first employed by the then London County Council.

1   Identify the social factors that were likely to adversely affect the health and well-being of the McPatricks.

2   Describe the likely impact of these factors on the health and well-being of the family.

3   Explain and evaluate the usefulness of the bio-medical and socio-medical models of health to account for their level of health and well-being.

[193]

7.12 Concepts of ill health: Mental illness

Student Book 1
pp 350–367

Prevalence of mental health problems, by gender (people aged between 16 and 64)

All figures are percentages.

Diagnosis and rate (past week)	Female		Male		All	
	1993	2000	1993	2000	1993	2000
Mixed anxiety and depression	10.1	11.2	5.5	7.2	**7.8**	**9.2**
Generalised anxiety disorder	5.3	4.8	4.0	4.6	**4.6**	**4.7**
Depressive episode	2.8	3.0	1.9	2.6	**2.3**	**2.8**
Phobias	2.6	2.4	1.3	1.5	**1.9**	**1.9**
Obsessive compulsive disorder	2.1	1.5	1.2	1.0	**1.7**	**1.2**
Panic disorder	1.0	0.7	0.9	0.8	**1.0**	**0.7**
Any neurotic disorder	19.9	20.2	12.6	14.4	**16.3**	**17.3**

Source: ONS, 2000, *Psychiatric morbidity among adults living in private households in Great Britain*

(Quoted on the Mind website: www.mind.org.uk)

1 What is meant by the term 'prevalence' in the title of the statistical table?

2 Define the term morbidity referred to in the table.

3 Identify two key trends presented by this data.

4 According to the statistics, which mental health condition is most commonly diagnosed?

5 According to the statistics, which mental health condition is least often diagnosed?

6 Why is it difficult to secure accurate figures for levels of mental illness? Include a consideration of the 'clinical iceberg' in your answer.

7 Talcott Parsons identified specific rights and responsibilities for people who were diagnosed as ill. Explain the concept of the 'sick role' as it applies to people with a mental illness.

- -

7.13 Mix and match: Understanding concepts of ill health

Student Book 1
pp 350–367

For this activity, your tutor will put you in pairs and give you a set of cards (showing concepts of ill health and their definitions), in random order. You need to match each concept with its correct definition.

7.14 Patterns of health and illness in different social groups

Student Book 1
pp 350–367

Working in pairs, think of reasons why people in the following groups may have poorer than average levels of health:

■ older people

■ babies and young children

■ people from the lower social classes

■ people from minority ethnic groups

■ people with disabilities

■ people with non-standard sexual orientations.

Then design a Mind Map® or a spidergram illustrating your main points. Show how these points interlink. Use your diagram as the basis for a five-minute presentation to the rest of the class, explaining the issues that you have identified.

7.15 Inequalities in health and well-being

Student Book 1
pp 350–367

1   Using the Internet and other library resources, work in groups to identify and explain differences in patterns of health and illness by:

■ social class

■ ethnic group

■ gender

■ age.

Remember to provide references and sources for all statistics and other information presented.

2   Produce a handout that can be distributed to all members of your class summarising your findings.

For learners attempting the distinction grade:

3   Evaluate how far the four sociological explanations for health inequalities described in the Black Report account for the differences identified.

7.16 Sociology and working in health and social care

**Student Book 1
pp 350–367**

Divide into small groups. Each group should prepare a five-minute talk explaining how a knowledge of the following sociological ideas and approaches could help you in social care practice:

■ the concepts of culture and diversity

■ one of the sociological perspectives introduced

■ the concepts of health and ill health

■ the different models of health

■ the models and approaches to ill health

■ patterns of health and illness within different social groups.

After each talk, the other groups should each agree on one question to ask the speaker.

8

Psychological perspectives for health and social care

unit overview

Unit 8 explores six core psychological perspectives: behaviourism, social learning, psychodynamic, humanistic, cognitive and biological. This unit is intended for students with no previous experience of studying psychology. It offers an exciting opportunity to look at some of the most interesting topics in psychology research, and apply them to practical scenarios.

Learning outcomes

On completion of this unit learners should:

8.1 understand psychological approaches to study
8.2 be able to apply psychological perspectives to health and social care.

Suggested activities

The At-a-glance activity grid shows how the activities in the Assessment and Delivery Resource (ADR) relate to the content of the unit. The activities include introductory and plenary activities and a variety of case studies, research tasks, discussions and presentations, using written, verbal and presentation skills. The activities may help learners prepare for assessment, and the grid indicates which assessment criteria are relevant for each activity. Copies of activity sheets can be given to learners.

Teaching Unit 8

This unit should be taught through a variety of tutor-led sessions and small group exercises, giving students a chance to get to grips with the theory before applying it to case studies. With the popularity of reality television series featuring psychologists helping members of the public, students are likely to find Unit 8 really interesting and enjoyable. By covering six different psychological perspectives, this unit gives learners an opportunity to consider and debate diverse aspects of psychology.

How this unit will be assessed

To reach Pass level, the evidence must show that the learner is able to:

P1 describe the application of behaviourist perspectives in health and social care
P2 explain the value of the social learning approach to health and social care provision
P3 describe the application of psychodynamic perspectives in health and social care
P4 describe the application of humanistic perspectives in health and social care
P5 describe the application of cognitive perspectives in health and social care
P6 describe the application of biological perspectives in health and social care.

To reach Merit level, the evidence must show that, in addition to the Pass criteria, the learner is able to:

M1 analyse the contribution of different psychological perspectives to the understanding and management of challenging behaviour

M2 analyse the contribution of different psychological perspectives to health and social care service provision.

To reach Distinction level, the evidence must show that, in addition to the Pass and Merit criteria, the learner is able to:

D1 evaluate the roles of different psychological perspectives in health and social care.

The content of the Learning outcomes

Unlike other units, the grading criteria for Unit 8 cannot be easily split according to Learning outcome. Both the Learning outcomes therefore need to be taught and assessed together. Students will need to explain and describe the way each psychological perspective is used in context for each part of their learning and assessment. All the activities have been designed to apply the six perspectives to health and social care. Tutors will need to ensure that students have access to books that explain the basic principles (e.g. D. Moxon, P. Emmerson and K. Brewer, *Psychology for AS Level*, published by Heinemann, 2003).

To fulfil the P1 criteria, students will need to complete Activities 8.1 and 8.2. These case studies will give learners an opportunity to discover how much they already use behaviourist principles, and then apply them to health and social care scenarios. The P2 criteria focus on social learning. Activity 8.3 applies the concept of role models to health promotion, and tutors should link this work to Units 1 and 20. P3 explores psychodynamic theory, an area that many students may find unfamiliar and difficult at first. Activities 8.4 and 8.5 apply psychodynamic theories to short scenarios, allowing a more concrete approach.

P4 deals with humanistic perspectives, ideas that many students on this course seem to find very natural. Activity 8.6 should follow a brief explanation of Maslow's hierarchy. P5 moves on to cognitive explanations. In Activity 8.7 learners use the behaviourist and cognitive approaches to complete a table of antecedents, behaviours and consequences. Activity 8.8 is a PowerPoint® presentation on the cognitive approach. Activity 8.9 allows students to put cognitive theories into action, using themselves as research subjects. P6 involves biological explanations. In Activity 8.10 students will apply the biological perspective to produce a leaflet on the problems caused by shift work and jet lag. Activity 8.11 requires learners to design a poster on developmental norms for young children. Finally, Activity 8.12 offers a light-hearted crossword to recap the content of the unit.

Assessment tasks

Assessment tasks should integrate both Learning outcomes, by outlining theory and then describing how it can be applied in practice. Assessment tasks can include essays, presentations, case studies and records of discussions or role plays.

Task 1 (relevant criteria: P1, P2, P3, M1)

Tutor information: This task should focus on the management and understanding of challenging behaviour. Students need to develop a case study of an individual with challenging and self-destructive behaviour. They should then use each psychological perspective to explain how the individual has developed this behaviour, and what interventions can be used to control the behaviour.

Task

Create a short case study of a health or social care service user with challenging behaviour. Remember to include *antecedents, behaviours and consequences.*

Then explain:

- what form the challenging behaviour takes
- how behaviourism can explain this behaviour
- a way that you can use social learning to address this behaviour
- how psychodynamic approaches can explain or change the behaviour
- how effective each of these approaches would be.

Task 2 (relevant criteria: P4, P5, P6, M2, D1)

Tutor information: This task should focus on the way psychological ideas can influence those who work in the health and social care sector. Students should be encouraged to create a handbook that explains how each perspective can help individuals understand and support service users in times of need.

Task

Part 1: Residential homes need to respond to the different needs of the people who live in them. Write an account of how humanistic perspectives can help *identify needs* and *plan for a fulfilling and satisfying life* for residents. **(P4)**

Part 2: Care and health workers need to understand *developmental norms*.

Explain:

- what *psychological developmental norms* are (hint: think PILES!)
- what we mean when we say someone has a *genetic predisposition* to a particular psychological illness or behaviour
- how *shift work* can be managed to reduce its impact on workers. **(P5)**

Part 3: Cognitive perspectives focus on the way people think and how they deal with information. Explain how cognitive approaches can be used to support either:

- individuals with *learning difficulties*
- or individuals with *psychiatric disorders*. **(P6)**

Part 4: Using your answers from the previous parts of this task together with activities from class, write a short essay (approximately 500 words long) that compares the advantages and disadvantages of applying psychological perspectives in health and social care. You may wish to include:

- any problems these approaches *cannot* help with
- the *practical difficulties* (e.g. cost, staff training, time, etc)
- whether each approach is *client-centred* or *practitioner-centred*
- problems with *labelling or stereotyping* service users. **(M2, D1)**

Please list below all the sources of information for this task (e.g. books, journals, websites, etc)

Scheme of work

BTEC National Health & Social Care
Unit 8 Psychological perspectives for health and social care

Academic year: ....

Broad aim: Successful completion of the unit

Teacher(s): ....

Sessions: 20 × 1.5 hours or 10 × 3hours

Guided learning hours: 30

Week/s	Topic/outcome	Tutor preparation	Student activity	Resources	Links to grading criteria
1–2	Introduction to Unit 8: Outline the six psychological perspectives	This PowerPoint® presentation introduces the key concepts and activities for both Learning outcomes	Learners can take notes on the content of the PowerPoint®, then carry out some independent research into the main psychological perspectives described	Introductory PowerPoint® presentation	All
3–4	Describe and apply behaviourist principles	Activity 8.1 should follow tutor-led work on behaviourism. It can be used as class work or homework. Activity 8.2 is broadly similar to 8.1, but requires students to use more independent analysis and synthesis skills	For Activity 8.1 learners can work in pairs or independently preparing answers, followed by researching further examples. For Activity 8.2 learners discuss issues arising from the case studies, and then research and suggest case studies of their own	Activity 8.1, Activity 8.2	P1
5–6	Describe and evaluate social learning approach	This activity involves preparing a public health video	Learners work in small groups preparing the material needed for the video, before creating a video covering these issues. This activity can be adapted using role play, with learners auditioning for roles in the video	Activity 8.3	P2
7–8	Describe and apply psychodynamic principles	Activity 8.4 involves analysing the roles of different parts of the personality (Ego, Superego, Id). Activity 8.5 is about identifying defence mechanisms in action	For both activities, learners need to understand the terminology before they start. Learners can discuss issues raised in Activity 8.4 in small groups before a full class discussion. In Activity 8.5 learners complete the examples in pairs before researching their own examples	Activity 8.4, Activity 8.5	P3
9–10	Complete Assessment task 1		Learners work individually on the assessment tasks, preparing written answers	Assessment task 1	P1, P2, P3
11–12	Describe and evaluate the humanistic approach	This activity introduces Maslow's hierarchy of needs, then applies it to several scenarios	Learners identify which needs are unfulfilled and suggest solutions, either alone, in pairs or small groups. Learners can discuss and research their own examples for each of the situations described	Activity 8.6	P4
13	Recognise and analyse antecedents, behaviours and consequences	This activity should reinforce work done on behaviourism, and show the relationship between behaviourist and cognitive approaches as found in CBT	Learners work to complete the table, before researching and developing their own examples and case studies	Activity 8.7	P5

Unit 8 Psychological perspectives for health and social care

Week/s	Topic/outcome	Tutor preparation	Student activity	Resources	Links to grading criteria
14	Describe the cognitive approach	Activity 8.8 is a PowerPoint® presentation with accompanying questions. Activity 8.9 deals with Kelly's personal construct theory.	For Activity 8.8, learners complete a gapped handout and work in pairs or small groups to answer the detailed questions. For Activity 8.9 learners create a small repertory grid and need to bear confidentiality issues in mind	Activity 8.8 (PowerPoint presentation and handout), Activity 8.9	P5
15–16	Describe and apply biological principles	Activity 8.10 involves designing a health information leaflet about shift work. For Activity 8.11 emphasis should be put on the psychological, rather than the physical, aspects of development	For Activity 8.10 learners create a leaflet based on information from independent research. For Activity 8.11, learners create a poster illustrating developmental norms in young children, again using information from independent research	Activity 8.10, Activity 8.11	P6
17–18	Complete Assessment task 2		Learners work individually on the assessment tasks, preparing written answers	Assessment task 2	P4, P5, P6
19–20	Upgrade assignments where necessary, and end-of-unit crossword	Activity 8.12 is a light-hearted crossword to recap and review the unit	Learners can work in pairs or alone on the crossword	Activity 8.12	All

At-a-glance activity grid
Unit 8 Psychological perspectives in health and social care

Activity	Title and description	Scheme of work	File/CD	Delivery notes	Additional resources	Links to grading criteria	Links to Student Book 1
Outcome 8.1 Understand psychological approaches to study **Outcome 8.2 Be able to apply psychological perspectives to health and social care**							
PowerPoint® presentation	Introduction to Unit 8: Outline the six psychological perspectives	Weeks 1–2	CD	This PowerPoint® presentation introduces the key concepts and activities for both Learning outcomes		All	pp 374–403
8.1	Behaviourism: Case study with accompanying questions	Week 3	File	This activity should follow tutor-led work on behaviourism. It can be used as class work or homework. The questions become more complex, allowing for differentiation by task. This activity could also link with other case studies on video etc.		P1, M1	pp 374–403
8.2	Applying behaviourism: Short case studies with questions	Week 4	File	This is broadly similar to Activity 8.1, but requires students to use more independent analysis and synthesis skills. The extension activity could be used as homework or to challenge more able students		P1, M1	pp 374–403
8.3	Social learning theory: Preparing a public health video	Weeks 5–6	File	You can adapt this activity using role play, with students auditioning for roles in the video	Video camera	P2, M2	pp 374–403
8.4	Analysing the roles of different parts of the personality: Id, Ego and Superego	Week 7	File	You will need to ensure that students have a reasonable definition of each term before they begin this activity. These definitions should then be revisited and refined at the end of the activity		P3, M1	pp 374–403
8.5	Identifying defence mechanisms in action	Week 8	File	Once again, learners will need definitions to hand before they begin. There are no right or wrong answers, as long as they can justify their decisions		P3, M1	pp 374–403

Activity	Title and description	Scheme of work	File/CD	Delivery notes	Additional resources	Links to grading criteria	Links to Student Book 1
8.6	Maslow's hierarchy: Recognising which needs are unfulfilled and suggesting solutions	Weeks 11–12	File	Students may wish to suggest solutions first, and this will make it easier to recognise the needs that are not met in the scenarios		P4, M2	pp 374–403
8.7	Know your ABCs: Recognising and analysing antecedents, behaviours and consequences	Week 13	File	This activity should reinforce work done on behaviourism, and show the relationship between the behaviourist and cognitive approaches as found in CBT		P1, P5, M1	pp 374–403
8.8	The cognitive approach	Week 14	CD, File	This is a PPT presentation with accompanying questions (Answers on CD)		P5, M2	pp 374–403
8.9	Kelly's personal construct theory: Creating a small repertory grid	Week 14	File	This activity should follow the Activity 8.8 PPT presentation. Students need to be aware of confidentiality issues when producing this grid		P5, M2, D1	pp 374–403
8.10	Shift work and jet lag: Producing a health information leaflet	Week 15	File	Some learners may need support identifying the correct resources for this activity. Leaflets could be used as evidence of key skills ICT, or tied in to other units		P6, M1	pp 374–403
8.11	Creating posters on developmental norms	Week 16	File	Emphasis should be put on the psychological, rather than the physical, aspects of development. Students should be encouraged to display and discuss their posters with the whole class	Materials needed to create posters (perhaps including one or two carefully selected pictures from magazines or catalogues)	P6, M1	pp 374–403
8.12	End-of-unit crossword	Weeks 19–20	File (Answers on CD)	This crossword is a light-hearted activity, suitable for the final session. You might like to have small prizes available for the first to complete, and for the correct solution!	Small prizes	All	pp 374–403

Unit 8 Lesson plan

Aims

- To introduce Unit 8
- To outline the six psychological perspectives.

This structure may be spread over a number of lessons as required.

Learning outcomes
• list the learning outcomes for this unit • describe the main features of each perspective • give examples of how each perspective may be applied.

Timing	Content	Teacher activity	Student activity	Resources	Individualised activity
5 mins	Introduction	Introduce unit: tutor to display lesson aims and objectives on flipchart		Flipchart	
20 mins	PowerPoint® to introduce Learning outcomes and grading criteria		Answering questions	PowerPoint®, Copies of simplified version of Scheme of work	Copies of PPT with note spaces to be made available for those who require them
30 mins	Snowball discussion	Tutor to put learners in pairs to discuss and note down what they know about psychology. After five minutes, pairs to become fours, then fours to become eights.	Answering questions in groups, contributing to discussion		Pairs and groups can be allocated according to ability. Tutor support for less able students, including suggestions as to media related to psychology (e.g. videos of *Supernanny* TV series, etc.)
20 mins	Class to feed back notes to tutor		Students to write responses on whiteboard using a different colour for each perspective. This should build to a spider diagram covering the six perspectives	Whiteboard, pens	Visual learners can be encouraged to make detailed spider diagrams. More confident learners can act as spokesperson for their groups
10 mins	Plenary: Whole group to discuss themes and issues raised	Tutor can guide students to add any key points that have been missed, and reinforce lesson themes	Spider diagrams can be handed in for assessment at the end of the session	Flipchart, pens	
5 mins	Recap: Whole class teaching to highlight where lesson objectives have been achieved	Directed questioning	Answering direct questions		

8.1   Behaviourism: Case study

Student Book 1
pp 374–403

Working in groups of three or four, read the following case study.

Fifteen-year-old Rashid loves football and chocolate. Rashid has learning difficulties and he regularly attends a youth club for young people with special needs. Recently his behaviour has become very difficult. During group activities Rashid shouts rude words or tells jokes. This makes the others in the group laugh, and disrupts the group activity. The youth workers tell Rashid to stop, and sometimes even have to shout at him, but this only seems to make him worse. Rashid's mum really wants him to continue coming to youth club, as she needs to spend time with Rashid's younger sister and brother, who have both been unwell recently. Also, she says Rashid really looks forward to youth club.

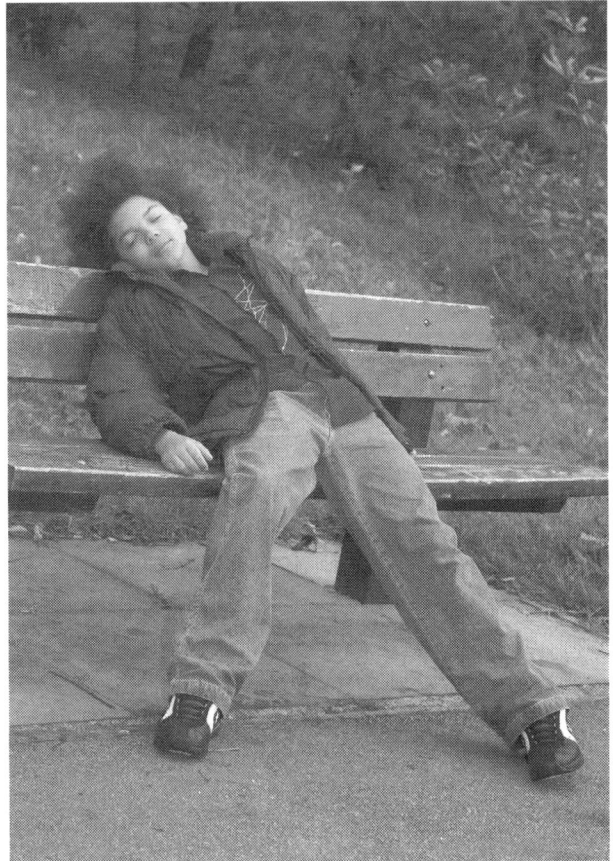

Now, using what you have learnt about the behaviourist perspective, answer the following questions:

- What inappropriate behaviour is Rashid showing?

- What reinforcement is he receiving?

- Rashid's brother and sister have both been ill. What impact has this had on Rashid's behaviour? Why would this happen?

- Are the youth workers right to ask Rashid to stop misbehaving?

- Are they right to shout?

- What reinforcements could you use to help Rashid behave appropriately?

Finally, write a checklist for the youth workers that will help them plan activities to keep Rashid behaving appropriately. Remember to include reinforcements and manageable aims.

8.2 Applying behaviourism: Case studies

Student Book 1
pp 374–403

Read the case studies below, and answer the questions that follow each one.

Billy, aged ten, was taken into care after his drug-addicted mother received a prison sentence. His home life has been chaotic. Since arriving at the care home two weeks ago, Billy has been very difficult to deal with. He refuses to eat with the other children, won't do any chores, and spends most of his time in the garden kicking a football. Billy does go to school, and his teachers say he is quiet and well behaved in class, but he has often been late or absent in the past. Billy is a very keen Arsenal fan.

■ How does behaviourism account for Billy's behaviour?

■ Using behaviourist techniques, how could you help Billy?

Ralph, aged 54, is currently an unemployed factory worker. Since his wife died a year ago, he has been the subject of several complaints from neighbours. Ralph's house is extremely dirty, and rats and other vermin have been breeding there. Ralph has a history of depression, but his new medication is helping. His social worker is keen to get him to look after himself and his home better.

■ How does behaviourism account for Ralph's behaviour?

■ Using behaviourist techniques, how could you help Ralph?

Sarah is terrified of lifts. This has not been a problem in the past, but she has MS and her symptoms are getting worse. She is now finding stairs more difficult to cope with, and she needs to overcome her fear of lifts.

■ Can behaviourism account for Sarah's fear?

■ Using behaviourist techniques, how could you help Sarah?

Extension task

If you have finished, you may wish to create some case studies of your own, analysing how behaviourism can help us understand and manage difficult behaviour.

8.3   Social learning theory and health education

Student Book 1
  pp 374–403

In groups, imagine that you are employed by a health charity that is working to reduce the incidence of sexually transmitted diseases among young people. The charity is going to make an information video to show in schools, colleges and youth centres. Your job is to find volunteers to appear in the video, and suggest what contribution they could make.

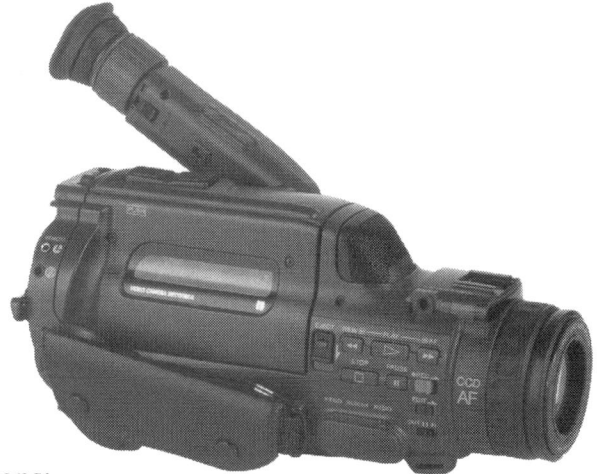

In your group, discuss the following questions:

- How would you select people to appear in the video?

- How would you use them in the video?

- Are there any celebrities you would approach? Why?

- Would you use actors?

- Or would you use health professionals, or young people?

Remember to consider:

- the qualities a good role model would need to have

- how you would use your video for observational learning

- how you could show vicarious reinforcement in action.

When you have finished your discussion, make your ideas into a poster, and be ready to share it with the rest of the class at the end of the session.

8.4 Analysing the roles of different parts of the personality: Id, Ego and Superego

Student Book 1
pp 374–403

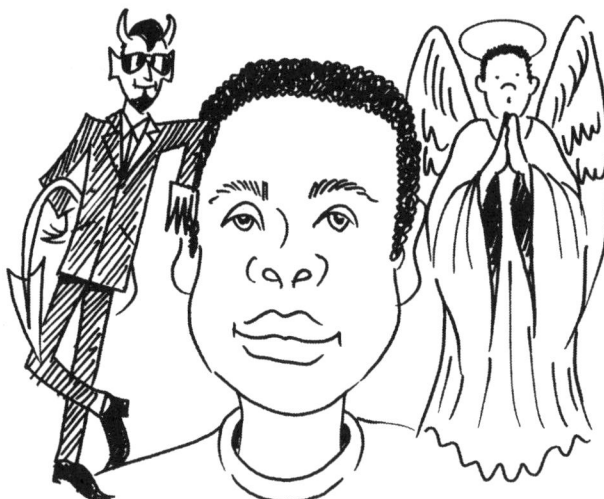

Working in small groups, start by writing down a short definition of each of the following three terms:

- Id

- Ego

- Superego.

Ask your tutor to check that your definitions are correct before you complete the rest of this activity.

Task

For each of the following situations, describe the roles of the Id, Ego and Superego.

Situation 1: You've been invited to dinner at your new neighbour's house. The dessert is your favourite pudding and there's one serving left. You could help yourself.

Situation 2: You've just discovered that Mr Nasty, the world's grumpiest customer, is going to receive the wrong delivery from you in about ten minutes. You could call him and explain, or you could go out to lunch and leave the new guy to answer the phone.

Situation 3: It's raining, you're running late to meet a friend, and you need to get some money from a cashpoint machine. There are always parking spaces a short walk away from the bank, but you've just spotted a disabled parking space right by the cashpoint machine.

Situation 4: As you walk in to your local health club you see the instructor (whose extremely tough class you are booked into) and you say hello. Just then, you see a friend, who suggests you go with her for coffee and a chat, and maybe one of those buns you really like.

8.5   Identifying defence mechanisms in action

Student Book 1
pp 374–403

Each of the following cases involves one or more defence mechanisms (Denial, Displacement, Projection, Regression, Repression and Sublimation). Can you identify them? Write the relevant defence mechanism/s after each example.

Alan is a doctor, working long shifts in a busy casualty department. Every week he plays three or four games of squash.

....

Geoff has been caught speeding again and may lose his licence. Angry and frustrated, he tells his wife that her complaints about his timekeeping are to blame.

....

Francine is a quiet, shy, easy-going student. When she was seen screaming and swearing at a shop assistant her friends were shocked, especially when she laughed off their concerned questions.

....

Melissa is always very smartly dressed and well groomed, apart from her fingernails. When she is feeling stressed she bites them almost to the quick.

....

Peter smokes thirty cigarettes a day. His doctor has warned him that this will make his heart condition worse, but P. says he's never felt better and he could give up any time.

....

Diane hates her job, and has been warned several times about her persistent lateness and the mistakes she has made. During her lunch break, she tells a friend that her colleague is lazy and incompetent, and should find herself another job.

....

When you have finished, create some case studies of your own that show defence mechanisms in action. Do you think they are an effective way to explain anxious or challenging behaviour?

8.6   Humanistic psychology: Maslow's hierarchy

Student Book 1
pp 374–403

Maslow believed that we all have needs that must be met in order to make us fulfilled and happy.

Maslow's hierarchy of needs

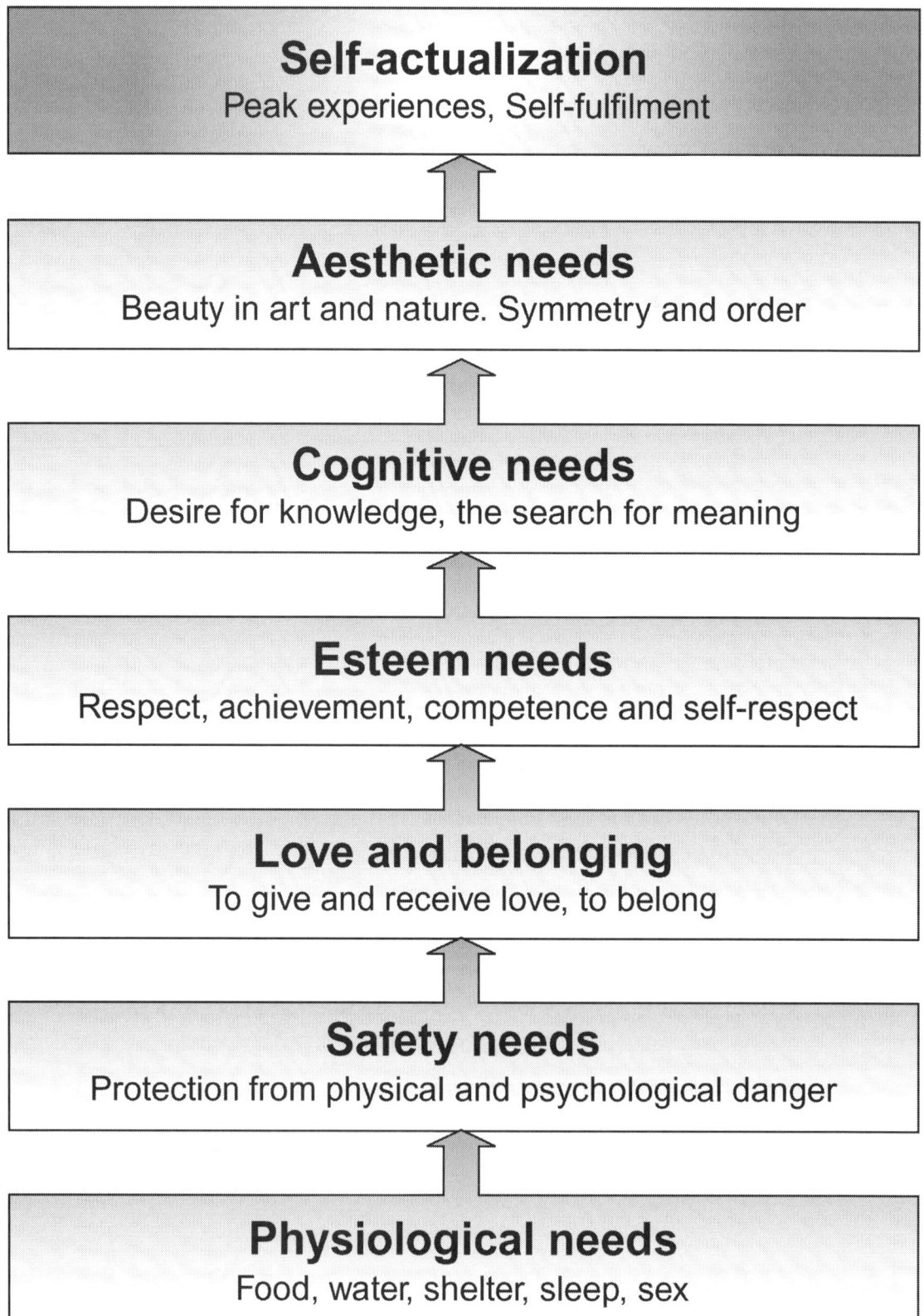

Self-actualization
Peak experiences, Self-fulfilment

Aesthetic needs
Beauty in art and nature. Symmetry and order

Cognitive needs
Desire for knowledge, the search for meaning

Esteem needs
Respect, achievement, competence and self-respect

Love and belonging
To give and receive love, to belong

Safety needs
Protection from physical and psychological danger

Physiological needs
Food, water, shelter, sleep, sex

Continued overleaf

8.6 Humanistic psychology: Maslow's hierarchy (*contd*)

For each of the examples below, decide which of these needs are not being met and suggest ways in which health or social care workers can help.

The problem	The need that is not being met	Possible solution
After being released from psychiatric care, Rosie lives on her own and feels lonely and isolated.		
Living in a care home has made Eileen bored and depressed. She misses her busy working life as a forensic scientist.		
Anna's boyfriend has a history of alcohol abuse and regularly physically and verbally abuses her.		
Despite his loving family, Doug feels that becoming disabled has made him less of a man, and he worries that no one has any respect for him any more.		
Clients of this day care centre are well looked after, but the scruffy, untidy building with its peeling grey paint seems to make everyone feel depressed.		
Charlie has been living on the streets since he ran away from home three months ago. He is dirty, exhausted and hungry.		

8.7   Know your ABCs: Antecedents, Behaviour and Consequences

Student Book 1
pp 374–403

Behaviourists and cognitive psychologists believe that much of what we do can be analysed by breaking it down into antecedents, behaviours and consequences. This approach can enable us to predict unacceptable behaviour and prevent it happening. Complete the table below by filling in suggested antecedents, behaviours and consequences. The final row has been left blank so that you can create your own case.

Antecedent	Behaviour	Consequence
Little brother Josh is bored: no one wants to play with him	Josh pushes Simone: Simone pinches Josh, Josh cries for Mummy	Seven-year-old Simone is sent to her room
		Thirteen-year-old Jimmy is receiving a police caution
		Fourteen-year-old Laura is pregnant
		Sam loses his TV privileges for a week
	Seventeen-year-old Vinny is smashing the glass in the bus stop	
	Twenty-year-old Maria has stopped talking to everyone at the day care centre she attends	

Continued overleaf

8.7 Know your ABCs (*contd*)

Now create some more examples, leaving two columns in each row blank. Pass them to someone else in your class to complete. Are their suggestions what you expected?

Antecedent	Behaviour	Consequence

Why do you think it is important to think about behaviour in this way?

Can this approach help in professional practice? How?

8.8 The cognitive approach

Student Book 1
pp 374–403

Watch the PowerPoint® presentation, and as you do fill in the gaps below.

Cognitive psychology is the study of _____

The Information-processing approach pictures the brain as being like a _____

Cognitive _____ is a way to study brain function using _____ _____

Irrational or illogical beliefs can be challenged using the techniques of _____

_____ _____ therapy, which was developed by _____ _____

Jean _____ was a developmental psychologist. He believed children's minds develop

in _____ .

George _____ produced a theory of how we _____ _____ other people.

This is called the _____ _____ theory.

The people in a personal construct are called _____

When three of these are selected together it is called a _____

When we identify a characteristic that we can use to measure each of the three it is called

a _____ .

When these are put into a table it is known as a _____ grid.

When you have finished watching the PowerPoint® presentation, spend some time discussing the cognitive approach. Here are some questions to consider:

- Is it helpful to think of the brain as being like a computer? Why (or why not)?

- Can you really change the way people think about things? And who should judge if a thought or belief needs to be changed?

- Do children really think differently from adults? Does this mean they should be treated differently?

- Is it possible to map out human relationships in the form of grids and tables? How can this help us understand each other more?

8.9   Kelly's personal construct theory

Student Book 1
pp 374–403

In this exercise, you will create a repertory grid that shows how you think of people in your life.

■ Write a list of the people who are most important to you, then pick three of them.

■ Of the three, decide which people are most alike, and which one is different. In what way is the person different? (For example, you might think two of your friends are very outgoing, but your brother is very shy.) This is a *construct,* a pair of opposites describing particular characteristics.

■ Do this again and again until you have about 10 constructs and no more than 25.

■ Look at your list, and for each person decide which of the pair of characteristics they are most like. (For example, your mum might be more outgoing.)

■ You can put your answers into a grid like the example below (see blank grid overleaf).

■ Now look at your grid. Does it accurately describe the people you put in it? Would you be happy to show it to them? What does it reveal about you?

Example grid

	My brother	Bill	Fred	Mum	Dad
Shy (/) Outgoing (X)	/	X	X	X	/
Intelligent (/) Unintelligent (X)	/	/	X	X	X
Attractive (/) Unattractive (X)	/	X	/	/	/
Organised (/) Disorganised (X)	/	X	X	/	X

Continued overleaf

8.9 Kelly's personal construct therory (*contd*)

Your grid

Shy (/) Outgoing (X)					
Intelligent (/) Unintelligent (X)					
Attractive (/) Unattractive (X)					
Organised (/) Disorganised (X)					

Repertory grids like this are used in therapy sessions to evaluate how people's perceptions of each other change over time, or to identify problems in the way clients think about other people. Can you suggest other ways in which they could be used?

8.10   Biological approaches: Shift work and jet lag

Student Book 1
pp 374–403

John Pinel, in his book *Biopsychology* (Allyn and Bacon, 1993), discusses research showing that nurses' shift work can cause a range of unpleasant symptoms, including:

■ insomnia

■ digestive problems

■ irritability

■ fatigue

■ depression.

Many psychologists argue that these symptoms are the result of a disruption of *circadian rhythms*. Similar effects are found amongst airline cabin crew, causing a condition often referred to as jet lag.

For this activity you need to create a short advice leaflet on the effects of shift work for workers in the health and social care sector. Your leaflet should include:

■ a brief definition of the term 'circadian rhythms'

■ one or more examples of research into circadian rhythms

■ an explanation of how and why these effects can cause problems for anyone working in health or social care settings

■ at least two ways in which individuals or organisations can avoid the harmful effects of shift work.

Use the resources in your library or LRC to help you. (Hint: it may be helpful to look into the effects of jet lag too, as it is very similar!)

8.11 Creating a poster on developmental norms

Student Book 1
pp 374–403

Psychologists and other health professionals use sets of developmental norms to check that children are growing and developing as expected. Your task is to work in small groups to research and create posters, informing parents of the developmental norms they can expect for their child.

Choose an age group from:

- 0–6 months

- 6–12 months

- 1–2 years

- 2–5 years

- 5–10 years

- 10–adult

Your poster should detail the expected stages in:

- social development

- emotional development

- intellectual development

- language development.

Remember to include points such as gender awareness, attachment to others, vocabulary and speech, and moral development.

You might want to use one or two carefully selected pictures you have created yourself, or taken from magazines or catalogues, to illustrate your posters. Make sure any illustrations are relevant and support the points you are making.

8.12 End-of-unit crossword

**Student Book 1
pp 374–403**

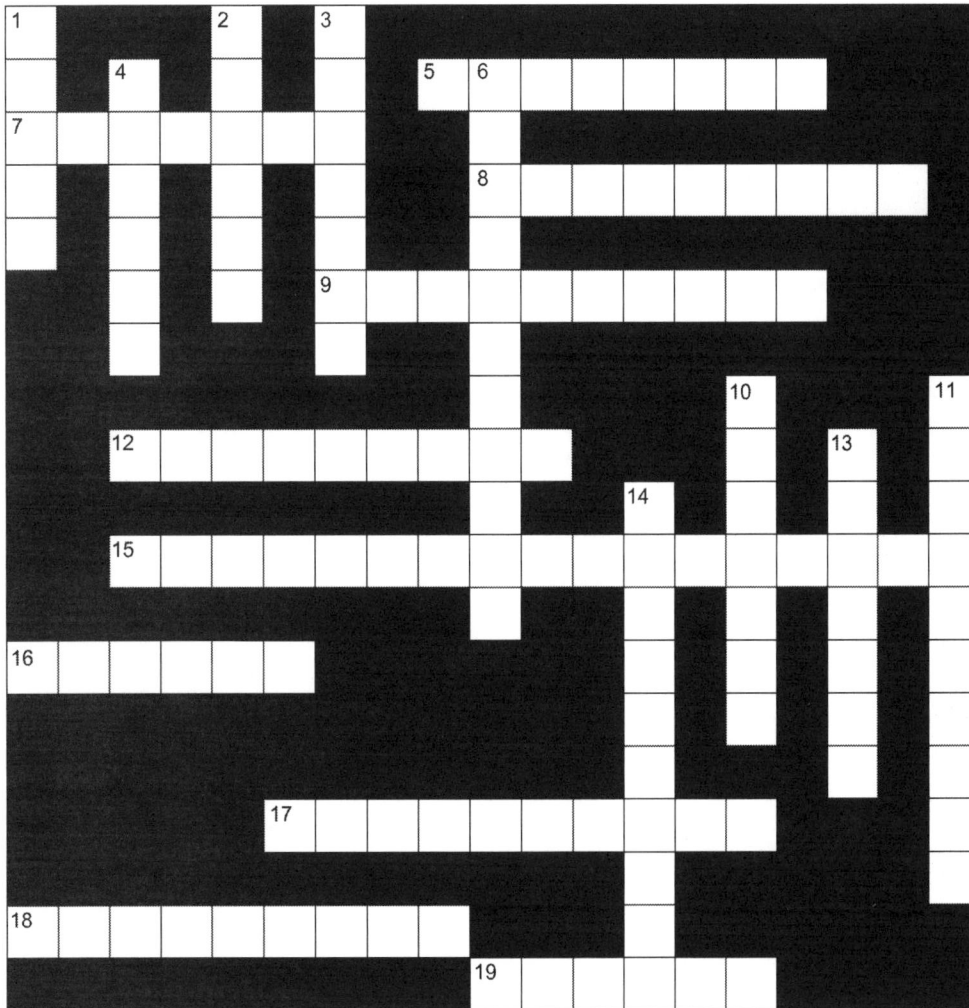

ACROSS

5 According to Freud, this is the last part of the personality to develop
7 Creator of the psycho-social stages of development
8 Branch of psychology concerned with thought processes
9 A 'reward' that shapes behaviour
12 Motivation from inside
15 The top of the humanistic hierarchy
16 Psychologist who developed the concept of maturation
17 The most commonly diagnosed psychiatric illness
18 Someone for social learners to look up to?
19 Barking mad endocrinologist?

DOWN

1 The so-called 'father of psychoanalysis'
2 Psychologist who introduced a hierarchy of needs
3 Academic who researched social learning theory
4 Swiss psychologist who described children's cognitive development
6 According to Freud, the hidden part of your mind
10 The ability to understand another's emotional state
11 Trained listener who helps those in distress
13 He worked with rats and pigeons
14 Approach to psychology which looks at physical factors

9

Values and planning in social care

unit overview

This unit explores the values and ethics of people involved in social care delivery as well as those of service users and their families. It has strong links with Unit 1 (Developing effective communication skills in health and social care), Unit 2 (Equality, diversity and rights in health and social care) and Unit 6 (Personal and professional development in health and social care). The unit is split into four Learning outcomes.

Learning outcomes

On completion of this unit learners should:

9.1 understand care planning principles and processes

9.2 understand the framework of legislation, policy and codes of practice that influence social care practice

9.3 understand the values that underpin social care practice

9.4 understand ethical principles in relation to social care.

Suggested activities

The At-a-glance activity grid shows how the activities in the Assessment and Delivery Resource (ADR) relate to the content of the unit. The activities include introductory and plenary activities and a variety of case studies, research tasks, discussions and presentations, using written, verbal and presentation skills. The activities may help learners prepare for assessment, and the grid indicates which assessment criteria are relevant for each activity. Copies of activity sheets can be given to learners.

Teaching Unit 9

Where possible Units 1 and 2 should be taught in year one of a two-year programme. Unit 9 should then be taught in year two, with Unit 6 being taught across both years. This will allow all underpinning knowledge regarding equality, diversity and rights and communication skills to be delivered before the introduction of care planning principles. Once learners have completed the first year of study and the relevant placements, it will be easier for them to relate the content of Unit 9 to practice.

Many activities in this unit focus on particular case studies. One of the most interesting aspects of these case studies is the challenge of balancing the needs and rights of service users with available resources and the legislative framework upon which social care is based. Interesting and thought-provoking discussions can be generated, allowing you, as tutor, to guide learners towards deeper consideration of the issues involved. You should encourage learners to keep drawing on their placement experiences to support their views and arguments. This will contribute to their development as reflective practitioners, as they reflect on such examples and consider their own roles and actions along with those of other professionals. The PowerPoint® presentations also offer many opportunities for discussion. In fact most of the real learning will take place during these discussions, as long as you encourage all learners to participate in them.

The content of each Learning outcome

Learning outcome 1: Understand care planning principles and processes (relevant criteria: P1, P2, M1, M2, D1)

The first Learning outcome lays the foundations for understanding the decision-making process in care planning. PowerPoint® 1 introduces the whole unit but focuses specifically on Learning outcome 1. Activity 9.1 involves a pair of case studies that can be used after or during the PowerPoint® presentation. Each case study looks at an individual for whom a care plan is to be developed. This activity 'sets the scene' for this unit and provides a fantastic opportunity to engage learners in deeper-level thinking with regard to decision-making processes. Activity 9.2 is a PowerPoint® presentation that explains the principles of care planning. This is accompanied by a creative poster task (Activity 9.3), in which learners can consolidate their knowledge of care planning principles. Activity 9.4 is a PowerPoint® presentation that takes a more detailed look at how care planning works. Activity 9.5 requires learners to start applying their knowledge of care planning to a case study. To achieve the relevant criteria for this Learning outcome, learners will need to explain the principles and processes of care planning. These include: assessment approaches, cycle of care planning, assessment tools, and approaches to implementing care plans and multi-disciplinary working.

Learning outcome 2: Understand the framework of legislation, policy and codes of practice that influence social care practice (relevant criteria: P3, M2, D1)

The second Learning outcome is very straightforward, as learners will already have gained the underpinning knowledge of key legislation, codes of practice, policy and standards in Units 2 and 6. However, learners still need to demonstrate an understanding of specific areas of regulation in relation to social care practice, specifically the process of care planning. PowerPoint® 2 introduces this Learning outcome and provides a 'gentle reminder' of the relevant legislation and policies. Learners will not be overly enthusiastic about this topic, as in some respects it is overdone. However, Activity 9.6 gives learners an opportunity to apply legislation, policy, codes of practice and standards to a case study that they create. They are required to consider all the ways in which legislation and other regulations affect care planning. This should be a group activity in order to encourage some 'group creativity' in an otherwise dry topic. I would recommend that you spend no more than two to three weeks on this outcome. To achieve the relevant criteria, learners must be able to describe key legislation, policy and codes of practice that influence social care, together with the impact of these regulations and the effectiveness of legislation in promoting care planning and multi-disciplinary working.

Learning outcome 3: Understand the values that underpin social care practice (relevant criteria: P4, M3, D2)

The third Learning outcome consolidates and extends learners' knowledge of promoting service users' rights (gained in Unit 2) and their knowledge of using effective communication skills (covered in Unit 1). PowerPoint® 3 introduces this Learning outcome and focuses on how the care value base influences the promotion of service users' rights, views and preferences. Activity 9.7 is a thought-provoking task that enables learners to see the huge differences between the rights they expect to have themselves, and their expectations about the rights of different service users. This activity can be particularly valuable in highlighting how and why care professionals do not always accord service users appropriate respect and privacy. Activities 9.8 and 9.9 provide opportunities for learners to consider the concept of dignity. Again, you should be able to generate excellent discussion around these case studies. Activity 9.10 is a PowerPoint® presentation that reintroduces the importance of confidentiality, but addresses it in more detail than previously in any of the other units. The accompanying case study (Activity 9.11) will engage learners in considering the different levels of confidentiality. To achieve the criteria for this outcome, learners need to demonstrate an understanding of the values underpinning social care practice, specifically the role of the care value base and the promotion of individual rights, together with an understanding of their own role.

Learning outcome 4: Understand ethical principles in relation to social care (relevant criteria: P5, M4, D2)

The fourth learning outcome addresses the difficulties learners may face in their future careers as social care professionals. PowerPoint® 4 introduces ethical dilemmas and is accompanied by two case studies (Activities 9.12 and 9.13) which provide examples of difficult ethical decisions. Encourage discussion whenever possible during this Learning outcome; learners will really enjoy the challenge of engaging with such an interesting topic. Activity 9.14 is a PowerPoint® presentation that introduces theories for ethical decision-making. This is followed by a case study (Activity 9.15) that requires learners to apply theoretical principles in order to reach a decision. Activity 9.16 is a PowerPoint® presentation covering conflicts of interest. This follows on from ethical dilemmas, and the Activity 9.11 case study used in Learning outcome 3 is utilised again, in Activity 9.17, as an example of conflict of interest. Activity 9.18 is a research task combined with a debate on the issue of euthanasia, which raises many controversial ethical issues. Finally, Activity 9.19 is a light-hearted crossword to review the unit content. In order to achieve the criteria for this outcome, learners must be able to describe the ethical principles related to social care and explain the roles of individuals and organisations in relation to ethical practice. They also need to be able to evaluate the impact of legislation and other forms of regulation on ethical practice. (This criterion is also partially covered in Learning outcome 3.)

How this unit will be assessed

To reach Pass level, the evidence must show that the learner is able to:

P1 describe the processes of care planning with reference to care planning principles
P2 identify the importance of multi-disciplinary and inter-agency working in the care planning process
P3 describe the key legislation, policies and codes of practice that influence social care
P4 describe the values that underpin social care practice
P5 describe ethical principles in relation to social care.

To reach Merit level, the evidence must show that, in addition to the Pass criteria, the learner is able to:

M1 explain care planning principles
M2 use examples to explain how multi-disciplinary and inter-agency working can improve the care planning process
M3 explain the impact of legislation on the concept of care planning
M4 explain the roles of individuals and organisations in relation to values and ethical practice.

To reach Distinction level, the evidence must show that, in addition to the Pass and Merit criteria, the learner is able to:

D1 evaluate the effectiveness of current legislation in promoting care planning and multi-disciplinary/inter-agency working
D2 evaluate the impact on social care practice of legislation, policies and codes of practice in relation to ethics and values.

Assessment tasks

Task 1 (relevant criteria: P1, P2, P3, M1, M2, M3, D1)

Write a case study about an imaginary service user who is about to be referred as part of the care planning process. Describe the process of care planning for this service user with reference to the following care planning principles:

- referral
- assessing holistic needs and preferences
- identifying current provision
- implementing, monitoring and reviewing
- considering service user empowerment, needs, choice, rights and confidentiality. **(P1)**

Explain the following care planning principles:

- empowerment
- rights
- potential use of advocates
- placing the service user at the centre of the process
- needs
- choice
- confidentiality. **(M1)**

Explain the importance of multi-disciplinary working (e.g. social workers, support workers, health visitors, etc) in the care planning process. Using examples from your placement, explain how multi-disciplinary and inter-agency working can improve the care planning process. **(P2, M2)**

Describe the key legislation, policies and code of practice that influence social care, and explain the impact of legislation on the care planning process. You should consider the impact of legislation on the use of different approaches and the handling of potential conflicts. **(P3, M3)**

Evaluate the effectiveness of current legislation in promoting care planning and multi-disciplinary/inter-agency working. Do you think current legislation effectively promotes care planning and multi-disciplinary /inter-agency working? What are the strengths and weaknesses? How does this impact on your imaginary service user? **(D1)**

Task 2 (relevant criteria: P4, P5, M4, D2)

Write an essay (approximately 2000 words) describing the values that underpin social care practice. Include:

- political values
- social values
- cultural values
- moral values
- and the values specified by professional bodies and the government. **(P4)**

Describe ethical principles in relation to social care. Then explain the roles of individuals and organisations in relation to values and ethical practice. Use examples from your own placements wherever possible to support the points you make. **(P5, M4)**

Evaluate the impact of legislation, policies and codes of practice on social care practice in relation to ethics and values. In other words, do laws, policies and codes of practice give clear guidance on how decisions should be made and which are the right decisions to make? Or do you think legislation, policies and codes of practice simply add to the conflicts of interest that can arise in ethical decision-making? What is the impact of legislation, policies and codes of practice on the service user? **(D2)**

Scheme of work

BTEC National Health & Social Care
Unit 9 Values and planning in social care

Academic year: ....

Broad aim: Successful completion of the unit

Teacher(s): ....

Number of weeks: 35

Duration of session: 1 hour 30 mins

Guided learning hours: 60

Week/s	Topic/outcome	Tutor preparation	Student activity	Resources	Links to grading criteria
1	Introduction to Unit 9 and Learning outcome 1: Care planning principles and processes	This PowerPoint® will help you to generate discussion. Use it in conjunction with Activity 9.1 (case studies)	Learners will discuss the first case study as a whole class, before splitting into smaller groups to discuss, and answer questions on, a second case study	PowerPoint® 1, Activity 9.1	P1, P2, M1, M2
2–3	Principles, approaches and rights of service users	Activity 9.2 is a PowerPoint®, which will introduce the underlying principles of care planning. Use it in conjunction with Activity 9.3 (the poster task)	Learners use information from the PowerPoint® to design a poster demonstrating the importance of the principles of care planning	Activity 9.2, Activity 9.3; paper, coloured pens	P1, P2, M1, M2
4–5	Processes of care planning; assessment and key people	Activity 9.4 is a PowerPoint®, which will address some of the issues involved in care planning. Use it in conjunction with Activity 9.5 (a case study)	Learners discuss themes arising from the case study, and demonstrate how the problems in it could be resolved	Activity 9.4, Activity 9.5	P1, P2, M1, M2
6–9	Introduction to Learning outcome 2: Legislation, codes of practice and policy standards	This PowerPoint® reinforces knowledge of relevant legislation, policy and codes of practice that has been gained in earlier units. Use it in conjunction with Activity 9.6 (group task)	Learners work in small groups preparing a care plan to match the case study, then present their ideas to the class for a full discussion	PowerPoint® 2, Activity 9.6	P3, M3, D1
10–12	Introduction to Learning outcome 3: Values and the care value base	This PowerPoint® reinforces knowledge of the care value base and the underpinning values. Use it in conjunction with Activity 9.7 (group task)	In small groups learners rank a series of rights according to a fixed viewpoint, then discuss their ideas with the rest of the class. This exercise could be extended with some role-play activities	PowerPoint® 3, Activity 9.7	P4, M4, D2
12–13	Individual rights, dignity, views and preferences	Activities 9.8 and 9.9 highlight the issue of individuals' dignity through two case studies	Learners discuss themes arising from case studies, and complete written responses to the questions. Learners can research further related examples from recent news stories to create their own case studies	Activity 9.8, Activity 9.9	P4, M4, D2

Unit 9 Values and planning in social care

Week/s	Topic/outcome	Tutor preparation	Student activity	Resources	Links to grading criteria
14–16	Workers' responsibilities; active support, communication and confidentiality	Activity 9.10 is a PowerPoint®, which reinforces the importance of confidentiality in promoting rights. Use it in conjunction with Activity 9.11 (a case study)	Learners discuss themes arising from the case study, and demonstrate how the problems in it could be resolved	Activity 9.10, Activity 9.11	P4, M4, D2
17–19	Introduction to Learning outcome 4: Ethical principles	This PowerPoint® introduces the concept of ethical dilemmas. Use it in conjunction with Activities 9.12 and 9.13 (two case studies involving ethical decision-making)	Learners can debate the scenarios in Activity 9.12 and Activity 9.13 and use this to reach a conclusion. You may wish to split the class into two teams, each arguing for a different solution	PowerPoint® 4, Activity 9.12, Activity 9.13	P5, M4, D2
20–24	Definition of ethics, reasons for ethical considerations	Activity 9.14 is a PowerPoint®, which introduces the theoretical framework for ethical decisions. Use it in conjunction with Activity 9.15	For Activity 9.15, learners consider their reactions independently, before taking part in a whole class discussion	Activity 9.14, Activity 9.15	P5, M4, D2
25–30	Situations care workers may face; Conflicts of interest	This PowerPoint® introduces conflicts of interest. Use it in conjunction with Activity 9.17 (a case study, linked to Activity 9.11)	Ask learners to review Activity 9.11 and discuss the different situations. Encourage learners to debate the merits of certain actions compared to others	Activity 9.16, Activity 9.17	P4, M1, D1
31–34	Euthanasia debate	Activity 9.18 is a research task combined with a debate on the issue of euthanasia, which raises many controversial ethical issues	Learners research euthanasia before working in groups to prepare for a whole class debate. To extend this activity learners could use role play or look for examples from recent news media	Activity 9.18	P5, M4, D2
35	Review of Unit 9 content	Activity 9.19 is a light-hearted crossword to consolidate learners' knowledge and complete the unit	Learners complete the crossword	Activity 9.19	All

At-a-glance activity grid
Unit 9 Values and planning in social care

Activity	Title and description	Scheme of work	File/CD	Delivery notes	Additional resources	Links to grading criteria	Activities for placement Links to other units	Links to Student Book 2
Outcome 9.1 Understand care planning principles and processes								
PowerPoint® 1	Introduction to Unit 9 and Learning outcome 1	Week 1	CD	This PPT will help you to generate discussion. Use it in conjunction with the Activity 9.1 case studies: Roger/Aleysha		**P1, P2, M1, M2**		pp 4–16
9.1	Case studies: Roger and Aleysha	Week 1	File	Use in conjunction with PowerPoint® 1		**P1, P2, M1, M2**		pp 4–16
9.2	Principles of care planning	Week 2	CD	This PPT will help you to generate discussion. Follow with Activity 9.3 Poster Task		**P1, P2, M1, M2**		pp 4–16
9.3	Poster task: Principles of care planning	Week 2	File	Learners create a poster which demonstrates their understanding of the principles of care planning	Large sheets of paper, coloured pens, brightly coloured paper, scissors, glue	**P1, P2, M1, M2**		pp 4–16
Activity 9.4	How does care planning work?	Week 4	CD	This PPT will help you to generate discussion. Follow it with the Activity 9.5 case study: Mr Brown		**P1, P2, M1, M2**		pp 4–16
Activity 9.5	Case study: Mr Brown	Week 4	File			**P1, P2, M1, M2**		pp 4–16
Outcome 9.2 Understand the framework of legislation, policy and codes of practice that influence social care practice								
PowerPoint® 2	Introduction to Learning outcome 2	Week 6	CD	This PPT consolidates knowledge of relevant legislation, policy and codes of practice gained in other units. Use it in conjunction with the Activity 9.6 group task: Legislation and care planning		**P3, M3, D1**		pp 17–18
9.6	Group task: Legislation and care planning	Week 6	File	Use this in conjunction with PowerPoint® 2		**P3, M3, D1**		pp 17–18

Activity	Title and description	Scheme of work	File/CD	Delivery notes	Additional resources	Links to grading criteria	Activities for placement / Links to other units	Links to Student Book 2
Outcome 9.3 Understand the values that underpin social care practice								
PowerPoint® 3	Introduction to Learning outcome 3	Week 10	CD	This PPT reinforces knowledge of the care value base and the underpinning values. Use it in conjunction with Activity 9.7 (group task)		**P4, M4, D2**	Learners to investigate the policies, codes of practice and procedures in their placements. They should ask if they can see the setting's policies and take copies, then record in their reflective journals how they see these policies in action. Are policies (e.g. the Health and Safety policy) adhered to all the time?	pp 19–29
9.7	Group activity: Whose right is it?	Week 10	File (Tutor information on CD)	Use this in conjunction with PowerPoint® 3	Whiteboard, flipchart or wall chart	**P4, M4, D2**		pp 19–29
9.8	Newspaper story: Over-protective mother	Week 12	File	This is an individual task with questions to encourage learners to consider the concept of dignity and how this links with this individual's rights. This task can be given to one half of group with 9.9 being given to other half		**P4, M4, D2**		pp 19–29
9.9	Case study: Child protection	Week 12	File	Individual task with questions to encourage learners to consider the concept of dignity and how this links with individual's rights		**P4, M4, D2**		pp 19–29
9.10	The role of confidentiality	Week 14	CD	Activity 9.10 is a PPT, which introduces the right of every person to have information about them kept confidential. Learner task included. Use in conjunction with Activity 9.11		**P4, M4, D2**	Is there a confidentiality policy in learners' placement settings? Learners to investigate and record in their reflective journals	pp 19–29
9.11	Case study: Sarah Evans	Week 14	File	Use this in conjunction with PPT 9.10		**P4, M4, D2**		pp 19–29

Outcome 9.4 Understand ethical principles in relation to social care

Activity	Title and description	Scheme of work	File/CD	Delivery notes	Additional resources	Links to grading criteria	Activities for placement Links to other units	Links to Student Book 2
PowerPoint® 4	Introduction to Learning outcome 4	Week 17	CD	This PPT introduces the concept of the ethical dilemma in care work. Use it in conjunction with Activities 9.12 and 9.13		**P5, M4, D2**	Learners to record in their reflective journals examples of when they have actively promoted anti-discriminatory practice. What are the strengths and weaknesses of each example and how could they improve? Links to Unit 6, Learning outcome 3	pp 29–34
9.12	Thought experiment: Runaway train problem	Week 17	File	Use this in conjunction with PowerPoint® 4		**P5, M4, D2**	Learners to ask themselves if staff in their placement (including themselves) are good role models. They should record their thoughts on this in their reflective journals. Links to Unit 6, Learning outcome 3	pp 29–34
9.13	Ethical dilemma: John and Michael	Week 17	File	Use this in conjunction with PowerPoint® 4		**P5, M4, D2**		pp 29–34
9.14	Theoretical frameworks for decision-making	Week 20	CD	Activity 9.14 is a PPT, which introduces the basic framework for decision-making. Use it in conjunction with Activity 9.15 (case study)		**P5, M4, D2**		pp 29–34
9.15	Case study: Kirsty and Simon	Week 20	File	Use this in conjunction with PPT 9.14		**P5, M4, D2**		pp 29–34
9.16	Conflicts of interest	Week 25	CD	Activity 9.16 is a PPT, which introduces the concept of conflicts of interest in care work. Use it in conjunction with Activity 9.17		**P5, M4, D2**		pp 29–34
9.17	Conflicts of interest activity	Week 25	File	Use this in conjunction with PPT 9.16 and Activity 9.11		**P5, M4, D2**		pp 29–34

Activity	Title and description	Scheme of work	File/CD	Delivery notes	Additional resources	Links to grading criteria	Activities for placement Links to other units	Links to Student Book 2
9.18	Euthanasia debate	Week 34	File	This is a research task followed by a debate	Internet access for research	**P5, M4, D2**		pp 29–34
9.19	End-of-unit crossword	Week 35	File (Answers on CD)	Consolidate knowledge gained in Unit 9 with this crossword		All		pp 29–34

Unit 9 Lesson plan

Aims

- To introduce Unit 9
- To introduce Learning outcome 1

This structure may be spread over a number of lessons as required.

Learning outcomes
• have an understanding of the content of Unit 9
• have gained an overview of the factors involved in care planning

Timing	Content	Teacher activity	Student activity	Resources	Individualised activity
5 mins	Welcome learners and register				
15 mins	Introduce Unit 9	Tutor to introduce Unit 9 by outlining topics to be covered. Moderate use of language to ensure full understanding of all learners	Learners to answer indirect questions to check understanding		
20 mins	Introduce Learning outcome 1	PPT presentation to be used as reference point/'backdrop' for teaching. Encourage discussion where appropriate. Moderate use of language to ensure full understanding of all learners	Learners to answer indirect questions to check understanding. Contribute to discussion	PowerPoint® 1	
15 mins	Activity 9.1: case studies	In groups of three or four, learners to read case studies and consider questions	Learners to relate to each other in groups of three or four, and answer indirect and direct questions to check understanding	Activity 9.1	Task to be explained using different levels of language. Circulate around class to check understanding and offer assistance or extension where needed
20 mins	Discussion: What factors should be considered when planning care for Roger and Aleysha?	Encourage learners to share ideas and views on the terminology in order to discuss issues around needs, and multi-disciplinary working and approaches. Ensure that all learners' contributions receive positive feedback	Learners to answer indirect and direct questions to check understanding. Contribute to discussion		
10 mins	Recap: Quick-fire questions about care planning	Check Learning outcomes. Ensure that all learners' contributions receive positive feedback	Learners to respond to questions		
5 mins	Thank you. Close				

9.1   Case studies: Roger and Aleysha

Student Book 2
pp 4–16

In groups of three, read the following case study:

Roger is 42 years old. He has recently been diagnosed with Motor Neurone Disease. He is having problems with his mobility and his speech. His physical decline appears to have been quite fast over the past few weeks. Roger is married and he and his wife have four children all under the age of ten. Roger is keen to stay at home and be part of his family's life for as long as possible, although he is not always able to climb the stairs to the bathroom or to get down the stairs. He has started to become very emotional – the slightest thing will make him cry. Roger's wife thinks this may be due to frustration, as he is not able to do all the things he used to do.

Now discuss the following questions:

■ What are Roger's needs?

■ Who are the key people involved in Roger's care?

■ Should anyone else's needs be considered in Roger's care planning?

■ What is the importance of a multi-disciplinary approach to Roger's care planning?

■ What are the implications of funding/cost for Roger's care?

In groups of three, read the following case study:

Aleysha is 20 years old, she has cerebral palsy and no mobility or speech. She lives with her parents in a three bedroom house. She attends a respite centre one weekend a month. Aleysha's parents are getting divorced and there is often a very tense atmosphere in the house, which upsets Aleysha. Her parents have asked that she attend the respite centre every week for the next few months.

Now discuss the following questions:

■ What are Aleysha's needs?

■ Who are the key people involved in Aleysha's care?

■ Should anyone else's needs be considered in Aleysha's care planning?

■ What is the importance of a multi-disciplinary approach to Aleysha's care planning?

■ What are the implications of funding/cost for Aleysha's care?

9.3   Principles of care planning poster task

Student Book 2
pp 4–16

Imagine that you work in advertising and you have been asked to promote the principles of care planning. Create a poster that clearly shows the importance of these principles to the service user. Make your poster bright, eye-catching and easy to read. This activity will help you achieve the P1 and M1 grading criteria.

9.5   Case study: Mr Brown

Student Book 2
pp 4–16

Mr Brown is 79 years old. He has recently suffered a stroke, which has left him unable to use the right side of his body. However, he is able to stand and shuffle along with the use of a Zimmer frame. He still has speech, although it is slurred. He is able to communicate with both his family and the carers. At present, he is being cared for in a nursing home after being discharged from hospital.

Mr Brown has a son and a daughter. His son is married with five children, and his daughter, who has two children, lives five minutes away from Mr Brown. Both Mr Brown's son and daughter say that he should not return home, as neither of them has time to care for him. Mr Brown owns his own home and feels that he should be allowed to return home if he wants to.

Consider the issues that might arise in this situation, and explore how Mr Brown could be cared for in the comfortable and familiar surroundings of his own home.

You will need to consider:

- Mr Brown's wishes and preferences
- Mr Brown's rights
- any possible risks to Mr Brown's health and well-being
- any possible benefits to Mr Brown's health and well-being
- availability of services such as occupational therapy
- the roles of carers, relatives, friends/neighbours
- costs
- other possible benefits
- any potential conflicts.

9.6   Legislation and care planning

Student Book 2
pp 17–18

In groups of two or three, create a scenario in which a service user needs a care plan. Start by writing a brief description of the service user, including age, family situation and physical abilities/disabilities, etc. You are the professional carer responsible for drawing up the care plan. Remember to go through each stage of the care planning process:

1   Referring the service user for assessment

2   Assessing the service user's needs

3   Deciding if the service user is eligible for services

4   Writing the care plan and identifying which services will be included in the care plan

5   Reviewing the care plan and service provision.

Most importantly, consider which pieces of legislation are relevant to and will affect each stage of the planning. It is your responsibility to ensure that the care plan meets all legal requirements.

Do you think the legislation you have identified encourages or discourages multi-disciplinary working?

When you have completed this task, share your scenario and care plan with the rest of the class and discuss them.

9.7   Whose right is it?

Student Book 2
pp 19–29

For this activity, your tutor will put you into small groups of three or four. Each group will receive a set of cards showing different rights (e.g. the right to stay up late, or the right to privacy).

You will be told whose viewpoint your group should take. It might be your own viewpoint, or it might be the viewpoint of a particular service user. Your group then needs to rank the various rights in order of importance from 1 to 20 (1 being most important and 20 being least important). Once your group has put the rights in order, according to your allocated viewpoint, you should put the cards on the board or flipchart provided.

9.8   Case study: Over-protective mother

Student Book 2
pp 19–29

The mother of 18-year-old Steven received a high court restraining order preventing her from interfering with his rights. The judge stated that, despite suffering from cerebral palsy, spastic quadriplegia and speech and learning difficulties, Steven was a mentally capable adult.

Steven's parents adopted him at three months old, but his mother became very over-protective of Steven and, in the words of the judge, 'exercised an increasingly close and intimate control over Steven's life'. Amongst other things, she prevented him from attending school and restricted his social life. This prevented Steven from achieving his full potential physically, socially, emotionally and educationally.

After being taken into care, Steven had gone to court seeking an order preventing his mother from running his life again by interfering with his rights to live where and with whomever he wanted. The judge declared there was 'a real risk of infringement of Steven's freedom'.

(Adapted from an article in the *Guardian*, 14 July 1995)

1   Do you think Steven was being treated in a dignified way?

2   Which of Steven's rights were not being respected?

3   Can you identify any areas that might have been difficult for the care professionals involved to make a decision about?

9.9   Case study: Child protection

Student Book 2
pp 19–29

Melissa has told her teacher that she has been sexually abused by her mum's boyfriend. The teacher followed the school's child protection policy and informed her head of department. The head of department also followed the child protection policy and informed the police.

The police questioned Melissa's mum, Sue, and Sue's boyfriend, as well as Melissa's two younger sisters. The police investigation found no evidence of abuse of any kind. Melissa and her sisters were allowed to continue living in the same house as their mum and her boyfriend.

However, Sue is really upset at what has happened to her family since the investigation. She claims that the police and the social worker seemed to actively deepen the rift between her and her daughters. This has made moving on, and dealing with the underlying issue of why Melissa made the allegation, much harder.

Sue says that she felt that she had lost control of her own life and her daughters' lives. She found herself at the mercy of a complex system, with people who seemed to want to keep her 'in the dark' and used a mass of difficult jargon.

In addition, the local newspaper printed a story about the alleged abuse. Although it did not name Melissa or the family, it included some graphic information about the allegations, together with 'other information' from 'another source'. It mentioned where they lived and gave the ages of the children. The family felt that these details identified them to anyone who wanted to know. When the article was printed someone painted the word 'paedophile' on the family's garage door.

Sarah, the younger daughter, became insecure, confused and afraid, and started having nightmares. She even began answering the phone with the question 'Are you the police or a social worker?'

After continual requests for help with the breakdown of her family, Sue was finally able to get a referral to a family therapist. The therapist concluded that there was no evidence of abuse but the whole family was suffering considerable stress from the investigation. Sue says that her partner Dave has needed treatment for depression and has suffered repeated panic attacks since his arrest and temporary imprisonment. She says that the social worker told Dave that he was not their concern, and that if he committed suicide as a result of the additional stress it would simply confirm his guilt.

About six months after the investigation Melissa began cutting herself with the edge of a coin and engraving patterns on herself with pins. She cut her wrists, took overdoses, and had to be hospitalised a number of times. She inhaled solvents, took various illegal substances, stole from home and was eventually arrested for shoplifting and possession of drugs.

Now consider the following questions:

1   Do you think Melissa and her family were treated in a dignified way?

2   Which of the family's rights were not respected?

3   Can you identify any areas that might have been difficult for the care professionals involved to make a decision about?

9.11 Case study: Sarah Evans

Student Book 2
pp 19–29

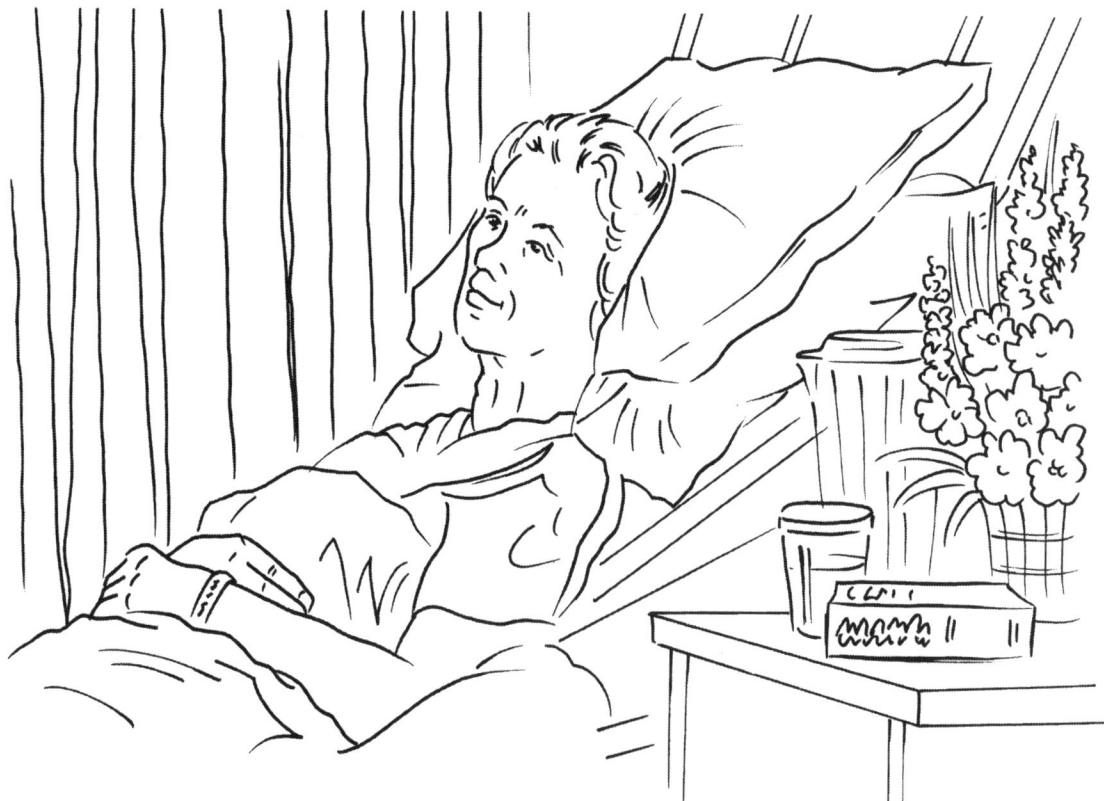

Sarah Evans is a 44-year-old married woman who lives on a housing estate on the outskirts of a large city. She has been admitted to the local hospital for a hysterectomy. She has been experiencing severe pain in her lower abdomen and has been found to have ovarian cancer. The hysterectomy will be followed by courses of radiotherapy and chemotherapy.

Sarah has three children and she is very concerned about her eldest son who is 19 years old. She recently became suspicious that he was using crack cocaine and this was later confirmed by one of the other children. Sarah has not told her husband of her concern but has confided in one of the nurses who was very sympathetic. Sarah is very worried about the hysterectomy, and this is made worse by her anxiety about her son's drug taking. She is also worried about the effect of the hysterectomy on her sexual relationship with her husband.

- Can you identify the four types of information about Sarah?

- Which information should the professional team caring for Sarah's medical needs have access to?

- Which information should other members of staff, such as receptionists and porters, have access to?

- Which information should be kept absolutely confidential?

9.12   Ethical dilemma: The runaway train

Student Book 2
pp 29–34

Imagine you are standing on a bridge overlooking a railway line and you can see that a runaway train is speeding down the track. You see that the track forks. On the left a small girl is playing on the track; on the right there are five children playing on the track. You realise that the train is heading towards the right and is going to kill the five children, who are unaware of its approach. You are too far away to warn the children, but there is a lever beside you on the bridge. You cannot stop the train with the lever but you can switch the points so that the train will head for the little girl instead. This will mean that only one child is killed, instead of five.

■ What would you do?

9.13   Case study: John and Michael

Student Book 2
pp 29–34

Read the following scenarios.

Scenario 1
John, 22 years old, stands to gain a large inheritance if anything should happen to his six-year-old cousin, Michael. One evening, while John is babysitting for him, Michael takes a bath. John sneaks up the stairs and into the bathroom and drowns the child. He arranges things so that it looks like an accident.

Scenario 2
John, 22 years old, stands to gain a large inheritance if anything should happen to his six-year-old cousin Michael. One evening, while John is babysitting for him, Michael takes a bath. John goes up the stairs to look into the bathroom, planning to check on the child. However, just as he enters the bathroom, he sees Michael slip, hit his head and fall face down into the water. John is delighted. He stands by, ready to push the child's head back under the water if necessary, but it isn't. With only a little thrashing about, the child drowns all by himself, accidentally. John watches and does nothing to help.

■ Is John's behaviour worse in Scenario 1 or in Scenario 2?

■ What are your reasons for coming to this conclusion?

9.15 An ethical dilemma: Kirsty and Simon

Student Book 2
pp 29–34

An ethical dilemma arises when there are conflicting interests between courses of action and a decision has to be made on whose rights should be upheld and whose rights should be overridden.

Kirsty is 24 years old and has Down's syndrome. She lives in supported housing and works part-time at Sainsbury's. Simon is also 24 years old and has severe learning difficulties. He recently moved into the same supported housing as Kirsty, after his mother died. Kirsty and Simon have become close and have started a sexual relationship. Imagine that you are the support worker for both Kirsty and Simon. You have been asked to 'manage' the situation. Would you attempt to offer advice or would you intervene?

Consider the following questions:

- Should Kirsty and Simon be able to choose whether to have a sexual relationship?

- Should their decision be respected, whether you agree with it or not?

- How will you demonstrate your non-discriminatory attitudes?

- Have you got Kirsty's and Simon's best interests at heart, taking into account the need to promote independence and autonomy?

- Will the decision about Kirsty's and Simon's relationship minimise harm in the future?

- How can you balance the need to protect vulnerable service users with the need to treat them with respect and positively promote their autonomy?

Spend about 10 minutes thinking and writing down your ideas and opinions regarding Kirsty's and Simon's relationship. Then discuss your ideas and opinions as a group.

9.17 Conflicts of interest

Student Book 2
pp 29–34

Look back at Activity 9.11, the case study about Sarah Evans. Then consider who else has a right to know Sarah's information.

In groups of three or four, consider the following situations and decide how you would deal with them:

1   Sarah's husband asks to see her medical records.

2   Sarah's best friend asks to see the ward sister and asks for detailed information on Sarah's medical problems.

3   Social Services are concerned about problems at home while Sarah is in hospital. They ask for more information about the family background.

4   Police are making enquiries about drug dealing in the local area. The nurse has told you about Sarah's son's crack cocaine use.

5   The local newspaper has discovered that Sarah's son is a suspect and they ask for detailed information about the family background and Sarah's condition.

Share and discuss your group's views and ideas with the rest of the class.

9.18 Euthanasia debate

Student Book 2
pp 29–34

The controversial subject of legalised euthanasia is never far from the news in the UK. There are various campaigns in favour of legalising euthanasia as well as campaigns that are firmly against it.

This is a difficult area for which the government has to legislate, as the issue of taking a person's life, with or without consent, raises many ethical considerations and provokes highly charged emotions. In the western world the sanctity of life is one of the guiding principles of conventions, policy and legislation. However, there has been massive public support for euthanasia in the Netherlands, where it has been legal to end a person's life, with the person's consent, for 25 years.

In the UK there have been landmark cases, such as those of Dianne Pretty and Annie Lindsell, who have pursued their 'right to choose' through the UK justice system, without success. There have also been cases of doctors who have deliberately administered drugs to end a suffering person's life, and have been cleared of any wrongdoing. These cases have been highly publicised and have tested the public's views in the 'right to life' debate.

Using the Internet, research the following:

■ Dr David Moor

■ Annie Lindsell

■ Mary Ormerod

■ Dianne Pretty

■ Pro Choice opinions

■ Pro Life opinions

■ euthanasia in the Netherlands

■ euthanasia in Australia.

If you were the government minister responsible, would you be able to make a decision as to whether to legalise euthanasia or not?

What are your views?

Bring your ideas back to the class and debate the issue.

9.19 End-of-unit crossword

Student Book 2
pp 29–34

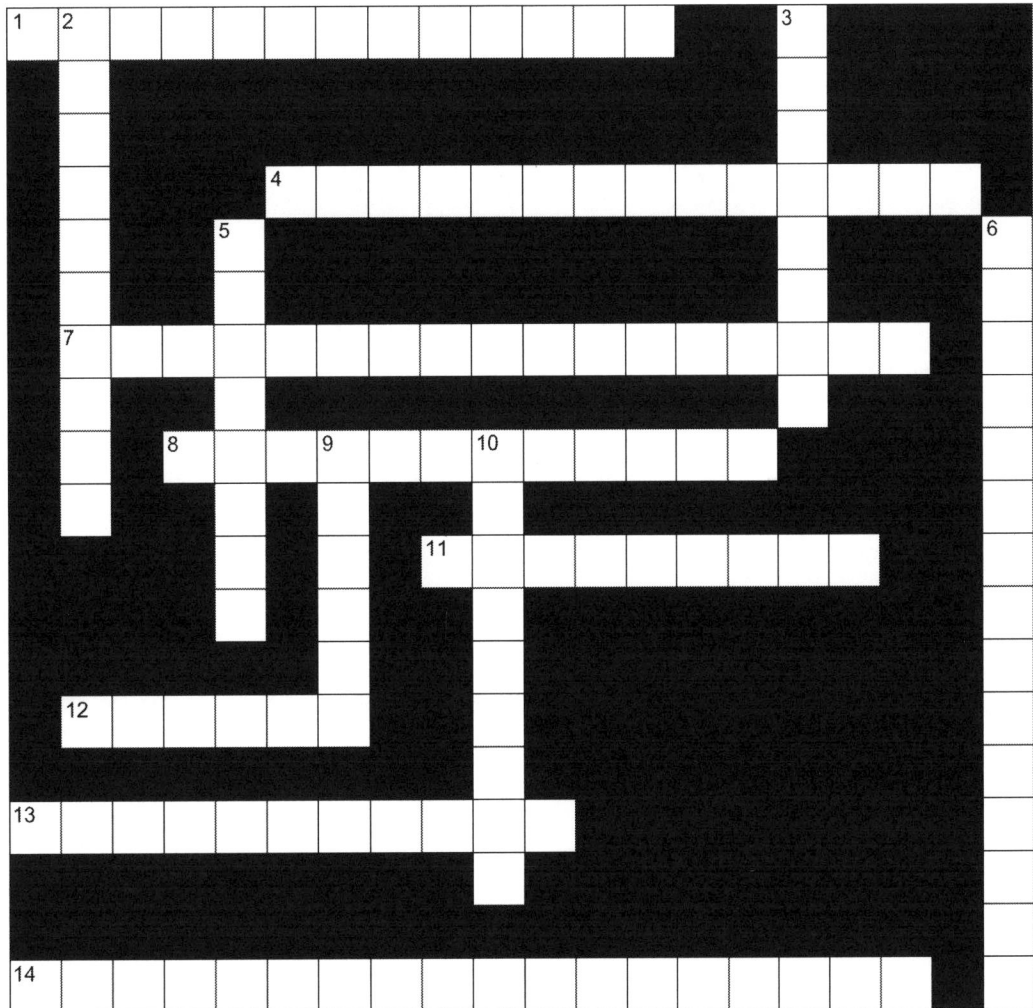

ACROSS

1 This sets out the values and principles necessary in social care

4 A very difficult situation where there is no right or wrong answer

7 Different professionals working together as a team

8 Freedom to do something

11 There are never enough!

12 Can be used as an alternative word to ethics

13 An approach that puts the availability of services at the centre

14 Ensuring that service users are safe

DOWN

2 The process of determining the needs of the service user

3 This is drawn up to ensure that a service user's needs are met

5 'Self rule': thinking, deciding and acting independently

6 Breaking this means disclosing information

9 Principles we adopt in order to make decisions

10 An approach that puts the service user at the centre

Note: In this crossword, you need to allow one square for the hyphen when the answer is a hyphenated word.

10

Caring for children and young people

unit overview

This unit looks at ways in which children and young people can be looked after within the health and social care sector. It covers sensitive subjects including fostering, adoption, family difficulties and abuse. The unit is divided into four Learning outcomes.

Learning outcomes

On completion of this unit learners should:

10.1 understand why children and young people need to be looked after

10.2 understand how care is provided for children and young people

10.3 understand the risks to children and young people of abusive and exploitative behaviour

10.4 know strategies to minimise the risk to children and young people of abusive and exploitative behaviour.

Suggested activities

The At-a-glance activity grid shows how the activities in the Assessment and Delivery Resource (ADR) relate to the content of the unit. The activities include introductory and plenary activities and a variety of case studies, research tasks, discussions and presentations, using written, verbal and presentation skills. The activities may help learners prepare for assessment, and the grid indicates which assessment criteria are relevant for each activity. Copies of activity sheets can be given to learners.

Teaching Unit 10

This unit needs sensitive handling, as one or more learners may have experienced being in the care of a local authority, being adopted, or being abused. If these subjects raise personal emotional issues for learners you will need to be able to deal with them, or make appropriate referrals for counselling. Students may also be emotionally affected by the course content if it reflects some of the experiences of their friends or relatives.

Covering the legislation related to this unit will provide learners with the underpinning knowledge required to meet professional standards. The issue of confidentiality may have been covered in other units but it is vital to discuss its importance again in relation to Unit 10. Personal issues, or issues relating to children or young people encountered during work placements, may have an adverse emotional impact upon students. Confidentiality is essential in all cases involving abuse or the personal care of children and young people, including the students on this course. Remind students that, while they are on work-related placements, they must follow the individual setting's polices and procedures, especially the maintenance of confidentiality relating to placement staff and service users. You will need to spend some time setting these ground rules in the first instance, and certainly before students attend their first placements.

You can add breadth to the students' learning by inviting guest speakers from children's homes, the NSPCC and voluntary organisations, as well as health visitors, social workers and youth workers. Speakers can inform learners about how they help to provide a service for children and young people. Students may also have an interest in their role as prospective employees.

There is a wealth of additional information available on websites, including VLE tutor resources (such as short videos introducing child protection for early years staff). It is worth spending time reviewing some of these websites, as they can add interest and variety to delivery of this unit. There are also activities on confidentiality in the Standards Unit Health and Social Care Resource Box.

The content of each Learning outcome

Learning outcome 1: Understand why children and young people need to be looked after (relevant criterion: P1)

For the first outcome, teaching will need to cover the rationale for care orders, fostering and adoption. Students should also learn to recognise situations, stresses and events that can affect a family's ability to look after their children (across the age range from 0 to 18 years old). In addition, this outcome covers disabilities, learning difficulties, abuse, health or behaviour problems faced by children and young people, as well as criminal offences that may lead to them needing to be looked after.

Learning outcome 2: Understand how care is provided for children and young people (relevant criteria: P2, P3, M1, M2, D1)

The second outcome focuses on the roles of the professionals who support children and their families when they are coping with permanent or temporary difficulties. The role of legislation in informing care policies, procedures and provision of services for children and young people is another important aspect of this Learning outcome.

Learning outcome 3: Understand the risks to children and young people of abusive and exploitative behaviour (relevant criteria: P1, P4)

In the third outcome, students cover some sensitive issues involving consequences, models, predisposing factors, indicators and recognition of abuse, direct and indirect exploitation, family functioning and different concepts of discipline.

Learning outcome 4: Know strategies to minimise the risk to children and young people of abusive and exploitative behaviour (relevant criteria: P5, P6, M3, D2)

The fourth outcome will help students understand the roles and responsibilities of those working to support children, young people and their families. The strategies used by these care professionals may include empowering and involving children and young people in keeping themselves safe, by reducing risks to their well-being, making decisions, expressing their feelings and building their self-confidence.

How this unit will be assessed

To reach Pass level, the evidence must show that the learner is able to:

P1   describe the main reasons why children and young people are looked after away from home
P2   identify the current relevant legislation affecting the care of children and young people
P3   describe health and social care service provision for looked-after children and young people
P4   describe signs and symptoms of child abuse
P5   describe appropriate responses where child abuse is suspected or confirmed, making reference to current legislation and policies
P6   identify the strategies and methods of supporting children, young people and their families.

To reach Merit level, the evidence must show that, in addition to the Pass criteria, the learner is able to:

M1   analyse how policies and procedures help children/young people and their families while the child is being looked after
M2   compare the care provided by at least two different organisations offering care to children and young people
M3   explain strategies and methods to minimise the risk to children and young people where abuse is suspected or confirmed.

To reach Distinction level, the evidence must show that, in addition to the Pass and Merit criteria, the learner is able to:

D1   evaluate the legal rights of the child/young person and the rights of their families, bearing in mind that the needs of the child/young person are paramount

D2   evaluate a range of strategies and methods to support children/young people and their families where abuse is suspected or confirmed.

Assessment tasks

The grading criteria can be broken down into three tasks. Task 1 only covers Pass and Merit criteria, but Tasks 2 and 3 will give students the opportunity to work through the levels from Pass to Distinction.

Task 1 (relevant criteria: P1, P3, M2)

Write a report explaining why children and young people may need to be looked after away from their families **(P1)**.

- Describe the type of health and social care provision available to look after and support children and young people who are not living with their families **(P3)**.
- Then compare the care provided for children and young people by two different organisations **(M2)**.

Task 2 (relevant criteria: P2, M1, D1)

Write an essay identifying current legislation affecting the care of children and young people **(P2)**.

- Analyse how policies and procedures help and support children, young people and their families while they are being looked after through care orders or fostering **(M1)**.
- Finally, evaluate the legal rights of children and young people as well as their families. Ensure that you reflect on the welfare and needs of children and young people remaining paramount **(D1)**.

Task 3 (relevant criteria: P4, P5, P6, M3, D2)

Produce an information booklet in three sections, aimed at people who are new to caring for children and young people.

- Use the first section to clearly explain the signs and symptoms of the four types of abuse used for registering children and young people at risk: physical, emotional, neglect and sexual **(P4)**.
- The second section should describe appropriate responses to suspected or confirmed cases of abuse, and outline the reporting process, which needs to be related to current legislation and policies **(P5)**.
- In the third section, identify strategies and methods of supporting children, young people and their families when abuse is suspected or confirmed **(P6)**.
- Explain how these strategies and methods are used to reduce the risks to children and young people where abuse is suspected or confirmed **(M3)**.
- Finally, evaluate a range of strategies and methods used to support children, young people and their families where abuse is suspected or confirmed **(D2)**.

Scheme of work

BTEC National Health & Social Care
Unit 10 Caring for children and young people

Academic year: ....

Broad aim: Successful completion of the unit

Teacher(s): ....

Number of weeks: 35
Duration of session: 1 hour 30 mins
Guided learning hours: 60

Week/s	Topic/outcome	Tutor preparation	Student activity	Resources	Links to grading criteria
1	Introduction to Unit 10, Holding confidential information	Introduce and explain the unit content and assessment process and discuss setting boundaries, confidentiality, dealing with own emotions, and information on counselling services	Learners need to consider the implications of secure information. You could expand this exercise through role plays or games that rely upon trust	Activity 10.1	P2, P5
2–3	Understand family-related stresses	Activity 10.2 is a PowerPoint® presentation, which will help learners gain an understanding of the family-related stresses and situations that may lead to children and young people being 'looked after'	Learners can take notes and record details and ideas throughout the presentation. Ask learners to discuss these with the class afterwards	Activity 10.2	P1, P3, P5, M2
4	Identify types of care	Learners explore how children and young people with disabilities and complex educational needs are cared for (e.g. specialist need for boarding educational establishments)	Learners work in small groups and match up situations and responses. Class discussion of issues raised would be a good conclusion to this topic	Activity 10.3	P1, P6, M2
5	Strategies for supporting children and young people: Counselling, anger management and behaviour modification	Explain strategies for supporting children and young people, the role of counselling, anger management and behaviour modification	Ask learners to research and prepare posters on the key strategies for dealing with children and young people	Internet access and materials to create posters	P3, P5, M2
6	Support available for children and young people: Therapy (i.e. art, music, drama), sport and youth activities	Activity 10.4 is a PowerPoint® presentation on support for children and young people	Learners to discuss support available for children and young people: the role of therapy (i.e. art, music, drama), sport and youth activities	Activity 10.4	P2, P3, P5, P6, M2, M3, D2

Unit 10 Caring for children and young people

Week/s	Topic/outcome	Tutor preparation	Student activity	Resources	Links to grading criteria
7–9	Different types of care provision for children and young people	Identifying different types of care provision for children and young people	Learners to research care available through the NSPCC, statutory provision of care (including social services role in providing and maintaining care facilities), voluntary and private provision of care (including foster care)	Internet access	P3, M2
10–11	Identify roles and responsibilities of those providing care	Introduce learners to the responsibilities of providing care.	This is an individual or small group-based case study activity to identify the role of observations in safeguarding children and young people	Activity 10.5	P3, M2
12	Assessment task 1	Set Assessment task 1, ensuring understanding and supporting students' planning to cover criteria of the first task			P1, P3, M2
13–15	Identify and discuss legislation	Identify relevant legislation (Children Act, Child Protection Act, Data Protection Act, and the Disability Discrimination Act)	Learners look at the role of legislation in providing care for children and young people in safe environments and discuss the need to write policies, follow procedures, and review and update on a regular basis	Activity 10.6	P2, M1, D1
16	Identify types of abuse	Activity 10.7 is a PowerPoint® presentation on identifying types of abuse and the categories used for placing children and young people on the 'At Risk Register'	Learners can take notes on the presentation and use these as a basis for discussion	Activity 10.7	P4
17	Recognise accidental and non-accidental injuries	Encourage learners to review factors that cause injuries	Learners consider and discuss in groups or pairs two case studies on recognising accidental and non-accidental injuries in relation to physical abuse	Activity 10.8	P4
18	Understand the term 'good enough parenting'	Explain the term 'good enough parenting' in relation to recognising neglect, and avoiding judging people by our own standards			P4
19	Sexual abuse		Learners to discuss different forms of sexual abuse according to the local area guidelines and including the use of Internet chat rooms		P4
20	Emotional abuse	Look at emotional abuse as a category in its own right as well as a secondary case of abuse when children are physically or sexually abused	Learners to consider the definitions of emotional abuse, in particular why it is not always linked to neglect		P4
21	Children and young people with communication difficulties	Activity 10.9 is a PowerPoint® presentation on communication difficulties in children, babies and young people	Learners to discuss their additional vulnerability, and research methods of overcoming this	Activity 10.9	P4, P6, M3, D2

|

Unit 10 Caring for children and young people

Week/s	Topic/outcome	Tutor preparation	Student activity	Resources	Links to grading criteria
22–23	Respond to suspected abuse	Ask learners to consider how they would respond to different examples of suspected abuse, while following procedures	Learners to complete the table, supplying a separate justification for answer. Learners can research examples to support their conclusions	Activity 10.10	P2, P5, P6, M1, M3, D1, D2
24	Report confirmed and suspected cases of abuse	Explain reporting process for confirmed and suspected cases of abuse, noting the differences when responding to cases of suspected sexual abuse	Learners to research examples of reporting processes		P2, P5, P6
25	Identify the consequences of abuse	Introduce the physical, emotional and social consequences of abuse for the abused child/ young person and their family	Learners to work in groups to identify the different consequences, and create a presentation on each		P6
26	Understand the case conference process	This activity explores the case conference process	A carefully managed role play may assist learners in their understanding		P2, P5, M1, D2
27	Record information	Identify the need for clear, factual and objective report writing	Learners to complete this activity as a preparation for drafting their own report	Activity 10.11	P5
28	Recognise predisposing abuse factors	This activity will give learners a greater understanding of the different stresses faced by families and the impact they can have on family life	Learners to discuss factors that may put children at higher risk of abuse, including the cycle of abuse	Activity 10.12	P1, P4, P6
29	Who may abuse?	Activity 10.13 is a PowerPoint® presentation on factors that may put children at higher risk of abuse	Learners to discuss the dangers of stereotyping and recognise that abuse occurs in all classes and cultures	Activity 10.13	P4
30	Discuss models of abuse	Discuss feminist, medical, psychological and sociological models of abuse	Learners can work in groups researching the different theories and then comparing them		P4
31	Understand risks of exploitation of children and young people	Look at the increasing use of children in prostitution and selling drugs	Learners to research how this problem has developed		P1, P4, M2
32	Support children and young people who have been abused	Discuss the role of counselling, support groups, and supervised contact with abusive family members to build positive relationships	A visiting speaker could talk to learners about the tasks involved in building positive relationships in families		P6, M3, D2
33	Identify parenting skills	Introduce the different needs of a child and the requirements of good parenting	In this activity, learners work in small groups to identify a child's needs, before preparing a short written account explaining why parental support is needed	Activity 10.14	P6, M3, D2

Unit 10 Caring for children and young people

Week/s	Topic/outcome	Tutor preparation	Student activity	Resources	Links to grading criteria
34	Explore need for support and possible counselling for those working with abused children/young people		Learners discuss the need for support and possible counselling for those working with abused children/young people		P6, M3, D2
35	Plenary activity: Create a 'Keeping safe' game	This activity is about raising awareness, and teaching children and young people to protect themselves	Learners work in small groups to create activities to suit a range of ages that will teach self-protection (e.g. body awareness and children's understanding of their rights)	Activity 10.15	P6, M3, D2

At-a-glance activity grid
Unit 10 Caring for children and young people

Activity	Title and description	Scheme of work	File/CD	Delivery notes	Additional resources	Links to grading criteria	Links to Student Book 2
Outcome 10.1 Understand why children and young people need to be looked after							
10.1	Introduction to Unit 10, Holding confidential information	Week 1	File	Explain the unit content and assessment process, and discuss setting boundaries, confidentiality, dealing with own emotions, and information on counselling services. Using Activity 10.1 at the start of the first lesson gives time for you to hold the students' personal information for a while. It's important to return the envelopes to the students. If possible, allow students to shred them at the end of the lesson	An envelope for every student, and a paper shredder if possible. There is a video showing this activity being carried out in the Health & Social Care standards unit resource box (DfES)	P2, P5	pp 40–44
10.2	Understand family-related stresses	Weeks 2–3	CD	Activity 10.2 is a PowerPoint® presentation. This will help students gain an understanding of the family-related stresses and situations that can lead to children and young people being 'looked after'. This activity may raise issues concerning students' own situations. A sensitive approach is required and boundaries need to be set clearly in relation to confidentiality	Contact details for counselling services	P1, P3, P5, P6, M2	pp 40–44
10.3	Identify types of care	Week 4	File (Tutor information and Answers on CD)	Learners explore how children and young people with disabilities and complex educational needs are cared for. Activity 10.3 is a matching game that is best used in small groups to allow discussion		P1, P6, M2	pp 40–44
Outcome 10.2 Understand how care is provided for children and young people							
10.4	Support available for children and young people: therapy (i.e. art, music, drama), sport and youth activities	Week 6	CD	Discuss support available for children and young people: the role of therapy (i.e. art, music, drama), sport and youth activities. Activity 10.4 is a PowerPoint® presentation on support for children and young people. Use the headings to lead the discussion	Local information leaflet on support available in the area	P2, P3, P5, P6, M2, M3, D2	pp 44–54
10.5	Identify roles and responsibilities of those providing care	Weeks 10–11	File	This is an individual or small group-based case study activity to identify the role of observations in safeguarding children and young people		P3, M2	pp 44–54

Activity	Title and description	Scheme of work	File/CD	Delivery notes	Additional resources	Links to grading criteria	Links to Student Book 2
10.6	Identify and discuss legislation	Weeks 13–15	File	Learners identify relevant legislation (Children Act, Child Protection Act, Data Protection Act, and the Disability Discrimination Act). This is a research activity to be carried out on an individual basis, within a set amount of time. A second task is included for more able students	Access to Internet and textbooks relating to legislation	P2, M1, D2	pp 44–54
Outcome 10.3 Understand the risks to children and young people of abusive and exploitative behaviour							
10.7	Identify types of abuse	Week 16	CD	Activity 10.7 is a PowerPoint® presentation on identifying types of abuse and the categories used when placing children and young people on the 'At Risk Register'. This is a very sensitive topic. The slides cover the key points, and further definition can be added	DfES publication ref: ppBel/D16-5981/0705/54 available free of charge	P4	pp 54–65
10.8	Recognise accidental and non-accidental injuries	Week 17	File	Learners consider two case studies on recognising accidental and non-accidental injuries in relation to physical abuse. The activity can be used individually or in small groups. There are questions at pass, merit and distinction levels	DfES publication ref: ppBel/D16-5981/0705/54 available free of charge	P4	pp 54–65
10.9	Children and young people with communication difficulties	Week 21	CD	Activity 10.9 is a PowerPoint® presentation on communication difficulties in children, babies and young people. Discuss their additional vulnerability, and identify strategies to overcome their difficulties		P4, P6, M3, D2	pp 54–65
10.10	Respond to suspected abuse	Weeks 22–23	File	Learners consider how they would respond to different examples of suspected abuse, while following procedures, ensuring the safety of the child or young person, and protecting themselves from accusations. This worksheet can be used individually but if used in small groups students will be more likely to analyse the information		P2, P5, P6, M1,M3, D1, D2	pp 54–65
Outcome 10.4 Know strategies to minimise the risk to children and young people of abusive and exploitative behaviour							
10.11	Record information	Week 27	File	Identify the need for clear, factual and objective report writing		P5	pp 66–75
10.12	Recognise predisposing abuse factors	Week 28	File	Discuss factors that may put children at higher risk of abuse, including the cycle of abuse. This activity will give learners a greater understanding of the different stresses faced by families and the impact they can have on family life		P1,P4, P6	pp 66–75
10.13	Who may abuse?	Week 29	CD	Activity 10.13 is a PowerPoint® presentation on factors that may put children at higher risk of abuse. This needs sensitive handling. Point out the dangers of stereotyping and encourage learners to recognise that abuse occurs in all classes and cultures		P4	pp 66–75

Activity	Title and description	Scheme of work	File/CD	Delivery notes	Additional resources	Links to grading criteria	Links to Student Book 2
10.14	Identify parenting skills	Week 33	File	Use Maslow's hierarchy of need as an introduction to this activity (see resources). Learners work in small groups to identify a child's needs and the requirements of good parenting	Maslow's hierarchy of need (available at http://www.learningandteaching.info/learning/motivlrn.htm)	P6, M3, D2	pp 66–75
10.15	Plenary activity: Create a 'Keeping safe' game	Week 35	File	This activity is about raising awareness, and teaching children and young people to protect themselves. Learners work in small groups to create activities to suit a range of ages that will teach self-protection (e.g. body awareness and children's understanding of their rights). Resources for making games need to be available at start of lesson. There are some electronic game makers available on the Internet. Students can locate these (using Google), if computers are available	Art and craft resources for making board games and books, soft materials for making teddy bears, puppets or dolls	P6, M3, D2	pp 66–75

Unit 10 Lesson plan

Aims

• To introduce Unit 10

This structure may be spread over a number of lessons as required.

Learning outcomes
• recognise topics to be covered
• identify the need for boundaries and confidentiality
• recognise the need to keep information safely
• list learning outcomes of Unit 10.

Timing	Content	Teacher activity	Student activity	Resources	Individualised activity
5 mins	Introduction to lesson	Write up and explain lesson aims and objectives. Use varied levels of vocabulary to ensure understanding and to extend vocabulary			
15 mins	Explanation of unit topics, method of delivery and assessment strategy	Give examples of how to attain high grades and ask open questions to confirm understanding	Learners make notes		
15 mins	Confidentiality envelope task	Highlight different possible interpretations of the task	Students complete task, putting required information in envelopes	Activity 10.1	
15 mins	Confidentiality	Encourage discussion of confidentiality issues relating to abuse	Learners work in small groups to consider possible difficulties in relation to confidentiality and to suggest boundaries	Flipchart	More able students can offer ideas on how to overcome the concerns raised, and make notes on flipchart paper
20 mins	Setting boundaries for the group	Clarify concerns about confidentiality and strategies that can be used to overcome the problems	Groups of learners offer feedback. Group feedback agreed and boundaries set		More confident students can give feedback for their group, offering reasons for the difficulties and asking questions of other groups
20 mins	Introduction of need for counselling	Explain how best to access counselling and note the phone number for Child Line: 0800 1111			

Timing	Content	Teacher activity	Student activity	Resources	Individualised activity
15 mins	Recap	Identify objectives met and give information on next lesson. Return envelopes to students and ask them to shred them if possible. Remember to use varied vocabulary and repetition to ensure understanding of all learners	Learners answer questions		

10.1 Holding confidential information

Student Book 2
pp 40–44

Take a moment to consider the amount of information about individuals that is collected and held by institutions. Some of the information is very personal, such as details of the person's health, financial or family situation. As a health and social care worker, there may be times when you will have access to such information about other individuals. You need to understand how vulnerable this can make people feel, and the level of trust they need to have in those using and holding this information.

Write some personal information below. This could include your home address, mobile phone number and/or date of birth. Fold your paper and seal it in the envelope provided. Now write your name across the seal. (This is often done to guard against confidential information being tampered with.)

....

....

....

....

....

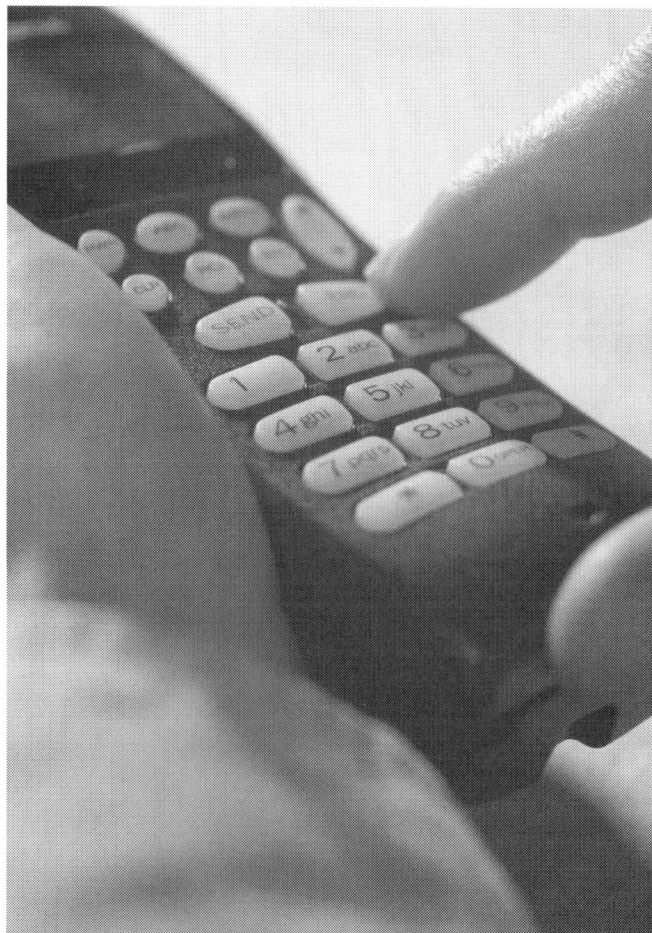

10.3 Type of care

Student Book 2
pp 40–44

Your tutor will put you into small groups for this activity, and give each group a set of cards. You need to match each family situation with a card showing the most appropriate type of care. In each situation the family members are experiencing difficulty in coping and have indicated that they need support.

- -

10.5 Identify the roles and responsibilities of those providing care

Student Book 2
pp 44–54

Read the following case studies. Then, for each case, identify who would be responsible for writing up reports and who should carry out the follow-up observations. Finally, identify whom the reports and possible observations will be shared with, and why those people should have access to the information included in the observations.

Case study 1

Jonathan has been in care since he was a baby. His mother was a drug addict who was unable to care for him. She had no extended family to support her. Jonathan was born with an addiction to cocaine and was placed in foster care. There is a care order in place and social services are now applying for an adoption order. The foster parents would like to adopt him, but the social worker does not feel that this is in his best interests. The case manager has asked for developmental and progress reports in order to make a decision on the foster parents' application to adopt.

Case study 2

The manager of a day nursery is concerned about a child who often misses nursery sessions after time spent with her father, since her parents' divorce. The child is nearly four years old. Until the divorce, she attended nursery regularly. Now she not only misses sessions but she also seems withdrawn when she comes back to nursery. The child's key worker has just informed the manager that the child has bruises on her inner thighs. These were noticed when the child was changing in the home corner.

Case study 3

Ben, the play leader at a youth centre, is concerned about a conversation he overhears as he comes up to a group of five teenage boys (aged 14 to 15). They are talking about their weekend and the amount of alcohol and unsafe sex they experienced. The boys have been known to exaggerate their stories before. However, Ben is really concerned, as the details sounded very believable.

10.6 Supportive legislation

Student Book 2
pp 44–54

There are a number of pieces of legislation that support the care, development and learning of children and young people. Identify at least three pieces of current relevant legislation.

List the key points in each piece of legislation, and explain how they support children and young people. For example, a key point from the Children Act 1989 was to recognise that children have rights and parents have responsibilities (remember that there is a more recent Children Act).

If you complete this task within the set time, you can go on to identify and review some relevant key reports as well.

10.8   Accidental and non-accidental injuries

Student Book 2
pp 54–65

Read the two case studies below and answer the questions that follow each one.

Josh

Josh is a four-year-old boy with Down's syndrome, who lives with his parents and younger sister. He readily makes friends with children and adults, and shows no fear of strangers. Josh suffers from repeated upper respiratory tract infections, catarrh and glue ear. He receives regular speech and language and occupational therapy. Sometimes the therapists visit him at his pre-school. Josh always enjoys his therapy sessions, although they can sometimes tire him.

Josh makes a good attempt at washing his hands and face. Dressing can be difficult, as Josh is unable to cope with buttons. However, he can undo press-studs and laces, and can pull zips up and down with assistance. Josh feeds himself with a spoon but still prefers to use his fingers. He drinks from a half-full un-lidded cup without spilling. Once Josh has had enough to eat, he will push his plate away and clap his hands, as he is unable to say he has had enough or is finished. Josh enjoys playing with small cars and musical instruments, and can complete a simple three-piece jigsaw puzzle. He plays alongside his peers at the local pre-school, which he has attended for four mornings a week since he was three years old.

Josh's comprehension is improving. He readily responds to instructions and will fetch common everyday objects. He has a vocabulary of around 20 words, and is picking up phrases from his younger sister, such as 'go away' and 'my juice'. He can use around 40 Makaton signs to make his needs known, although he gets frustrated when he is not understood and this can lead to him throwing his toys or any objects he can pick up. When Josh is faced with new or challenging tasks, he often pretends that he's asleep by folding his arms, laying his head on them and closing his eyes.

When Josh's mum collected him from pre-school yesterday he was crying, which was unusual for him. When they got home he sat in the corner of the lounge and pretended to be asleep. He was 'grumpy' all afternoon, and he would not eat his tea. His mum thought he might be coming down with a cold. When undressing him for his bath she was shocked to see two large bruises on the back of his leg. When she looked more closely the bruises were the size of an adult's hand. Josh does not have the language skills to explain what happened.

When she touched his leg and asked 'how?', he frowned and signed 'lady'. The next day Josh's mother told the pre-school supervisor about the bruises and said she wanted an explanation from the supervisor. After all the children had gone home the supervisor asked the staff about what Josh had been doing at pre-school but did not tell them about his mother's visit. Josh's key worker said he had been fine and had spent most of the morning playing on his own alongside the other children. He then became difficult when another child would not let him have a car. He threw toys and knocked down towers of blocks that other children had made. To calm him down, the new student took him out of the main room into the quiet side room to read to him. He was kicking and screaming as she carried him out but he stopped screaming shortly after the door between the two rooms shut.

Continued overleaf

10.8 Accidental and non-accidental injuries (*contd*)

■ Consider how you would handle this situation and describe your responses.

■ With the above information, what steps would you take if you were the mother?

■ What steps would you take if you were the supervisor?

■ Explain how the setting's policies and procedures may help in this situation.

Jane

Jane is six years old and is the only child of Linda, a single parent. They live in a rundown area of town. While Jane is at school, Linda works part-time to try and make ends meet. Jane's father only sees her once a month, as he lives some distance away. He has a new partner and twin babies a few months old.

Jane attends the local primary school and during a PE lesson on a Monday morning her teacher noticed bruises under both her knees. When asked how she got them Jane said 'daddy did it'. The teacher said 'that's not nice' but was then distracted by another child who started screaming. When the teacher returned to talk to Jane again about the bruises Jane said she fell on to the doorstep at daddy's house. The teacher asked if Jane had told her mummy about the bruises. Jane said her mummy had said it was her own fault.

The teacher has reported Jane's comments verbally to the deputy head who is the named person for child protection. The teacher thinks they should contact social services.

■ With the above information, what steps would you take if you were the deputy head?

■ Write a short report explaining your opinion of the situation.

■ Now take on the role of the 'named person for child protection' and decide what your next steps would be. Explain how the setting's policies and procedures would support your actions.

■ Justify your decisions and the actions to be taken.

10.10 Responding to suspected abuse

Student Book 2
pp 54–65

Read the following situations and responses, and say whether each response is appropriate or inappropriate. On a separate sheet of paper, write a statement justifying your answer in each case.

	Situation	Response	Appropriate / Inappropriate?
1	A child at your work placement setting tells you the room supervisor kisses him	Ask a work colleague if the child has ever told them the same thing	
2	A child discloses that they are being abused	Ask the child questions to get more information	
3	A child tells you that the babysitter is abusing her	Telephone the child's parents/carer and tell them what the child has told you	
4	Two children are playing 'mummies and daddies' in the home corner. They act out a violent argument	Write down everything that is said and describe any actions	
5	When taking a little boy to the toilet he asks if you will hold and shake his penis for him like his key worker	Tell the child he is clever enough to do it all by himself, then leave the child alone while you think about what he has said	
6	At group time a child tells his news: 'Mummy went to hospital because Daddy hit her'	Tell the child not to make up stories, as it will get him into trouble. You know and respect the family	
7	When helping a child to take off his jumper, his T-shirt lifts up with the jumper, and you notice what appears to be an adult-sized bite on his back	Leave the child and fetch the 'named person for child protection' to come and talk to him	
8	You are changing a child's clothes because she has spilt her drink when you notice a large striped bruise on her upper thighs and across her bottom	Contact the child's parents and ask them to come to the school immediately	

10.11 Recording information

Student Book 2
pp 66–75

When you are working with children and young people, information often needs to be recorded. All information should be held securely and kept confidential, and should only ever be shared on a 'need to know' basis. Remember to inform the children and young people you are working with that you have a duty of care to them. Explain that, in order to protect them or others, your duty of care could mean that you have to share information about them with another professional.

Complete the following tasks in relation to recording and keeping information.

Task	Information
Read through the statement opposite. When you see two words together, in italics, cross out the less appropriate word.	When undertaking observations to support allegations of abuse you need to be *subjective / objective*. All reports must be *clear / interesting* to read. If hand-written, they should be in *blue / black* ink. Reports should *always/never* be shared with the parents. When arranging meetings to discuss a child or young person, you *must / must not* invite them or their parents.
Is the information opposite true or false?	Personal records of children and young people who have been or are at risk of being abused are kept on a central register. This register can be accessed by anyone who works with children and/or young people by phoning social services. *True/False*
Fill in the missing words opposite.	All personal records should be kept in a _____ filing cabinet. Only those involved in a child or young person's _____ should have access to their care plan.
Is the information opposite true or false?	1 Children and young people are never allowed to attend case conferences held to discuss their risk of abuse. *True/False* 2 Parents are always informed that a detailed assessment of their parenting skills will be undertaken. *True/False* 3 Children and young people can ask for a change in their appointed key worker. *True/False* 4 The Data Protection Act ensures that everyone can have access to anyone else's information. *True/False* 5 The United Nations Convention on The Rights of The Child is law in England. *True/False*

10.12 Recognising predisposing factors

Student Book 2
pp 66–75

Factor no.	Predisposing factor	Rationale of risk
1	Living in poverty	
2	Drug-addicted parents	
3	Member of the family suffering from mental illness	
4	Reconstructed family (step-siblings)	
5	Both parents were neglected and physically abused as children	
6	Child or young person is disabled	
7	Domestic violence	
8	Both parents are unemployed	
9	Alcoholic mother	
10	Father with drug and/or gambling addiction	

■ Explain why the above factors may put children at higher risk of being abused. (You can use additional paper for your responses.)

■ Then identify supporting strategies that may assist families to reduce the risk of abuse to children across the 0 to 16-year-old age range.

10.14 Parenting skills

Student Book 2
pp 66–75

Children are often neglected because their parents don't understand their needs. This may be because the parents have learning difficulties, or they had poor parenting experiences when they were growing up, or because they have not adapted to their children's needs as they have grown older.

Working in small groups, identify the needs of a child and the responsibilities of good parenting. After each item below, write 'C' (for a child's needs) or 'P' (if you think it's a parent's responsibility).

Meeting/supporting/supervising hygiene needs ….

Giving love and affection ….

Stable family set-up ….

Ensuring feelings of self-worth ….

Providing a balanced diet ….

Stimulation to develop and learn ….

Sleep and rest ….

Routines/structure to their day ….

Social interaction with their peers ….

Access to education ….

Household budgeting ….

Cooking ….

Free time ….

Suitable clothing ….

Now write a short account explaining why parents may need support to meet the needs of children and young people and to provide them with a safe and secure home environment.

....

....

....

....

....

....

....

10.15 Creating a 'Keeping safe' game

Student Book 2
pp 66–75

Working in groups of four, plan and produce a game that will teach children to keep themselves safe from abuse. You will need to consider the following points:

- the age range the game will be aimed at

- possible type or types of abuse you intend to safeguard against

- rules for the game

- how the game may be used

- who would supervise the game

- resources required to make the game and the cost implications.

Once you have produced your game, try it out!

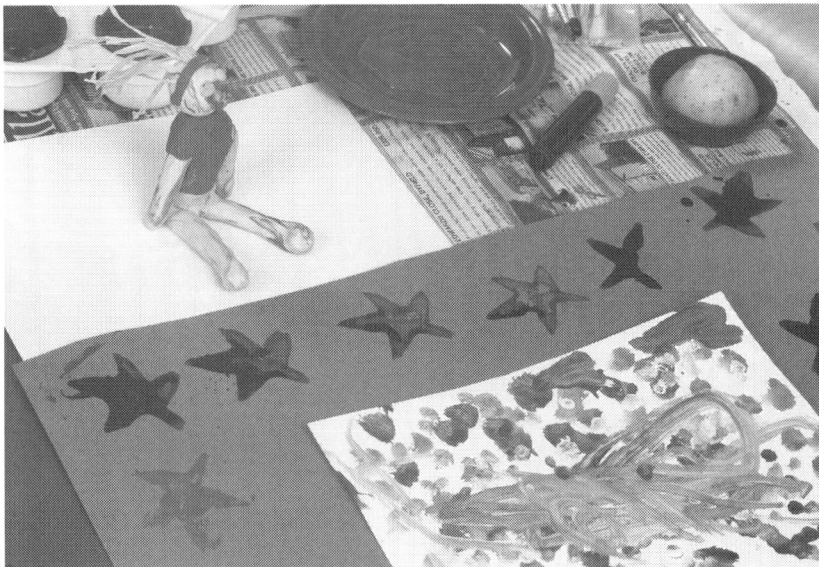

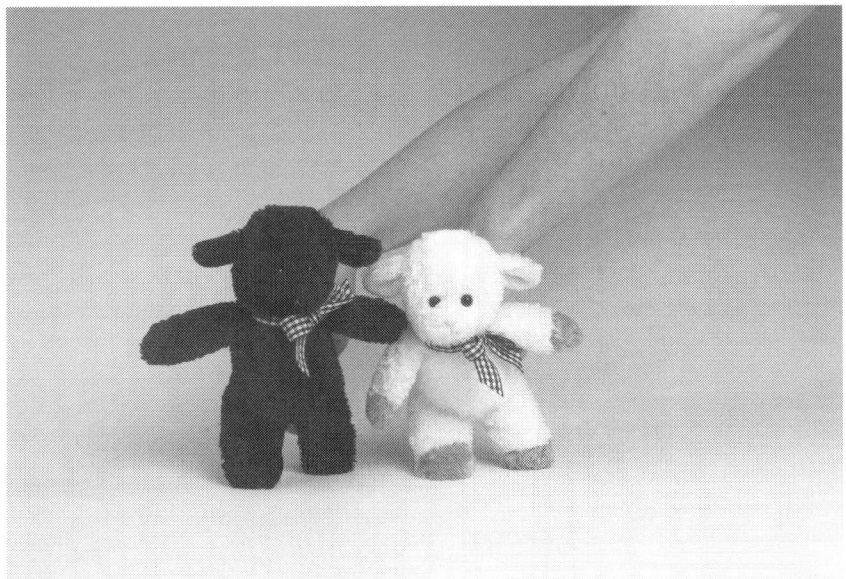

11

Supporting and protecting adults

unit overview

This unit looks at ways in which adults are supported and protected within the health and social care sector. It covers sensitive subjects including physical, psychological, sexual and financial abuse. The unit is divided into four Learning outcomes.

Learning outcomes

On completion of this unit learners should:

11.1   know how to develop supportive relationships with adult users of health and social care services

11.2   understand types of abuse and indicators of abuse in health and social care contexts

11.3   understand the potential for abuse in health and social care contexts

11.4   understand working strategies to minimise abuse.

Suggested activities

The At-a-glance activity grid shows how the activities in the Assessment and Delivery Resource (ADR) relate to the content of the unit. The activities include introductory and plenary activities and a variety of case studies, research tasks, discussions and presentations, using written, verbal and presentation skills. The activities may help learners prepare for assessment, and the grid indicates which assessment criteria are relevant for each activity. Copies of activity sheets can be given to learners.

Teaching Unit 11

This unit needs careful delivery in order to protect the emotional welfare of students. From this point of view, it may be best to teach Unit 11 quite late in the course, when students have gained a mature understanding of professional practice and the importance of confidentiality. Exploring the vulnerability of adults with particular care needs can be difficult for students whose elderly relatives or close family friends may be dealing with similar issues.

The topic of abuse may also raise sensitive issues relating to students' personal experiences. Students who have been abused themselves often find it extremely difficult to write about abuse, especially its consequences. To overcome this difficulty and to enable such students to complete the unit, tutors may need to consider appointing an assigned scribe and allowing additional time for completion of the Assessment tasks. In such instances it is extremely important that support is offered confidentially, as group awareness can increase the distress experienced by the abused student. During the last five minutes of each lesson students should be given the opportunity to 'de-stress' as the topics covered may evoke strong emotions. The first six weeks are less stressful than the rest of the unit, and this should allow the students to start feeling comfortable with each other and to bond as a group.

Confidentiality is covered in several units on the course, but it is still necessary to remind learners of the importance of boundaries, especially in relation to information gained during work placements. Ensure that you discuss confidentiality and personal support in the first few lessons in order to establish a safe teaching environment for both students and staff.

Legislation, which forms the backbone of policies and procedures in health and social care settings, is constantly being reviewed. It is therefore vital to check before delivering this unit that the information on legislation is up to date. Giving students a brief outline of the legislative history will help them understand the process of legislative change and the need for formal review of legislation.

Inviting guest speakers (e.g. social workers, health professionals and voluntary workers providing residential services or care in the community) to talk to the students about their experiences will bring an extra dimension to the delivery of this unit. The general term 'health and social care settings' has been used throughout the text. However, when delivering this unit, the tutor should refer to specific settings including hospitals, residential care/nursing homes, hostels, community homes and service users' own homes.

The content of each Learning outcome

Learning outcome 1: Know how to develop supportive relationships with adult users of health and social care services (relevant criteria: P1, M1, D1)

For the first Learning outcome, students need to investigate how to develop supportive, enabling relationships and how to promote individual rights. Communication skills, confidentiality and setting clear boundaries for professional relationships are all key elements. This Learning outcome also offers a good opportunity to introduce students to available counselling services and the concept of support for staff who identify abuse. It begins with a PowerPoint® presentation on the rights of service users. This is followed by Activity 11.1, a word search on human rights. Activity 11.2 explores trust and respect in relationships between service users and service providers, and Activity 11.3 gives learners a chance to understand communication difficulties by communicating information without using words.

Learning outcome 2: Understand types of abuse and indicators of abuse in health and social care contexts (relevant criteria: P2, P3)

The topics covered in the second Learning outcome are extremely sensitive and care is essential when introducing the concept of abuse. Students learn how to set clear boundaries of confidentiality. They also learn how to recognise the signs and symptoms of abuse, including domestic violence. This outcome begins with a PowerPoint® presentation on different types of abuse. Activity 11.4 is a detailed case study on the subject of possible psychological abuse. This is followed by Activity 11.5, in which learners identify possible financial abuse in six different care situations. This is followed by Activity 11.6, a PowerPoint® presentation on emotions evoked by abuse. Activity 11.7 is a crossword on domestic violence, and this outcome finishes with a gapped handout (Activity 11.8) on providing support following abuse.

Learning outcome 3: Understand the potential for abuse in health and social care contexts (relevant criteria: P4, M2)

The third Learning outcome covers the potential for abuse within the community, and in day-care and residential settings. It begins with a PowerPoint® presentation looking at the vulnerability of those who rely on others for their personal care. This may raise personal issues for some students, especially those who have vulnerable relatives or friends. In Activity 11.9, learners identify the risks to both service users and professionals of bullying, abuse, system abuse and invasion of privacy. Activity 11.10 is a matching game, in which students match job titles with the services provided by particular health and social care professionals. This is followed by Activity 11.11, in which students use the multi-disciplinary wheel to identify team members who may be involved with five different cases.

Learning outcome 4: Understand working strategies to minimise abuse (relevant criteria: P5, P6, M3, D2)

The fourth Learning outcome covers legislation, codes of practice, national standards, and the policies and procedures that are in place to help protect vulnerable adults as well as those who care for them. It is essential for students to become familiar with the reporting procedures for disclosures and suspected cases of abuse. This Learning outcome begins with a PowerPoint® presentation on policies and procedures in health and social care settings. Activity 11.12 is a research task on legislation to protect vulnerable adults. In Activity 11.13, students learn about the procedures used when recruiting people to work with vulnerable adults. This is followed by Activity 11.14, in which students consider clinical supervision in relation to four case studies. Finally, in Activity 11.15, learners review the unit content by devising their own quiz to be played in teams.

How this unit will be assessed

To reach Pass level, the evidence must show that the learner is able to:

P1 explain how individual rights can be respected in a supportive relationship
P2 describe different forms of abuse which may be experienced by vulnerable adults
P3 describe different indicators of abuse in vulnerable adults
P4 describe the potential for abuse in health and social care contexts
P5 describe strategies and working practices used to minimise abuse
P6 identify the legislation, policies and procedures that protect adults receiving health and social care services.

To reach Merit level, the evidence must show that, in addition to the Pass criteria, the learner is able to:

M1 explain how supportive relationships can enhance the life experiences of individuals receiving health and social care services
M2 analyse the potential for abuse in four health and social care contexts
M3 explain how legislation, policies and procedures contribute to the protection of vulnerable adults.

To reach Distinction level, the evidence must show that, in addition to the Pass and Merit criteria, the learner is able to:

D1 use examples to evaluate the role of supportive relationships in enhancing the life experiences of individuals receiving health and social care services
D2 analyse the role of multi-agency working in minimising the risks of abuse in health and social care contexts.

Assessment tasks

These three Assessment tasks will give students the opportunity to work through from pass to merit and on to distinction level.

Task 1 (relevant criteria: P1, M1, D1)

* Produce an information leaflet for new staff in health and social care settings explaining how to build supportive relationships with service users and respect individual rights. **(P1)**
* Explain how such an approach could enhance the life experiences of those they will be caring for. **(M1)**
* Include examples evaluating how the relationships have enhanced the life experiences of those receiving health and social care services. **(D1)**

Task 2 (relevant criteria: P2, P3, P4, M2)

* Describe the different forms of abuse that can be experienced by vulnerable adults. **(P2)**
* Identify different indicators of abuse. **(P3)**
* Now describe the potential for abuse, including system abuse, in relation to vulnerable adults. **(P4)**
* Finally, select four different health and social care settings and analyse the potential for abuse in these particular settings. **(M2)**

Task 3 (relevant criteria: P5, P6, M3, D2)

* Write a report on the legislation, policies, procedures and codes of practice that are in place to protect vulnerable adults receiving health and social care services. **(P6)**
* Give a detailed description of the strategies and working practices used to reduce the risk of abuse. **(P5)**
* Finally, complete your report by analysing the role of multi-agency working in reducing the risk of abuse in health and social care settings. **(D2)**

Scheme of work

BTEC National Health & Social Care
Unit 11 Supporting and protecting adults

Academic year: ....

Broad aim: To give an awareness of the risks of abuse and the vulnerability of adults who receive health and/or social care and to identify professional responses to abuse

Teacher(s): ....

Number of weeks: 35

Duration of session: 1 hour 30 mins

Guided learning hours: 60

ADR = Assessment and Delivery Resource

Week/s	Topic/outcome	Tutor preparation	Student activity	Resources	Links to grading criteria
1	Understand the importance of confidentiality	Explain the importance of confidentiality for both service users and the student group, recognising the rights of the individual. Begin with the PowerPoint® presentation on the rights of service users	Learners complete Activity 11.1, a word search on human rights. Ask learners to discuss the themes connected to the solutions.	PowerPoint® 1, Activity 11.1	P1, M1, D1
2	Explore the social model of disability	Explore the social model of disability	Learners to discuss advocacy, empowerment and promoting the rights of the individual through a humanistic approach		P1, M1, D1
3	Understand different types of relationships and the importance of mutual respect	Activity 11.2 highlights the importance of mutual respect between service providers and service users	Discuss different types of relationships, noting the differences between family relationships, friendships and professional relationships. Learners to rewrite a series of statements to reflect how relationships affect communication	Activity 11.2	P1, M1, D1
4	Understand the benefits of consistency of care	Look at how consistency of care can offer security of delivery and care practice for service users			P1, M1, D1
5	Explore ways of overcoming communication difficulties	Introduce different types of non-verbal communication e.g. gestures and facial expressions	In Activity 11.3 learners work in pairs to describe situations to each other without speaking. Ask learners to discuss particular problems they found in communication	Activity 11.3	P1, M1, D1
6	Understand equality of service and respect for individual needs and rights	Introduce equality of service, respect for individual needs and rights, and delivery of service through joint care plans	Learners to discuss and carry out research into different individual needs and processes used to fulfil these needs		P1, M1, D1
7–8	Complete Assessment task 1	Learners work on Assessment task 1 with support from you, as tutor, due to the sensitive nature of the task			P1, M1, D1

Unit 11 Supporting and protecting adults

Week/s	Topic/outcome	Tutor preparation	Student activity	Resources	Links to grading criteria
9	Recognise specific categories of abuse	This is a PowerPoint® presentation on specific categories of abuse	Learners can take notes on the presentation and use these as a basis for researching the indicators for types of abuse	PowerPoint® 2	P2, P3
10	Identify the signs and symptoms of physical neglect		Students learn to recognise signs and symptoms of physical neglect and lack of care and/or medical treatment		P2, P3
11	Identify the signs and symptoms of psychological abuse	Discuss how to recognise the signs and symptoms of psychological abuse (e.g. threats, bullying and belittling/humiliation)	Activity 11.4 is a case study that helps learners identify these signs by preparing a written account	Activity 11.4	P2, P3
12	Deal with disclosure, and recognise the signs and symptoms of sexual abuse	Introduce learners to disclosure procedures, and how to recognise the signs and symptoms of sexual abuse	Learners to research and prepare a presentation on how sexual abuse is identified		P2, P3
13	Identify the signs and symptoms of financial abuse	Introduce the signs of financial abuse (e.g. making use of service users' funds without permission and the misuse/claiming of benefits by carers)	In Activity 11.5 students identify the signs and symptoms of financial abuse	Activity 11.5	P2, P3
14	Identify the signs and symptoms of institutional abuse	Introduce the signs of institutional abuse (e.g. unsafe and abusive practices, and intentional misuse of theory and/or medication)	Students learn to recognise the signs and symptoms of institutional abuse		P2, P3
15	Recognise discrimination	Activity 11.6 is a PowerPoint® presentation on the emotions evoked by abuse	Students learn to recognise discrimination on the grounds of gender, age, health, disability, sexuality, religion or ethnicity in relation to service users or care/health professionals	Activity 11.6	P2, P3
16	Discuss domestic violence/abuse and recognise the problem of gender stereotyping	Activity 11.7 is a crossword on domestic violence	Learners discuss domestic violence/abuse (including physical, sexual and psychological) and recognise the problem of stereotyping, i.e. always placing the woman in the role of the victim and the man in the role of abuser	Activity 11.7	P2, P3
17	Identify the signs and symptoms of self-harming	This topic requires sensitive handling, as some students may have personal experience of these issues	Students learn to recognise the signs and symptoms of self-harming, as in the form of physical injuries, medication, alcohol, drugs or substance abuse		P2, P3
18	Look at power within relationships	Introduce imbalances of power (e.g. through levels of knowledge/ understanding, and position or professional status as care giver/receiver)	Learners look at imbalance of power within relationships. Ask learners to role play situations that show an imbalance of power and then discuss the implications		P2, P3, M2

Unit 11 Supporting and protecting adults

Week/s	Topic/outcome	Tutor preparation	Student activity	Resources	Links to grading criteria
19	Support caring relationships in the health and social care sector	Introduce providing and supporting caring relationships through key worker systems, information sharing, and including service users in decisions about the provision and delivery of care packages	Learners complete a gapped handout, and then use this as a basis for whole class discussion	Activity 11.8	P2, P3
20	Recognise predisposing factors that may increase the risk of abuse	This is a PowerPoint® presentation on the predisposing factors that may increase the risk of abuse of all types	Learners to take notes throughout presentation and use this as the basis for completing a written report (with research) on the key factors	PowerPoint® 3	P2, P3, P4, M2
21	Recognise the potential for abuse within health and care services, and identify risks to both service users and professionals	Introduce learners to recognising the potential for abuse within health and care services and identify risks to both service users and professionals of bullying, abuse, system abuse or invasion of privacy	Learners work in pairs or small groups to complete a table of actions to take in certain situations, and then report their decisions back to the rest of the class. Encourage a debate in which differing ideas are presented	Activity 11.9	P4, M2
22–23	Complete Assessment task 2	Learners work on Assessment task 2 with support from you, as tutor, due to the sensitive nature of the task			P2, P3, P4, M2
24	Identify the different roles and responsibilities of health and social care professionals and how they can work together	Identify the different roles and responsibilities and how they interlink	In Activity 11.10 students identify the different roles of health and social care professionals with the services they provide. Activity 11.11 is a diagram that students complete to show how various team members can work together to provide care packages	Activity 11.10, Activity 11.11	P5, P6, M3, D2
25	Identify good working practices that help protect clients from abuse and staff from false accusations	Learners are introduced to good working practices that help protect service users from abuse and staff from false accusations (e.g. keeping clear written records on contact with service users)	Invite a visiting speaker to explain working practices to learners and the importance of following these. Learners can complete a written report on the talk		P5, P6, M3
26	Understand policies and procedures that help to protect service users and service providers	This is a PowerPoint® presentation on the policies and procedures that help to protect service users and service providers in different health and social care settings	Learners to complete notes during the presentation and use these as a basis for discussion	PowerPoint® 4	P5, P6, M3

Unit 11 Supporting and protecting adults

Week/s	Topic/outcome	Tutor preparation	Student activity	Resources	Links to grading criteria
27	Recognise the strategies used to protect vulnerable adults	Students learn about strategies used to protect vulnerable adults and to assist service users to protect themselves and make them aware of their individual rights			P5, P6, M3
28	Identify the key points of the Data Protection Act, Care Standards Act, Mental Health Act, and NHS and Community Care Act	Introduce learners to the key points of the legislation	Learners carry out research into the legislation, working independently and completing a written report	Activity 11.12	P5, P6, M3
29	Identify the key points of the Disability Discrimination Act, Special Educational Needs Act and Human Rights Act	Identify the key points of the Disability Discrimination Act, the Special Educational Needs Act, and the Human Rights Act			P5, P6, M3
30	Understand Codes of Practice for nursing and social workers and care home regulations 2003	Identify the Codes of Practice for nursing and social workers and National Standards for Care, care home regulations 2003			P5, P6, M3
31–32	Complete Assessment task 3	Learners work on Assessment task 3 with support from you, as tutor, due to the sensitive nature of the task			P5, P6, M3, D2
33	Understand safe employment practices	Introduce safe employment practices	Learners prepare a role play covering procedures for employing vulnerable adverts, carrying out research and group work to prepare for mock interviews of candidates	Activity 11.13	P4, M3
34	Understand the reasons for the introduction of clinical supervision, following the Beverly Allott case	Prepare material for learners covering the reasons for introduction of clinical supervision	Activity 11.14 provides four case study situations in which care has gone wrong. Learners discuss issues arising from case studies and how to respond to concerns about professional malpractice	Activity 11.14	P4, P6, M3
35	Review Unit 11	Help learners devise appropriate questions and answers if necessary	Learners review the unit content and Learning outcomes covered by devising their own quiz	Activity 11.15	All

At-a-glance activity grid
Unit 11 Supporting and protecting adults

Activity	Title and description	Scheme of work	File/CD	Delivery notes	Additional resources	Links to grading criteria	Links to Student Book 2
Outcome 11.1 Know how to develop supportive relationships with adult users of health and social care services							
PowerPoint 1	Understand rights	Week 1	CD	This PPT presentation looks at a couple of 'human rights' and how they can be used to protect vulnerable adults. The activity can be extended by asking students to research human rights in general, and their implications in relation to care	Internet resources on human rights	P1, M1, D1	pp 82–90
11.1	Human Rights Act word search	Week 1	File (Answers on CD)	This word search should be used on an individual basis. The activity can be extended by asking learners to research further information on the Human Rights Act	Internet resources on the Human Rights Act	P1, M1, D1	pp 82–90
11.2	Relationships: Respect through language	Week 3	File	This individual-based task could also be used when covering communications. It can be extended through role play		P1, M1, D1	pp 82–90
11.3	Communication: Expressing specific information without using verbal communication	Week 5	File (Tutor information on CD)	This activity is best used in pairs, so that students gain an understanding and increased awareness of the frustration felt by those with poor communication skills	Information from http://www.makaton.org/about/ss_how.htm on MAKATON signing vocabulary	P1, M1, D1	pp 82–90
Outcome 11.2 Understand types of abuse and indicators of abuse in health and social care contexts							
PowerPoint 2	Recognise specific categories of abuse	Week 9	CD	This PPT presentation explains specific categories of abuse	Useful contact numbers for counselling and support	P2, P3	pp 90–96
11.4	Identify psychological abuse	Week 11	File	This is a case study for group discussion. Due to the sensitive nature of the topic, this is best worked on in small groups. You should move between groups while they discuss each aspect of the case. You can extend this activity by making links with other types of abuse and identifying the reporting process that would be used		P2, P3	pp 90–96
11.5	Identify financial abuse	Week 13	File	This activity includes six situations for group discussion. Again, you should move between the groups while they discuss each issue. You can extend it by getting the students to discuss how a line manager would respond to the information		P2, P3	pp 90–96

Activity	Title and description	Scheme of work	File/CD	Delivery notes	Additional resources	Links to grading criteria	Links to Student Book 2
11.6	Understand the emotions evoked by abuse	Week 15	CD	This is a PPT presentation on the emotions evoked by abuse. This is a sensitive topic and is therefore best discussed as a group. It is important not to highlight any one person's responses	Counselling services information to give out to students as a group	P2, P3	pp 90–96
11.7	Understand vocabulary related to domestic violence	Week 16	File (Answers on CD)	This is a crossword to be completed on an individual basis. You can extend this activity by asking students to create their own crosswords		P2, P3	pp 90–96
11.8	Identify appropriate support for victims and staff following abuse	Week 19	File (Answers on CD)	This gapped worksheet can be used on an individual basis or as a small group activity. It can be extended by researching local support available and counselling options	Internet resources for research	P2, P3	pp 90–96
Outcome 11.3 Understand the potential for abuse in health and social care contexts							
PowerPoint 3	Identify predisposing factors that may increase the risk of abuse	Week 20	CD	This PPT presentation summarises the predisposing factors that may increase the risk of abuse of all types. You can use this presentation to lead the discussion, then extend the activity with a role play to promote empathy		P2, P3, P4, M2	pp 96–99
11.9	Identify ways in which service providers need to protect themselves from suspicion of abuse	Week 21	File (Answers on CD)	For this activity, the students work in small groups, then feed back their group's findings to the whole class. This can be extended by asking each group of students to create a PPT presentation on their findings	Access to computers to create PowerPoint® presentations	P4	pp 96–99
11.10	Match health/social care professions with the services they provide	Week 24	File (Tutor information on CD)	The cards for this matching game can be used on an individual or small group basis and should generate discussion of different professional roles. The cards can also be used to make a dominoes game. The activity can be extended by asking students to research job roles in more detail and discover training route and qualifications required	Internet resources for research	P5, P6, M3, D2	pp 96–99
11.11	Identify multi-disciplinary team support needed to meet specific needs of service users	Week 24	File	This may be used as an individual or group task. As each local area has different support services and teams, no answer is provided on the CD	Information on multi-disciplinary teams from Activity 11.10	P5, P6, M3, D2	pp 96–99

Outcome 11.4 Understand working strategies to minimise abuse

Activity	Title and description	Scheme of work	File/CD	Delivery notes	Additional resources	Links to grading criteria	Links to Student Book 2
Power Point® 4	Understand policies and procedures that help to protect service users and service providers	Week 26	CD	This PPT presentation explains the policies and procedures that help to protect service users and service providers in different health and social care settings		P5, P6, M3	pp 100–109
11.12	Research current legislation	Week 28	File	For individual or small group work on Data Protection Act, Care Standards Act, Mental Health Act, and NHS and Community Care Act. Can be extended by selecting specific Acts of supportive law to be investigated by each group and then asking the groups to give feedback to the whole class	Internet resources for research	P5, P6, M3	pp 100–109
11.13	Understand safe employment practices	Week 33	File	Students can work on this activity in pairs or small groups. You may want to spread it over a two-week period and carry out the interviews in the second week. Extend it by carrying out mock interviews and evaluating interviewee responses	A supply of sample job application forms	P4, M3	pp 100–109
11.14	Understand the reasons for the introduction of clinical supervision, following the Beverly Allott case	Week 34	File	These discussion-based case studies are intended for small group work. Even if groups have the same case study they may have different responses. The activity can be extended by asking students to research the Beverly Allott case and the inquiry that followed	Internet resources for research	P4, P6, M3	pp 100–109
11.15	Unit review quiz	Week 35	File	This is a group activity, in which students devise their own quiz to recap the unit content	Spare paper for questions and answers	All	pp 100–109

Unit 11 Lesson plan

Aims

• To introduce Unit 11

This structure may be spread over a number of lessons as required.

Learning outcomes
• recognise topics to be covered and list Learning outcomes of Unit 11
• identify emotional responses to abuse, and the need for boundaries and confidentiality
• recognise the need for safe keeping of information.

Timing	Content	Teacher activity	Student activity	Resources	Individualised activity
5 mins	Introduction	Write up and explain lesson aims and objectives. Use varied vocabulary to ensure understanding and to extend vocabulary			
10 mins	Explanation of the Learning outcomes and topics to be covered	Discuss the sensitivity of the material covered in this unit. Give examples of how to attain high grades. Ask open questions to confirm understanding	Learners to answer open questions	Copies of the unit criteria, or BTEC course specifications handbook	
15 mins	Importance of confidentiality	Discuss confidentiality issues that may affect the group. Clarify students' concerns and suggest strategies to overcome them	Learners contribute to whole class discussion		
15 mins	Definition of service users' rights	Work through the PPT presentation, using slides to lead the discussion	Learners contribute to whole class discussion	PowerPoint® 1	Extend students through stepped questions in relation to their perspective on rights
20 mins	Word search on the Human Rights Act	Ask learners to complete word search on an individual basis, then get into groups to relate the words to their meanings and discuss individual rights. Move between groups to support discussions	Learners complete word searches, then contribute to group discussions	Activity 11.1 (Answers on CD)	More able students can extend their understanding of the Human Rights Act by carrying out secondary research
20 mins	Recap	Identify objectives met and give information on next lesson to prepare students. Use varied vocabulary and repetition to ensure understanding	Learners to answer open questions		

Timing	Content	Teacher activity	Student activity	Resources	Individualised activity
5 mins	End	Give students the opportunity to 'de-stress' for the last five minutes of the lesson, as the topics covered are very sensitive and may evoke emotional responses related to their personal experiences			

11.1 Human Rights Act word search

Student Book 2
pp 82–90

Hidden in the grid below are words related to the Human Rights Act. The words may be horizontal, vertical, diagonal and spelt in either direction. See how many you can find, and tick each one in the list below the grid. Once you have discovered all the words, make a note of what each word means to you in relation to providing health and social care services.

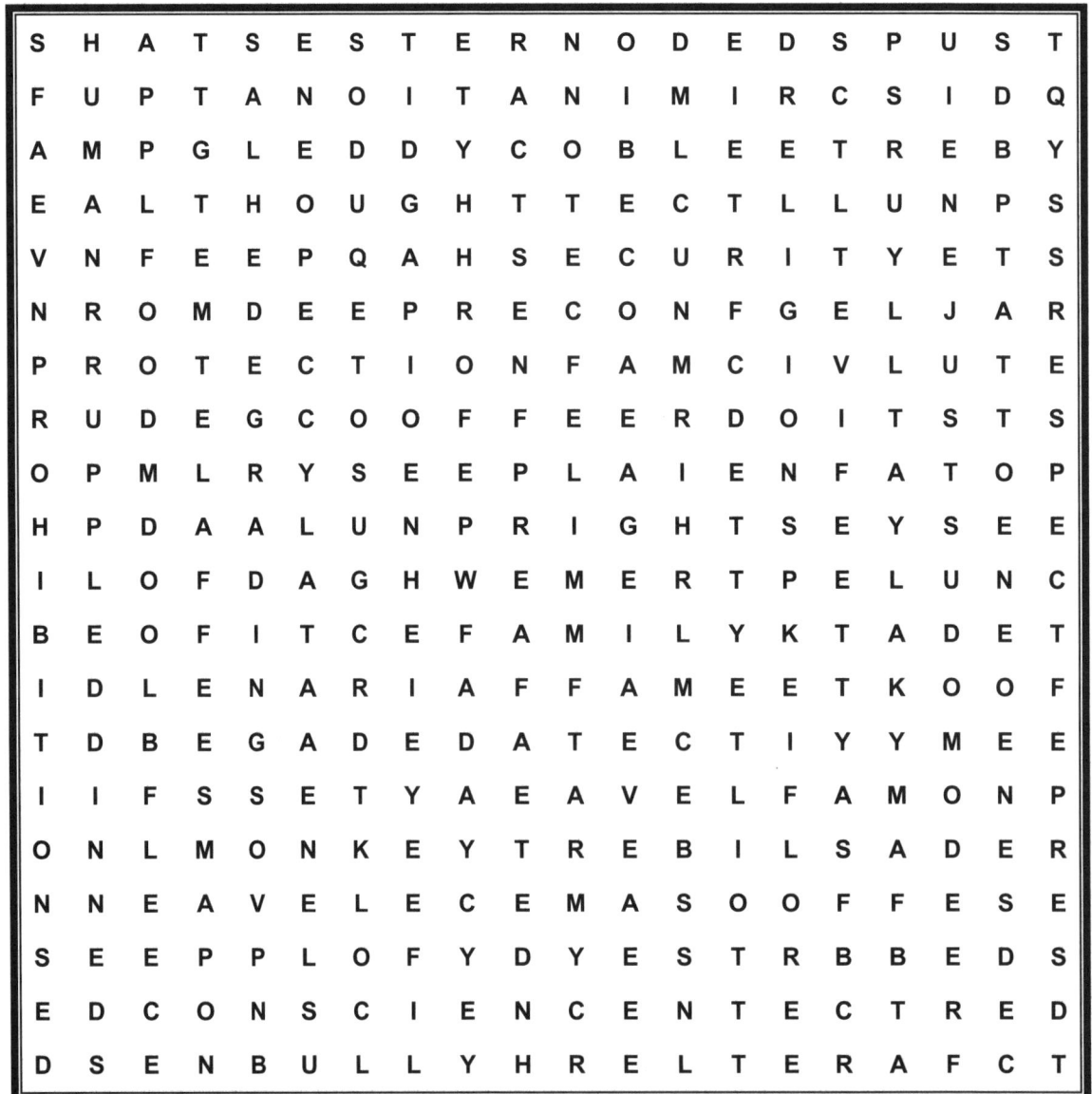

S	H	A	T	S	E	S	T	E	R	N	O	D	E	D	S	P	U	S	T
F	U	P	T	A	N	O	I	T	A	N	I	M	I	R	C	S	I	D	Q
A	M	P	G	L	E	D	D	Y	C	O	B	L	E	E	T	R	E	B	Y
E	A	L	T	H	O	U	G	H	T	T	E	C	T	L	L	U	N	P	S
V	N	F	E	E	P	Q	A	H	S	E	C	U	R	I	T	Y	E	T	S
N	R	O	M	D	E	E	P	R	E	C	O	N	F	G	E	L	J	A	R
P	R	O	T	E	C	T	I	O	N	F	A	M	C	I	V	L	U	T	E
R	U	D	E	G	C	O	O	F	F	E	E	R	D	O	I	T	S	T	S
O	P	M	L	R	Y	S	E	E	P	L	A	I	E	N	F	A	T	O	P
H	P	D	A	A	L	U	N	P	R	I	G	H	T	S	E	Y	S	E	E
I	L	O	F	D	A	G	H	W	E	M	E	R	T	P	E	L	U	N	C
B	E	O	F	I	T	C	E	F	A	M	I	L	Y	K	T	A	D	E	T
I	D	L	E	N	A	R	I	A	F	F	A	M	E	E	T	K	O	O	F
T	D	B	E	G	A	D	E	D	A	T	E	C	T	I	Y	Y	M	E	E
I	I	F	S	S	E	T	Y	A	E	A	V	E	L	F	A	M	O	N	P
O	N	L	M	O	N	K	E	Y	T	R	E	B	I	L	S	A	D	E	R
N	N	E	A	V	E	L	E	C	E	M	A	S	O	O	F	F	E	S	E
S	E	E	P	P	L	O	F	Y	D	Y	E	S	T	R	B	B	B	E	D
E	D	C	O	N	S	C	I	E	N	C	E	N	T	E	C	T	R	E	D
D	S	E	N	B	U	L	L	Y	H	R	E	L	T	E	R	A	F	C	T

1	CONSCIENCE	
2	DEGRADING	
3	DISCRIMINATION	
4	FAIR	
5	FAMILY	
6	FREEDOM	
7	HUMAN	
8	JUST	
9	LIBERTY	

10	LIFE
11	PROHIBITION
12	PROTECTION
13	RELIGION
14	RESPECT
15	RIGHTS
16	SECURITY
17	THOUGHT
18	TREATMENT

11.2   Respect in relationships

Student Book 2
pp 82–90

Relationships between service users and service providers are a key component in providing positive care packages. Professional relationships should be based on mutual trust and respect. As a professional, you need to ensure that you respect service users' right to:

1   make their own choices
2   have their own beliefs and preferences
3   have privacy and confidentiality.

Read the following statements made by service providers, identify the area of respect violated (as in the numbered list above), and then rewrite the statements showing respect.

Negative statement	Area violated	Positive statement
Here is an example: 'Time for your bath, Tom. It needs to be quick, as I have a meeting to go to.'	Area 1	'Tom, I have a meeting to go to in 30 minutes, so would you like to have a quick bath before I go, or wait till later?'
'Jane only has her benefits to live on. The poor thing has no savings.' (talking to Jane's neighbour)		
A Muslim resident is told, 'There's not much bacon with the liver and it is lamb's liver, so just eat the liver and leave the bacon bits on your plate.'		
'Let's open the windows and let some fresh air in. You can put a jumper on if it's cold.'		
'The newspaper man will be here shortly. I'll take a couple of pounds from your purse and get you a paper.'		
'There's a letter for you. It's from your daughter in Australia, I'll read it for you.'		
'I'll put the television on. It's time for the news on the BBC. You like to hear what is happening in the world.'		
'I've got your clothes out ready for you. The student is going to watch how I wash and dress you, so she can learn.'		
'Time for your vitamin tablets. I know you think they are a waste of time, but we like everyone to have them.'		
'You really do need a shave. It will make you feel and look better.'		
'Leave the bathroom door open, so I can see when you are finished.'		

11.3 Communication difficulties game

Student Book 2
pp 82–90

Your tutor will put you in pairs for this activity, and give you a set of cards with communication tasks written on them. Place the cards face down and divide them equally. Take it in turns to describe each situation to your partner without using verbal communication. You can use gestures, facial expressions and body language but no words. You can use the blank cards for your own ideas, if you wish. If your partner can understand what you are describing, you get a point. Count up the points at the end, and see which of you has won.

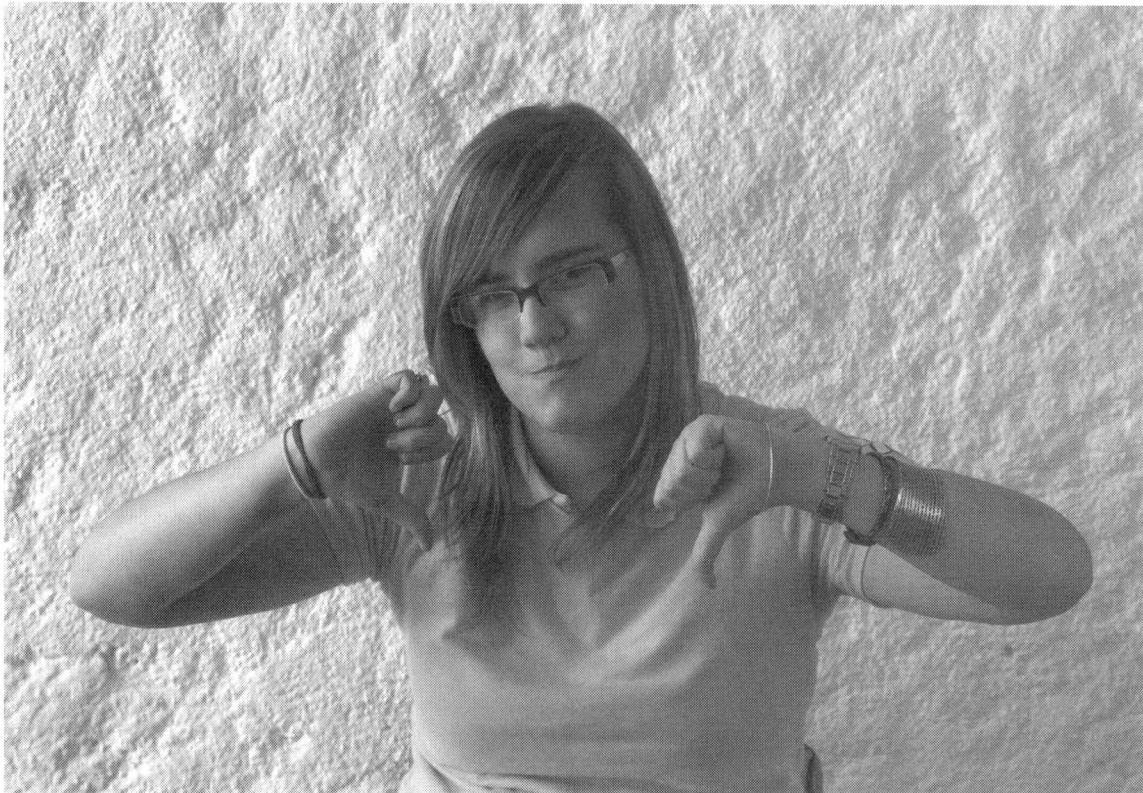

11.4 Recognising psychological abuse

**Student Book 2
pp 90–96**

Read the following case study.

James is 35 years old and has considerable physical difficulties following a motorcycle accident when he was 17 years old. He receives disability living allowances at the highest level for both mobility and care. James has always lived in his family home with his parents. A little over three years ago, James underwent brain surgery. Unfortunately his soft palate was damaged so he is now tube-fed via a 'peg' in his abdomen. His feeding regime includes two multivitamin milkshakes injected through his 'peg' and a 1-litre bottle of complete food supplement delivered through the night using a pump on a timer connected via tubes to the 'peg'. He used to attend an adult centre twice a week, a disability horse riding facility once a week and a special club two evenings a week. He had a good social life, with family and friends visiting regularly and his mother taking him on visits.

His mother used to be his main carer. She used to shower him daily, dress and undress him, and manage his feeding regime. She also drove him to and from his activities and kept him company on the days he was at home. His mother received a carer's allowance and also managed James's finances. Unfortunately his parents' marriage fell apart and his mother moved out of the family home. James went with her. He started attending a new day centre, as they were some distance away from his previous centre, but the rest of his social life continued as before.

However, James did not like change and missed his fully adapted room, so he moved back to live with his father and his father's new partner. His father did not want to take up the role of carer and applied to social services for support. Within a short time it was noted that James had lost weight, he seemed slightly withdrawn, he stopped going to the evening clubs and did not attend his horse riding every week. After a month he asked both family and friends not to visit him as it made his father's partner uncomfortable. James had always been very generous with his nephews and nieces but their birthdays were missed and there were no Christmas presents.

The only family contact that was maintained was with his sister, who visited him, and his father would occasionally drop James off at her house when he was going out. His mother had also given James a mobile phone with preset numbers for herself, his sister, brother and a favourite aunt. However, when his sister visited, their father kept coming in and out of James's room, he never knocked and when he was in the room he stared at James intently. When his sister mentioned to her father that James was losing weight, he told her he was attending a gym. When she asked James if he wanted to go shopping with her for birthday gifts, the father answered, 'No, his money is not sorted.'

His sister was concerned, as the atmosphere changed whenever their father came into the room; James became tense and stopped talking. Every time his mother phoned to arrange a visit his father said they were busy. Three months went by without anyone seeing James;

Continued overleaf

11.4 Recognising psychological abuse (*contd*)

his father said that they had flu in the house. One Sunday afternoon his sister popped over to the house to see James. She found him still in bed. He had not been washed and was unshaven. There was no one else at home. His sister showered and dressed him and helped him to shave. She noticed a few bruises on his upper arms and back when she was washing him. When she asked how he got them he shrugged and said he didn't know.

When their father returned it was obvious that both he and his partner had been drinking. The sister asked how James had managed to bruise himself so badly and his father stared at James and shouted, 'You remember, you fell in the shower yesterday.' He then said to the daughter, 'You know how stupid he is, always walking into the wall. Stupid aren't you,' he said, moving towards James. James pulled himself back on the chair and looked at the floor. His sister told her father he shouldn't talk like that. He told her to get out and not come back, it was his house and she was no longer welcome. James's sister was now really concerned. She did not want to worry her mother who was currently in hospital having surgery. She also knew that if she told her older brother he would lose his temper and make the situation worse. She had already left a message with social services to say she was concerned for her brother's welfare.

When you have finished reading the case study, consider whether the evidence suggests that psychological or any other type of abuse is taking place. If you think it does, write a report that clearly indicates your concerns. Identify what action needs to be taken in order to assess the situation and ensure James's well-being.

11.5 Identifying financial abuse

Student Book 2
pp 90–96

Read the following situations. For each situation, decide whether financial abuse is taking place or if it is a case of poor practice. Give reasons for your decision.

Situation	Abuse	Poor practice
1 A home carer does some shopping for a service user, even though this is not a designated part of her job. When shopping she buys a number of items that are 'buy one, get one free' offers. She keeps all the additional free items for herself. The service user pays the total cost.		
2 A family carer takes all of her middle-aged disabled daughter's disability allowance and gives her £5 a week pocket money. The daughter is not very good with money and has been known to give it away. The family carer uses the allowance to cover all of the daughter's living expenses.		
3 A nurse takes money from a patient's purse to pay for the patient's newspaper and some chocolates. The patient was in the X-ray department at the time and had mentioned to the nurse that she might miss the trolley and she wanted a newspaper and some chocolates. However, she did not ask the nurse to get them for her.		
4 A private care home manager takes all residents' pension books for 'safe keeping'. She gets the residents to sign the books and she collects the pensions for them. She deducts £20 from each resident's pension for this service.		
5 An occupational therapy assistant is responsible for adapting equipment in service users' homes. The service is provided free of charge by the local health authority. However, he is often asked how much the bill is and his normal response is: 'It will be just over £100 if they invoice you. But if you give me £50 cash, it will save you £50.' Everyone takes him up on the offer.		
6 A social worker assistant completes a service user's benefit claim forms. She accidentally fills in her own bank details instead of the service user's details. Two weeks later, the service user contacts the social worker assistant to say she is not getting her benefits. When checking, the assistant notes her error, and put in a new form with the service user's details. She contacts the service user and says there has been an error and she will drop off a cash payment. She withdraws the right amount of money from her own account, puts it in an envelope and takes it to the service user's home. She does not tell her line manager what has happened.		

11.7 Domestic violence crossword

Student Book 2
pp 90–96

Complete the crossword.

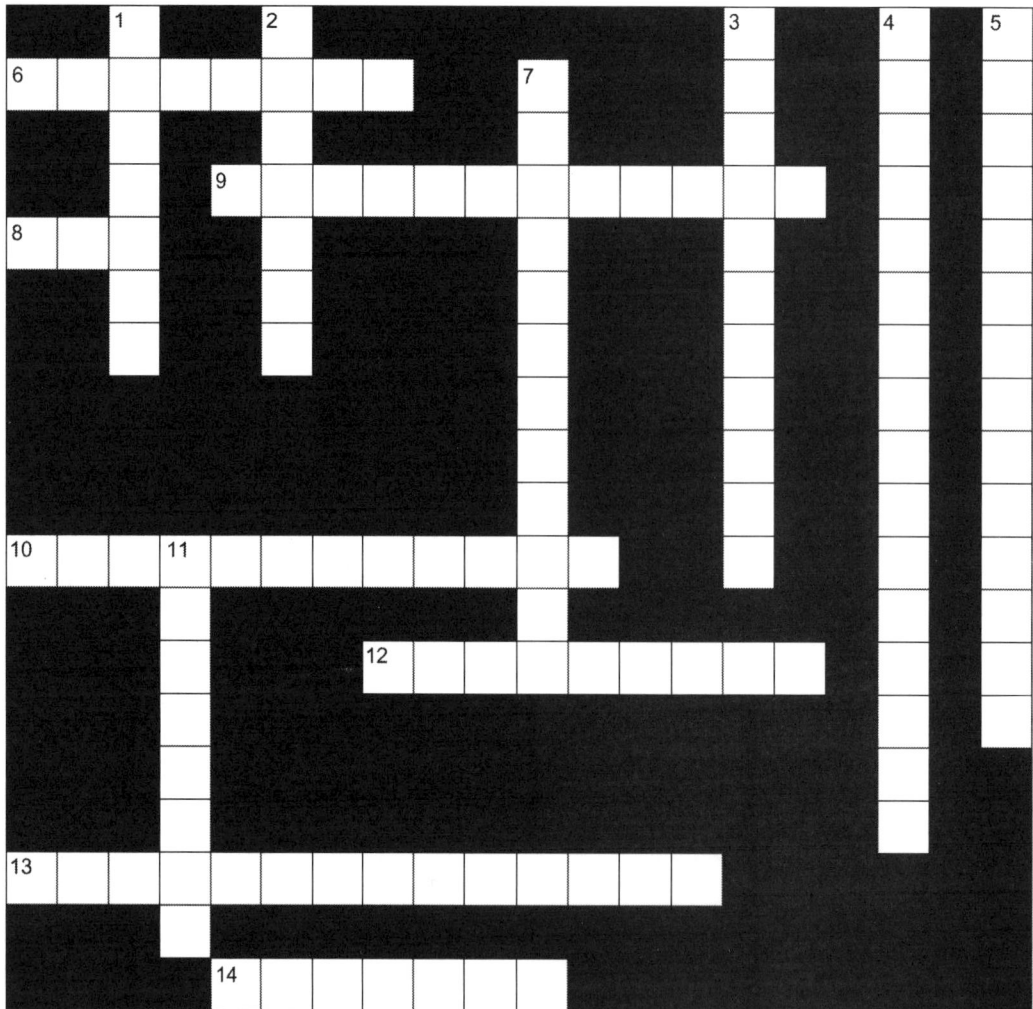

ACROSS

6 Less able
8 Police unit for dealing with domestic violence
9 Person who needs help and support from a care service
10 Needs to be built on trust
12 Unsafe
13 Being biased towards a particular group of people
14 Being vulnerable

DOWN

1 Crime of physical injury
2 Advancing in years
3 Able to live on their own
4 Where a vulnerable person may live
5 Care given to people in their own home
7 A factor that is present that may have an impact
11 Having another person talk and act on your behalf

Note: In this crossword, you need to allow a blank sqaure between separate words in two- or three-word answers.

11.8 Support following abuse

Student Book 2
pp 90–96

Identify the appropriate support for victims and staff who have been involved in suspected or confirmed cases of abuse. Write the missing words in the gaps that describe the best type of support for each case mentioned.

A residential care home has been closed and all the residents have been moved to new care facilities as near to the previous location as possible. Before the closure an investigation took place because a member of staff had reported system abuse. A large number of the staff (but not all) were party to the abuse, which included physical, sexual and psychological abuse of residents. There was also sexual harassment of some staff members. Six members of staff are awaiting prosecution for their actions. The remaining 11 members of staff are seeking new employment, but two of them have decided to leave the care industry.

All residents and staff involved were offered individual ……………………, which they

could choose to take up as ……………………… or as ……………………… counselling.

Service users who were sexually abused were also offered small group classes in

…………………………………. and their right to say ………… . All residents were given

a safe ……………………… worker of their own choice, so they could raise any issues

with them. Service users who were psychologically and/or physically abused were also

given the option of attending classes to help build their………………………..

11.9 Potential for abuse

Student Book 2
pp 96–99

Health and social care staff are often in a position of power over service users. Their professional relationships rely on them being trusted not to abuse this power. How can professionals and staff prove their trustworthiness in cases of doubt? Consider the following statements and then decide what action staff could take to protect their integrity and trustworthiness. Remember that policies and procedures are there to protect staff as well as service users. Discuss your options within your group, and note the most appropriate actions to take in each situation.

	Situation	Action
1	Service user has claimed neglect of care, stating that care staff have not been meeting their daily hygiene needs. How could the care worker prove she had undertaken the required tasks?	
2	Patient refuses a tetanus injection following a severe wound caused by falling onto rusty metal. Patient then complains that he was not given the correct treatment. How could evidence be provided that the treatment had been offered?	
3	Every time a carer arrives at a young male client's home, he is in a state of undress and exposes himself to her. How should she respond and whom should she inform?	
4	When booking clients into a residential home it is normal practice to record their valuables. It has been noted that the deputy manager does not complete the required paperwork. How would you address this as the manager?	
5	The fire brigade has responded to a number of false alarms at a care home for teenagers with behaviour difficulties. The manager has called a staff meeting to discuss the problem and has suggested that they disarm the smoke detectors in the building. As a staff member, how might you respond to his suggestion?	

11.10 Roles and responsibilities

Student Book 2
pp 96–99

Your tutor will give you one set of job title cards and another set of cards showing roles and responsibilities. You need to match each job title with the relevant role or responsibility.

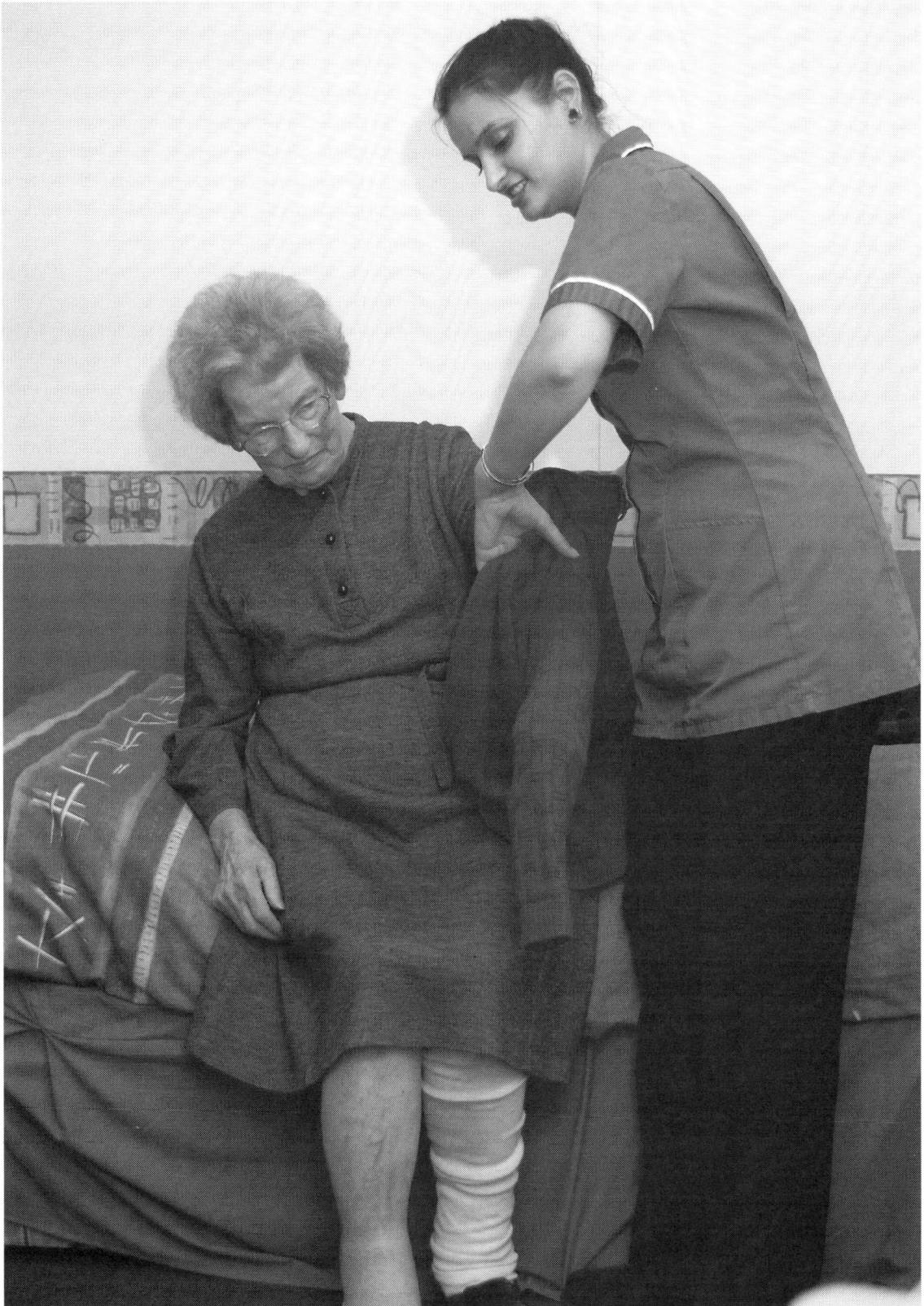

11.11 Multi-agency and multi-disciplinary support

Student Book 2
pp 96–99

The multi-disciplinary team

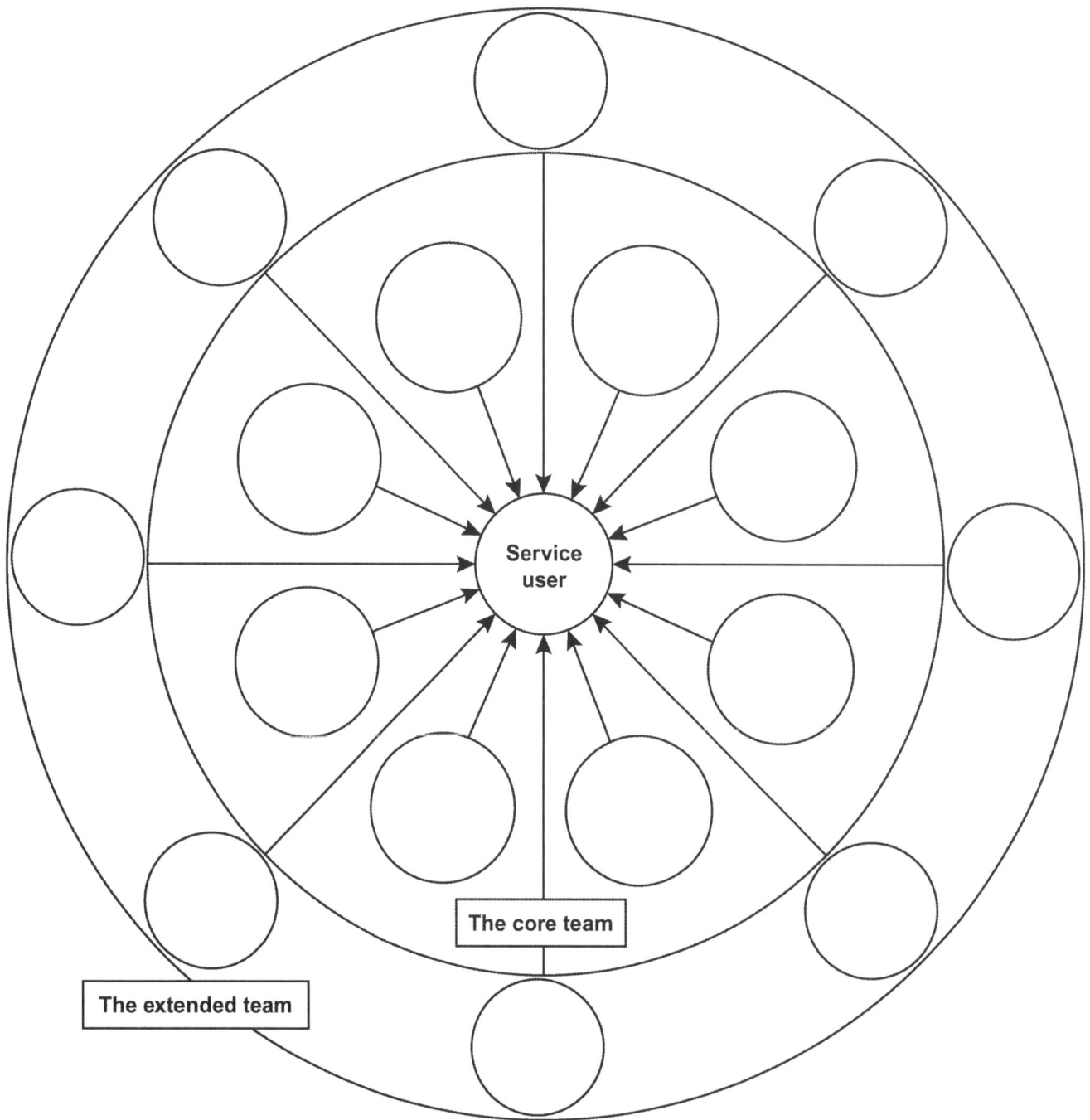

The core team

The extended team

Service user

Using the multi-disciplinary team wheel above, identify the team members who may be involved with the following cases:

1   an elderly man with dementia in a residential nursing home
2   a road traffic accident victim in a coma in an intensive care unit
3   a single man living alone, who is wheelchair-bound due to multiple sclerosis
4   a young woman with severe learning difficulties living in a shared community home
5   a single mother who is terminally ill with AIDS (acquired immune deficiency syndrome), who has three young children.

11.12 Understanding legislation

Student Book 2 pp 100–109

As a health and social care worker, you will need to understand the key points of legislation and which Act is relevant in any given situation. Legislation protects service users, staff that provide services, and organisations that provide health and social care facilities. Over the past five years, the government has brought in several new pieces of health and social care legislation. Health and care settings refer to this legislation when producing policies and procedures. Identify two key pieces of legislation that health and care settings use to protect vulnerable adults. Remember to include the dates of the Acts you mention. Then briefly explain how the legislation actually helps to protect vulnerable adults.

11.13 Understanding safe employment practices

Student Book 2 pp 100–109

When health and social care settings consider employing people to work with vulnerable adults they need to carry out a number of checks. All settings have an employment policy and procedure that is based on current employment regulations. Getting references, obtaining a Criminal Records Bureau check, checking qualifications and thorough interviewing are basic elements in this process.

How would you ensure that such procedures are carried out and that the results can be trusted?

- Draw up a checklist that can be used to ensure that checking procedures are carried out thoroughly and reliably.

- Design an advert for a local newspaper and professional magazine for a post of your choice in a health or social care setting.

- Write a list of interview questions that will help you gain an insight into the personality and suitability of candidates as well as revealing their previous experiences of working with vulnerable adults.

- Select an interview panel. Ensure that there is at least one person to represent personnel and the direct line manager. You may decide to have one or two more people, depending on the post you are interviewing for.

- Circulate your advert and issue application forms to members of your class.

- To complete this activity, carry out mock interviews and evaluate the interviewees' responses.

11.14 Clinical supervision

Student Book 2
pp 100–109

The term 'clinical supervision' refers to paired, small group and management support that is offered to all staff working within the National Health Service (NHS). Staff members are normally allocated a set amount of clinical supervision time per month, pro-rata to the hours they work. The time is used to discuss, confidentially, any issues relating either to another member of staff or to their own practice. Staff who facilitate clinical supervision have to undertake specific training to do so.

The clinical supervision system was brought in following the case of Nurse Beverly Allott, as several health care team members at the hospital where she worked had concerns about her practice and her responses to patients and families. This system allows staff to discuss issues relating to practice confidentially. It also offers support to staff in cases where poor practice has been identified. Dangerous practices clearly need to be reported without delay. However, a number of situations are referred to as 'grey areas'. It is these cases where support is most needed and group discussions involving professionals from different disciplines within the NHS can reveal different viewpoints.

In small groups, read the following case studies.

Case study 1: Concern raised by a staff nurse

Jane is a new member of the ancillary support team at a community hospital. Her duties include helping to meet patients' hygiene needs, serving food and drinks to patients, and keeping all the working areas tidy. Jane has no medical qualifications and is currently undertaking an NVQ in Care on a part-time basis. The staff nurse feels uneasy because she believes that Jane may be reading patients' medical notes and discussing medical issues with the patients. Twice in the last week the staff nurse has noted that the curtains have been pulled around a patient's bed. As there were no doctors on the ward at the time, she went to investigate. On each occasion Jane was sitting on the edge of the patient's bed with their observation notes, talking quietly with the patient. Jane got up and immediately hung the notes back on the bottom of the bed, saying 'Sorry, I knocked them down when I pulled the curtains', and left. There appeared to be no reason for the curtains to be pulled around the bed and the patient made no protest when they were drawn back. The second occasion was exactly the same, word for word, which made the staff nurse feel uneasy and so she asked why the curtains had been pulled. Jane said the patient asked for some privacy but then quickly moved away. The patient looked at the staff nurse and said 'She is a clever girl.'

Case study 2: Concern raised by a community home care worker

Jimmy has been working at a community home for over five years. The home has four female residents, all in their late twenties with various forms of learning difficulties. Staff work on a shift basis and this includes weekends and sleep-ins. Over the past couple of weeks Jimmy has seemed short-tempered and has started raising his voice when discussing issues with the residents. This is not like him at all. When asked if anything is

Continued overleaf

11.14 Clinical supervision (*contd*)

wrong he just says it's fine. When he was told he was shouting he looked upset and said he wasn't. The home is noisy most of the time, as the television is nearly always on and turned up loud. He has also started getting in to work late.

Case study 3: Concern raised by new health visitor (Pam)

Jill, the senior health visitor, never seems to visit any of the families in her case load that live in the poorer areas of the town. However, she appears to make regular visits to the families in the wealthy areas. During a staff meeting, when the team were discussing the new health promotion work they had to undertake by visiting different areas in the community, Pam noted that she was given one of the roughest areas and that Jill had not actually allocated herself an area at all. Pam said that she was nervous about going out on her own and asked if Jill could go with her. The rest of the team started to laugh and made comments about that being too low an area for Jill. Pam is concerned that this is discrimination, in relation to the families and to herself.

Case study 4: Concern raised by a community care worker (Julie)

Julie works in the community, visiting the elderly and disabled. Her morning duties include helping service users to get out of bed, get washed and dressed, and prepare breakfast. She returns to the same people in the evening and helps them get undressed, washed and into bed. Julie works Monday to Friday; the weekends are currently covered by agency staff. Julie is concerned because the past couple of Monday mornings, when she returned to one of her elderly service users, she noticed that she had bruises on her wrists. The elderly woman is not sure how she got them. Last Friday the woman asked Julie to tell the agency that she did not need anyone as her grand-daughter was coming to stay for the weekend. When Julie visited the woman on the Monday morning she could tell that she had not been washed and her nightwear had not been changed since those Julie used on the Friday. When talking with the woman it became clear that there was no planned visit from the grand-daughter. The service user just did not want the agency staff.

As a group, discuss each situation and draw up an action plan to address the issues. Remember that you are not managers so you cannot arrange training to send the member of staff on. However, you can make suggestions and involve the manager.

11.15 Unit review quiz

Student Book 2
pp 100–109

Working in groups of four or five, look back over the unit content and prepare a quiz. You will need 10 questions (and answers) for each round.

Each group should prepare 20 questions, just in case your question has already been used by another group. Then, in your teams, undertake the quiz on a Round Robin basis.

Remember to keep your questions clear and easy to understand. Build the difficulty level of the questions, and have a tie-breaker question ready in case of a tie.

Learning outcome 2: Understand the research methodology that is relevant to health and social care (relevant criteria: P2)

Although the second Learning outcome only has one pass criterion, it gives students a framework with which to complete the rest of the unit, and therefore requires a thorough approach. This outcome should focus on relevant examples and practical work in small groups. Students could set up and run some mini projects to explore the methodologies. These might include:

- comparing the experience of structured and unstructured interviews (Activity 22.4)
- creating a small questionnaire and using it to gather data (Activity 22.5)
- setting up and running experiments in class on learning and memory
- completing observations in placement (an excellent chance to link with Unit 44).

Other activities for this outcome include a simple quiz, which checks students' learning (Activity 22.3), and a game that prepares students for the complexities of conducting their own research (Activity 22.6).

Learning outcome 3: Be able to identify a suitable research project and produce a plan for a research proposal (relevant criteria: P3, M1)

The third Learning outcome deals with planning the research project. Students should start collecting articles on health and social care as soon as possible for their literature search. They should keep copies of anything interesting or relevant, including newspaper and magazine articles, recordings of TV or video programmes, websites, leaflets, textbook references, etc. Tutors should also collect materials, and use them to trigger class or group discussions. Activities 22.9 and 22.10 will help learners select relevant material. Discussing ideas like this can help students who are unsure about a topic to make an appropriate choice. Activity 22.7 focuses on choosing a manageable topic. This is often a very popular part of the unit, as it allows students to express their opinions on a number of issues that interest them. Many articles include references to other reports, and students should be encouraged to follow these up wherever possible. Journalists and authors often publish their email addresses, and this can be a very useful resource, as well as adding excitement! Activity 22.8 is a PowerPoint®-led activity which guides learners through the process of turning ideas into functional hypotheses.

At this stage, students will need to consider the practical limitations of their chosen research method. Wherever possible, they should run a pilot in order to iron out any problems. Learners will find it easier to plan their research projects if they use a checklist like the one in Activity 22.11. If they wish, students could use a project planning package to show evidence of their planning.

Learning outcome 4: Be able to conduct the research and present the findings (relevant criteria: P4, P5, M2)

The fourth Learning outcome is the practical component. This provides an excellent opportunity for students to achieve key skills criteria; and a team teaching approach with key skills tutors would work very well. At this stage, classes should run as clinics, with students able to call on one-to-one support from the tutor. Whole class teaching can be used to solve common problems, and to explore particular themes or ideas. Again, the Activity 22.11 checklist provides an invaluable tool, and learners should be encouraged to refer to their notes from Activities 22.2 to 22.5. Students will need good access to IT facilities in order to deal with statistical analyses and to produce their final report. Activities 22.15 and 22.17 provide students with worked examples that will guide them through some of the more common difficulties. At this stage, input from colleagues with maths, application of number and IT skills will be extremely useful.

Learning outcome 5: Be able to evaluate the research project (relevant criteria: P6, M2, M3, D1, D2)

Once their research is complete, many students may be disheartened if it has not gone exactly to plan. However, any flaws in their projects provide great opportunities to analyse their work and valuable evidence for the fifth learning outcome. If things do start to go wrong, you should encourage students to look at any problems as good learning opportunities. Activities 22.14, 22.16 and 22.18 will give students a chance to understand and apply the concepts needed to analyse their work objectively. Activity 22.20 brings all these themes together and allows students to share their experiences positively.

Learning outcome 6: Understand the implications of, and ethical issues related to, using research in health and social care (relevant criteria: P7, M4)

The sixth Learning outcome gives students a chance to reflect on their own and others' work, and place their work in a wider context. Students should be encouraged to debate and discuss the topics, especially controversial issues such as euthanasia or obesity. Activity 22.13 and 22.16 will allow for discussion of the issues, and tutors and learners may like to revisit Activity 22.1 for examples of how research results can affect current practice.

How this unit will be assessed

To reach Pass level, the evidence must show that the learner is able to:

P1   explain the purpose and role of research for the health and social care sectors
P2   describe the key elements of research methodology
P3   identify a research topic and carry out a literature search
P4   carry out the primary research and collect and record appropriate data
P5   present and report findings in a relevant format, identifying sources of bias or error
P6   discuss the findings of the research in relation to the original hypothesis
P7   outline any possible improvements to the research, referring to any relevant implications and ethical issues.

To reach Merit level, the evidence must show that, in addition to the Pass criteria, the learner is able to:

M1   justify the choice of topic and hypothesis
M2   review the research methods chosen in relation to the results obtained, any sources of bias or error and ethical considerations
M3   analyse the findings of the research in relation to the original hypothesis
M4   discuss the possible implications that the research results may have for current practice.

To reach Distinction level, the evidence must show that, in addition to the Pass and Merit criteria, the learner is able to:

D1   discuss how the methodology of the research project could be altered to reduce bias and error
D2   analyse the purpose and role of research in the health and social care sector, drawing on the piece of research undertaken.

Because of the large amount of work this unit requires, you need to ensure that students are managing their workload effectively. Students can use the Activity 22.11 checklist to keep track of each task, with projected and actual completion dates.

The research report will necessarily be a long piece of written work. Other Learning outcomes should therefore be assessed using other methods. This allows for differentiation across abilities and learning styles, and ensures that students remain fully engaged throughout the unit.

Assessment tasks

There are four Assessment tasks for this unit, as outlined below.

Task 1 (relevant criteria: P1, P2)

In groups, prepare a short PowerPoint® presentation (approximately 8 to 10 minutes long) to explain how and why research is carried out into health and social care. Alternatively, you could produce a set of information leaflets or posters.

Make sure you include:

- the purposes of research (at least three)
- the roles of research (at least five)
- qualitative and quantative research
- primary research, including questionnaires, experiments, interviews and observations
- secondary research, including the Internet, professional journals, books and the media.

Task 2 (relevant criteria: P3, M1)

For this task, you need to plan a suitable research project on a topic related to health and social care, and create a research hypothesis. Produce a suitable timeline for the project, including dates and plans for contingencies. This can be handwritten or produced using a software package. You should also have a literature file, containing properly referenced and indexed data. For the M1 criteria, you must include a short statement explaining why you have selected this topic, and how you have formed your hypothesis. This could be included at the front of the literature file.

In order to achieve the criteria, you will need to hand in:

- an indexed literature file, with appropriate notes and summaries
- a timeline, which details the tasks you need to complete, the dates you think you will complete them, and details of whatever resources or help you will need.

You will also have to hand in a statement of hypotheses. This should be about two A4 pages long, describing the secondary research you have undertaken, the key ideas you want to find out about, the method you plan to use, and what your research hypothesis will be.

Task 3 (relevant criteria: P4, P5, P6, M2, M3, D1)

This task involves carrying out the actual research, and producing a formal research report. This should include a range of evidence, including charts and graphs, and raw data in relevant appendices.

In order to achieve the criteria, you must:

- follow your plan from Task 2
- carry out your research project
- present your findings in a report.

Your report should be about six pages long, arranged in the following sections:

- abstract (a short description of the whole project)
- introduction (the background to your topic)
- method (what you actually did).

Make sure you include copies of all your data, including tally charts, completed questionnaires and interview notes. **(P4)**

Your findings refer to what you found out, and how this relates to your hypothesis. Your report should include graphs or charts, and detail any statistical calculations (e.g. percentages or proportions) you have used. **(P5)** Make sure you note down any problems you have had – you will not lose marks if you have made a mistake!

Restate your hypothesis and state whether you have accepted or rejected it, and say what this means. **(P6)**

Is it what you expected? **(M3)** Explain your answer in your findings section.

In your conclusions, say what it all means, and how you tackled any errors, bias or ethical issues.

Describe what you did to avoid bias, error and ethical problems. **(M2)**

Describe how changing the way you conducted your research could eliminate all bias, error or ethical problems in your project. **(D1)**

Task 4 (relevant criteria: P7, M4, D2)

For this task, you need to analyse and evaluate your research, focusing on how it could be improved and applied in practice. Students can provide evidence by keeping a journal as they carry out their project. The journal should describe the difficulties they have faced, and the ways in which they have overcome them.

To meet the criteria, write an essay entitled 'Implications of My Research'. This essay should be no more than 2000 words long.

Include the following questions:

- How could you make your research more useful?
- What would need to happen to make your findings relevant to current practice? **(P7)**

List all the weaknesses or difficulties you have identified in your research. For each difficulty or weakness, describe:

- what effect this could have on your participants (especially the ethical implications)
- what effect this could have on your results.

What has your research taught you that could be used in health or social care settings? Describe ways in which your research findings could be used in practice, and discuss any factors that could prevent this happening. **(M4)**

What have you learnt about the way research is used in the health and social care sector? **(D2)**

You may like to discuss:

- new skills you have learnt
- the limitations of research in this sector
- the ways in which research could be misused
- the problems of carrying out research in this sector
- the effect this type of research can have on participants, health and social care workers, and service users.

Scheme of work

BTEC National Health & Social Care
Unit 22 Research methodology for health and social care

Academic year: ....   **Number of weeks:** 35
Broad aim: Successful completion of the unit   **Duration of session:** 3 hours
Teacher(s): ....   **Guided learning hours:** 90

Week/s	Topic/outcome	Tutor preparation	Student activity	Resources	Links to grading criteria
1	Introduction of Learning outcomes 1 and 2	Whole class teaching for PowerPoint® presentation (explaining the purposes and roles of research)	Learners discuss the sample newspaper article and debate in what ways the article could be reliable or unreliable. Ask learners to debate whether they would accept the article or not	PowerPoint® 1, Activity 22.1	P1, P2
2–5	Gain an overview of research methodology	See Tutor information on CD for these two activities	Learners work in small groups to draw up a draft timeline (schedule) for a project. On completion, learners should justify their time decisions to the rest of the class. Learners can then individually, or in pairs, complete the timeline	Activity 22.2, Activity 22.3, flipchart, paper, pens	P1, P2
6–7	Learn how to conduct interviews	This task assumes learners have been on placement. If not, the task may need adapting accordingly (see CD)	Learners conduct role play interviews in pairs, first structured then unstructured, after which they complete a report	Activity 22.4	P2
8–9	Analyse questionnaire items	You may like to provide other examples of questionnaires for learners to consider	Learners can discuss the issues raised, and then prepare some questions of their own – some open, others subtly biased	Activity 22.5	P2
10–11	Consolidate knowledge and complete Assessment task 1	You can use the board game in Activity 22.6 to consolidate learners' knowledge (see Tutor information on CD)	Learners can also use this time to make their presentations for Assessment task 1	Activity 22.6	P1, P2
12–13	Choose a topic and write a hypothesis	You may wish to have a list of possible research topics	Learners can take notes on the presentation, before working with a partner or alone to decide on a research topic. Learners should discuss initial ideas with the rest of the class	PowerPoint® 2, Activity 2.7, Activity 22.8	P3, M1
14 (and ongoing)	Find research literature	You may need to arrange for learners to get help from library staff, and time in the library	Learners work in groups to prepare an initial literature file, before reporting their ideas back to the rest of the class	Activity 22.9, Activity 22.10	P3, P4, M1

[321]

Unit 22 Research methodology for health and social care

Week/s	Topic/outcome	Tutor preparation	Student activity	Resources	Links to grading criteria
14–15	Create a plan for the research project and complete Assessment task 2	Check that learners' plans include SMART objectives	Learners draw up an initial plan for their research project. They also check and record their progress on Assessment task 2, using the Activity 22.11 checklist	Activity 22.11	P4, P5, P6
15 (and ongoing)	Create and pilot instrument	Sessions should be run in clinic style	Learners create and pilot the instrument. They also check and record their progress on Assessment tasks 2, using the checklist	Activity 22.11	P4, P5, P6
15 (and ongoing)	Distribute questionnaires or complete interviews	Sessions should be run in clinic style	Learners distribute questionnaires or conduct interviews. They also check and record their progress on Assessment task 2	Activity 22.11	P4, P5, P6
16–17	Understand validity and reliability	Talk students through the research examples on this worksheet	Learners complete worksheet	Activity 22.12	P5, P7
18–19	Know how to deal with vulnerable client groups	Introduce concepts behind vulnerable client groups	Students should be encouraged to spend time discussing all the possible ethical issues in these three case study examples	Activity 22.13	P7, M2
20–21	Apply ethics	Split learners into groups of varying ability to work on the case studies	Activity 22.14 offers progressively more complex case studies for discussion	Activity 22.14	P7, M2, D1
22–27	Collate and analyse data	These activities deal with calculating averages and collating data. Support may be needed from application of number tutors	Ask learners to discuss the data issues in whole class situations, before splitting into groups to work through the examples	Activity 22.15, 22.16, 22.17	P4, P5, P6
28–30	Learn how to evaluate research, write up report and complete Assessment task 3	Sessions should be run in clinic style	Learners can take notes on the presentation before preparing written responses to the Activity 22.18 questions	PowerPoint® 3, Activity 22.18	P4, P5, P6
31	Explore findings and suggest improvements	Prepare by providing a range of current newspapers for learners to use, and encourage learners to share their work	Learners to work in groups and prepare a written report or presentation on the differences between two articles before a whole class discussion	Activity 22.19	P7, M4
32–33	Analyse research	You may wish to use witness statements or a video recording of this activity as evidence for the grading criteria	This activity gives students a chance to share their experiences and combine all the unit themes.	Activity 22.20	P4, P5, P6, M2 M3, D1
34–35	Recap unit and complete Assessment task 4	See crossword solution on CD	Learners to complete unit review crossword	Activity 22.21	P7, M4, D2
35	Upgrade and finalise Assessment tasks	Finalise Assessment tasks 1, 2, 3, 4	Learners to prepare individual answers to the assessment tasks		All

At-a-glance activity grid
Unit 22 Research methodology for health and social care

Activity	Title and description	Scheme of work	File/CD	Delivery notes	Additional resources	Links to grading criteria	Links to Student Book 1
Outcome 22.1 Understand the purpose and role of research within health and social care **Outcome 22.2 Understand the research methodology relevant to health and social care**							
Power Point® 1	Introduction of Learning outcomes 1 and 2	Week 1	CD	Introduce the purpose, role and methodology of research in health and social care	Tutors may wish to provide hard copies of the PPT presentation	P1, P2	pp 408–427
22.1	Identifying the role of research	Week 1	File	This activity includes a short article on smoking, followed by a set of questions and discussion points. Students can work alone or in pairs, reading the article and noting down their answers	Tutors can provide alternative articles	P1, M4	pp 408–427
22.2	Planning research	Weeks 2–3	File (Tutor information on CD)	In this small group activity learners create a research timeline by putting task cards in the correct order. Tutors may wish to record final timelines to distribute to the class later	Two sets of cards per group (prepared as described in the Tutor information on the CD)	P2, P3	pp 408–427
22.3	Research methodology quiz	Weeks 4–5	File (Tutor information on CD)	This simple quiz can be administered as photocopied sheets or orally. This would be an effective end-of-section activity		P2	pp 408–427
22.4	Conducting interviews	Weeks 6–7	File (Tutor information on CD)	Put students in two groups, then get them to compare their findings in order to compare and evaluate the two interviewing techniques (structured and unstructured)	Two classrooms, or a large room	P2	pp 408–427
22.5	Critical analysis of questionnaire items	Weeks 8–9	File	Students may wish to find more examples as homework. This activity should help students to design effective questionnaires for use in their own research project	Tutors may like to collect extra examples of flawed questionnaire items for discussion	P2	pp 408–427
22.6	The research game	Weeks 10–11	File (Tutor information on CD)	This is a light-hearted trip through the research process in the form of a board game. Students should play in teams, with either the tutor or another student as question master. Tutors may wish to have small prizes at the ready!	Game board, dice, a token per team, and category cards (prepared as described in the Tutor information on the CD), small prizes (optional)	P2	pp 408–427

Activity	Title and description	Scheme of work	File/CD	Delivery notes	Additional resources	Links to grading criteria	Links to Student Book 1
Outcome 22.3 Be able to identify a suitable research project and produce a plan for a research proposal **Outcome 22.4 Be able to conduct the research and present the findings**							
Power Point® 2	Introduction of Learning outcomes 3 and 4	Week 12	CD	Introduce the planning and presentation of research	Tutors may wish to provide hard copies of the PPT presentation	P3, P4, P5, M1, M2	pp 428–452
22.7	Choosing a topic	Weeks 12–13	File	Students learn how to turn a topic into a research question		P3, M1	pp 428–452
22.8	Writing hypotheses	Week 13	CD	This activity is a PPT presentation with accompanying questions. Tutors should print hard copies that include the questions	Hard copies of the PPT presentation	P3, M1	pp 428–452
22.9	The literature file	Week 14 and ongoing	File	This activity gives guidance on collecting appropriate literature or research. It should be paired with Activity 22.10. Following this activity, students should be encouraged to visit their LRC and begin collecting data. Once students have begun to collect data, tutors should organise one-to-one sessions to enable them to decide on a single topic for their project	LRC resources	P3, M1	pp 428–452
22.10	Finding literature	Week 14	File	This is a group task that explores different sources of secondary information	LRC resources	P3, P4, M1	pp 428–452
22.11	Project checklist	Week 15 and ongoing	File	This checklist breaks the project into manageable tasks with time-specific outcomes This is an ongoing task, which should be used to help plan and support students' work		P4, P5, P6	pp 428–452
22.12	Validity and reliability	Weeks 16–17	File	Tutors should talk students through the research examples on this worksheet		P5, P7	pp 428–452
22.13	Vulnerable client groups	Weeks 18–19	File	This activity involves three case study examples. Students should be encouraged to spend time discussing all the possible ethical issues, and may like to produce their own hypothetical research situations		P7, M2	pp 428–452
22.14	Applying ethics	Weeks 20–21	File	Activity 22.14 offers progressively more complex case studies for discussion		P7, M2, D1	pp 428–452
22.15	Means, modes and medians	Weeks 22–23	File	This worksheet explains how to calculate means, modes and medians using simple worked examples. Tutors may want to link this with work from Key skills: application of number	Calculators	P4	pp 428–452
22.16	Bias and error	Weeks 24–25	File	This activity should provide a framework for a tutor-led discussion on bias and error		P7	pp 428–452

Activity	Title and description	Scheme of work	File/CD	Delivery notes	Additional resources	Links to grading criteria	Links to Student Book 1
22.17	Using Excel®	Weeks 26–27	File	This practical activity uses a worked example of simple graph drawing. It should be adapted to differentiate between more able and less able learners. Students should be encouraged to use their own project results	Access to computers with Excel®	P4	pp 428–452
Outcome 22.5 Be able to evaluate the research project Outcome 22.6 Understand the implications of, and ethical issues related to, using research in health and social care							
Power Point® 3	Introduction of Learning outcomes 5 and 6	Week 28	CD	Introduce the evaluation of research	Tutors may wish to provide hard copies of the PPT presentation		pp 452–463
22.18	Drawing conclusions	Weeks 28–30	File	This activity gives some example results to illustrate how to draw out the meaning from data. Questions become gradually more complex to allow differentiation by ability		P6, P7, M3, D1	pp 452–463
22.19	The role of the media	Week 31	File	Activity 22.19 compares the way research is reported by different media. Tutors should prepare by providing a range of current newspapers for learners to use	Current newspapers		pp 452–463
22.20	Evaluation	Weeks 32–33	File	This activity gives students a chance to share their experiences and combine all the unit themes. Tutors may wish to use witness statements or a video recording of this activity as evidence for the grading criteria		P6, P7, M4, D2	pp 452–463
22.21	End-of-unit crossword	Weeks 34–35	File (Answers on CD)	Tutors might like to use this crossword twice (once at the start and once at the end of the unit) to demonstrate attainment		All	pp 452–463

Unit 22 Lesson plan

Aims

- To introduce Unit 22
- To relate the unit aims to examples of recent research.

This structure may be spread over a number of lessons as required.

Learning outcomes • be able to list the Learning outcomes for this unit • be able to describe examples of research in health and social care • be able to discuss key issues in research.					
Timing	**Content**	**Teacher activity**	**Student activity**	**Resources**	**Individualised activity**
5 mins	Introduction to Unit 22	Tutor to display lesson aims and objectives on flipchart		Flipchart	
20 mins	PowerPoint® presentation	Ask questions to check understanding	Learners to answer questions and contribute to discussion	PowerPoint® 1	Copies of PPT with note spaces to be made available for those who require them
30 mins	Small group work	Tutor gives each group an article to discuss, from Activity 22.1	Learners answer worksheet questions on article, and produce a flipchart poster about it	Activity 22.1, materials for making posters, flipchart	Groups can be allocated according to ability. Other articles can be selected according to complexity to match group ability. Group roles (e.g. scribe, spokesperson, artist, etc) can reflect learning styles
20 mins	Presentaton of posters		Each group to describe their article to the whole class using their poster		Visual learners can be encouraged to make flipchart posters. More confident ones can speak for the group
10 mins	Plenary discussion of issues and themes raised	Tutor can guide learners to add any key points that have been missed, and reinforce lesson themes	Learners hand worksheets in for assessment at the end of the session		
5 mins	Recap	Whole class teaching to highlight where lesson objectives have been achieved. Ask directed questions to check understanding	Learners to answer direct questions		

22.1 Research example: Smoking in the workplace

Student Book 1
pp 408–427

The question of whether or not people should be allowed to smoke at work raises a number of controversial issues. Read the article below and then answer the following:

1   Where is the article from?

2   Is this a reliable source of information?

3   Who is interviewed in this article?

4   What was the purpose of this research?

5   Which organisation conducted the research?

6   Is this organisation likely to be biased?

7   What has been changed by this research?

8   How could this research affect health and social care policies in the UK?

9   How could this affect small businesses?

10   How could this research affect smokers and non-smokers?

Firms urged to give smokers time off with pay to try to kick habit

People who smoke should be allowed to take time off work to attend smoking clinics to help them give up without any loss of pay, according to new public health recommendations.

The National Institute for Health and Clinical Excellence has issued the guidelines for every workplace in England, in preparation for the smoking ban in enclosed public places starting on July 1.

The independent organisation claims the proposal will cut the £5bn annual cost of loss of productivity, absenteeism and fire damage caused by employees who smoke and believes businesses will save money based on the increased productivity by helping employees to stop smoking.

This is the first time the institute has issued guidance that applies beyond the NHS, effectively including every workplace in England, all of which will be bound by the July 1 ban whether they be offices, factories or pubs.

The recommendations include making information on local stop-smoking services widely available at work and, where there is sufficient demand, providing on-site support for stopping smoking.

The institute believes a business with 20 employees, of which typically five would smoke, could spend £66 providing advice and make an overall saving of £350, which is based on increased productivity.

Andrew Dillon, chief executive of the institute, said the advice was the best way of achieving smoke-free environments that would benefit both employers and employees. "Our advice is based on the best evidence of which workplace approaches are effective for smokers and make business sense for employers."

In the first year after a smoking ban was introduced in Scotland in March 2006, figures revealed that smokers had made more than 46,000 attempts to quit, and more than a third of those who had tried to give up cigarettes said they had not smoked a month after quitting.

Smoking costs the NHS an estimated £1.5bn a year. It provides stop-smoking sessions which usually last 14 hours and run for a six-to-seven week period. Those who attend the course spend two weeks preparing to stop, with meetings of two hours once a week. Once they quit, there are a further five meetings to attend and figures show that one in two people have given up smoking by the end.

Amanda Sandford, research manager at the charity Action on Smoking and Health, said: "Providing employees are offered help and directed to services with a good track record, this seems to be a very sound policy and will reap benefits for the individual and the employer."

But Simon Clark, director of Forest, the Freedom Organisation for the Right to Enjoy Smoking Tobacco, said it was "absolutely ridiculous" that workers should attend stop-smoking clinics during working hours.

"It's wrong to expect employers to accept employees taking time off, and I imagine their non-smoking colleagues will be very unhappy about it," he said.

"It's generally acknowledged these quit-smoking courses are not very successful – it's a matter for willpower."

Lee Glendinning, the *Guardian*, 25 April 2007 (Copyright © Guardian News & Media Ltd 2007)

22.2 Planning a research project

Student Book 1
pp 408–427

For this activity, you will be working in small groups. Your tutor will give each group two sets of cards. One set of cards shows stages in the planning of your research project. The other set of cards shows weeks numbered from 1 to 20. You will also need some flipchart paper and pens.

You need to arrange the tasks in order, and work out how long each task will take. The end result should be a timeline, including all the tasks needed to complete the research project.

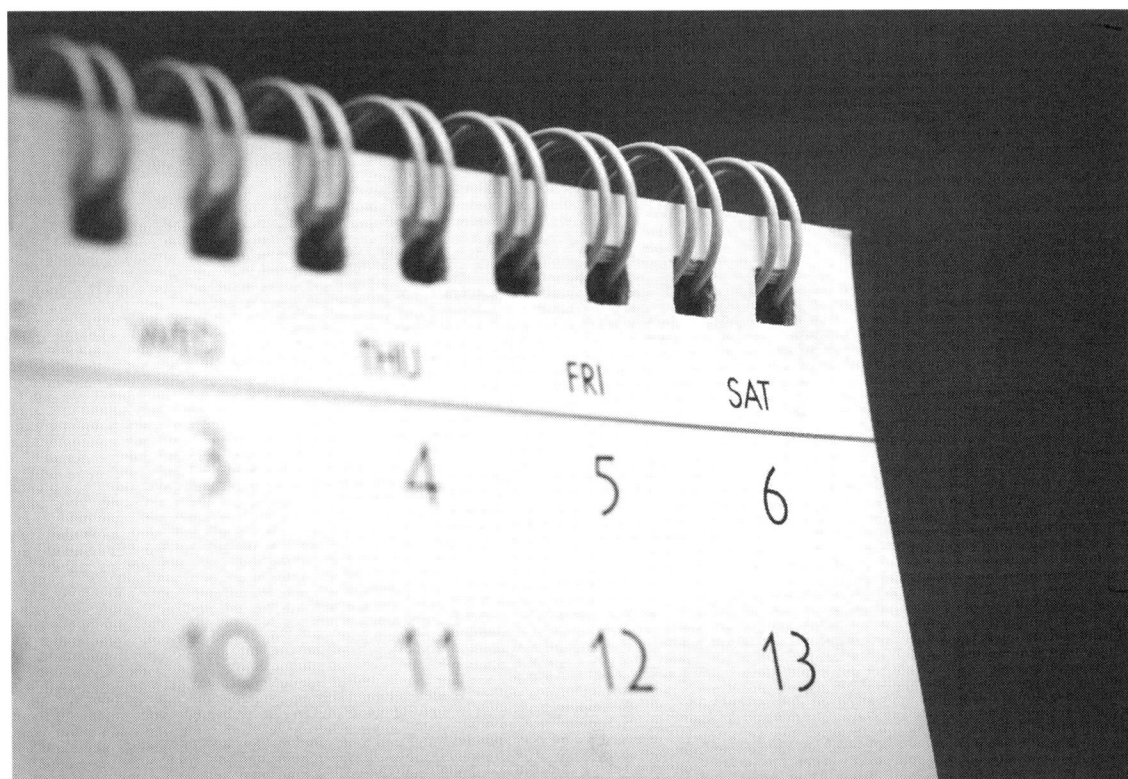

22.3   Primary research methodology: A quiz

Student Book 1
pp 408–427

Part 1: Methods

1   Which research method would you use to ask lots of people the same questions?

2   Which research method studies how people behave under controlled conditions?

3   Which research method involves watching people carefully?

4   What type of interview carefully follows a list of questions?

5   What type of interview allows the interviewer to ask any question they choose?

6   Name three ways in which a questionnaire can be conducted.

7   Which method would you use to investigate care home residents' diets?

8   Which method would you use to investigate how people's reaction times slow down with age?

Part 2: Methods in practice

1   Who should be asked permission before you can conduct research with hospital patients?

2   Which method is best for gathering lots of people's opinions?

3   What is the term used for a test run of a questionnaire or interview schedule?

4   In an experiment, what is the 'independent variable'?

5   In an experiment, what is the 'dependent variable'?

6   How many questionnaires should you use to have a good-sized sample?

7   Why is it important to plan observations carefully?

8   What details should you record during an observation?

9   What do we mean when we say research will be kept confidential?

10   How would you keep participants' identities anonymous?

Part 3: Identifying problems

1   What does it mean if research is described as 'reliable'?

2   What does it mean if research is described as 'valid'?

3   What is a 'confounding variable'?

4   What is a 'correlation'?

5   Which method claims to show cause and effect?

6   Define 'ecological validity'.

7   Can you give an example of a 'leading question'?

8   What is an 'experimenter expectancy effect'?

9   What should you do if a participant does not want to be in your study any longer?

10   Why should questionnaires and interview schedules be piloted?

11   What is a code of ethics? Can you give an example of a code of ethics?

12   Why do we need to use statistical tests?

22.4 Conducting interviews

Student Book 1
pp 408–427

For this activity, your tutor will put you in two groups and allocate one of the following interview schedules to your groups. Within your groups, you need to get into pairs to conduct interviews.

Group 1: Interview schedule

Carry out a structured interview with your partner. Please read the following questions carefully. Then ask them, in order, and take notes of the answers in the spaces below.

1   What is your current placement?

2   Do you find placement enjoyable?

3   What is the best thing about your placement?

4   What is the worst thing about your placement?

5   What is the most important thing you have got from your placement?

6   What could college do to improve your experience of placements?

7   Would you recommend your current placement to other students?

8   Are there any other comments you would like to make about placement?

Continued overleaf

22.4 Conducting interviews (*contd*)

Group 2: Interview schedule

Carry out an unstructured interview. Ask your partner about their current placement, and do your best to get as much qualitative information from them as you can. Make whatever notes you feel are appropriate on a separate piece of paper.

Interviews: Task feedback

As the class discusses the interview task, complete the table below with the points raised.

Method	Advantages	Disadvantages
Structured interview		
Unstructured interview		

Do you think there is another way to conduct an interview that would combine the advantages of both methods? Make some notes on a separate piece of paper about how you could do it.

22.5 Constructing questionnaires

Student Book 1
pp 408–427

According to the *Oxford English Dictionary*, a questionnaire is:
'A formulated series of questions by which information is sought from a selected group, usually for statistical analysis; a document containing these'.

This activity looks at some common problems in creating questionnaires. It provides good background and structure for the P4, M2, P7 and D1 criteria. The questions you use on a questionnaire need to be simple to understand, and simple to answer. Here are some examples of possible survey questions. See if you can identify any problems with them. Can you write better versions?

---

1 The dangerous and filthy habit of smoking is becoming far too widespread nowadays.
   Do you:
   a) Agree
   b) Disagree

2 How much alcohol do you drink each week?
   a) None
   b) 1–5 units
   c) 5–15 units
   d) 15+ units

3 Excluding domiciliary standing charges, normal rate taxation and privately owned investment income, what was your pro rata annual income last financial year?

4 When flying, would you prefer it if the passenger in front could not lower their seat back into your personal space?
   a) Yes
   b) No

5 Please select the person who should run your college from now on:
   a) Coco the Clown
   b) Barney the Dinosaur
   c) Hannibal Lecter
   d) Mickey Mouse

6 On average, how often do you have sex?
   a) Never
   b) Once a month
   c) Once a week
   d) Every day

Questions on a questionnaire are usually called 'items', and the questionnaire is often called the 'instrument'. When you write questions, it is important to make sure they are not:

- **Biased:** Question 1 is obviously biased, but what about question 4? This is very similar to a real item used by a low-cost airline. They wanted to save money by putting fixed seats in all their aircraft. They knew many people would prefer seats that reclined, so they gave customers this carefully worded question in order to prove that people really wanted fixed seats. Can you reword the question in favour of those people who like to lie back and relax on aeroplanes?

Continued overleaf

22.5 Constructing questionnaires (*contd*)

■ **Too technical:** Question 2 looks simple enough at first. But it assumes the respondent (the person answering the questions) knows what a unit of alcohol is. What could happen if the respondent did not know the meaning of a unit of alcohol?

■ **Jargon:** Question 3 is confusing, and unlikely to get an accurate answer, or any answer at all!

■ **Too limited**: It's very likely that you wouldn't want any of the people in question 5 running your college, but there is no option to say none of the above. It is often wise to give respondents an open-ended question such as 'other – please give details'. That way you get responses you had not anticipated, that you might otherwise have missed.

■ **Too personal**: Question 6 is likely to cause offence. It might also cause other difficulties. If you gave this question to men you would probably get a very different set of answers from the ones you would receive from women. There are times when you may need to ask personal questions like this, but you must be sure you have done everything possible to protect your respondent's confidentiality.

Most questionnaires try to measure two things. For example, you might want to investigate how the use of prescription medicines varies according to people's age or social group. In that case it is best to ask people easy questions first. You might want to start by asking about age, occupation, postcode and income, then move onto questions about visits to the doctor and number of prescriptions. (Bear in mind that many people lie about, or simply don't know, their annual income!) Starting with easy questions prevents people being put off by the questionnaire, and they are therefore more likely to complete it.

22.6 The research game

Student Book 1
pp 408–427

Your objective is to complete a research project by collecting a card for every category on the board.

Throw the dice and follow the numbered squares on the board. When you reach a question square, your tutor will ask you a question related to the category on the square. When you have gone round the board and collected a card for every category, you can move into the centre and answer a final question to win.

The game board is a circular shape, with 'spokes' pointing to a central hub. Around the edge are the following categories:

- choosing a topic

- hypotheses

- samples

- methods

- analysis

- bias and ethics.

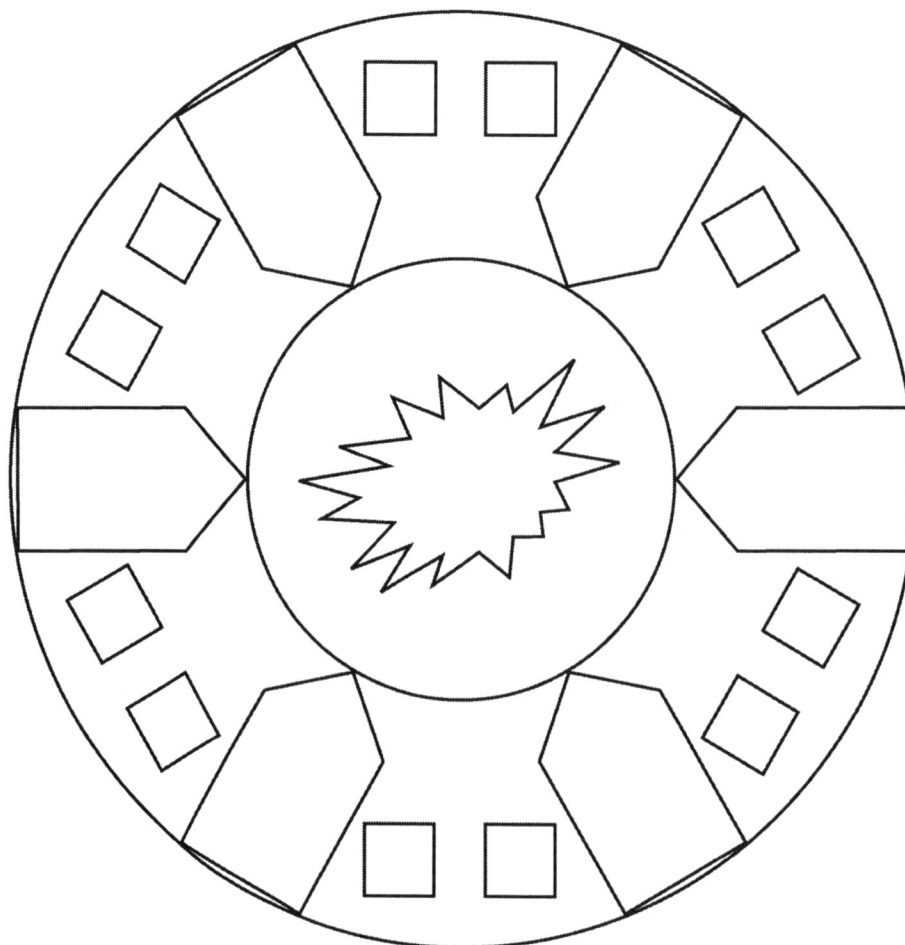

22.7   Choosing a research topic

Student Book 1
pp 428–452

This activity will help you select a suitable research topic. First work on your own and write down as many health and social care research subjects as you can think of.

Your tutor will then write everyone's answers on the board, and show you how to turn a topic into a research question. For example, the topic 'childhood obesity' could be turned into one of the following research questions:

■ Are children's diets different today from the way they were twenty years ago?

■ Are obese children bullied more?

■ Do children understand what makes a balanced diet?

Next, pick two or three topics that you think are interesting. You don't have to choose a final topic yet; just choose some that you like the sound of.

Working alone, or with a partner, fill in the following table for each topic.

Topic	How interesting is this to me?	What question(s) will I ask?	Possible sources of information	Possible problems I will face	Ethical concerns that might arise

Now look at the completed table. Does any topic seem easier to work on? Perhaps, as you filled in your answers, one topic seemed easier than the others? Use your reflections to help you choose a suitable topic.

22.9 Compiling a literature file

Student Book 1
pp 428–452

Assessment task 2 (see p 319) requires you to carry out a literature search, and produce a research hypothesis. To do this you will need to gather literature from a range of sources. Your first task is to gather information about the topic you want to study. At this stage you can be very wide ranging, and include *anything* that gets you thinking about your topic.

Here are some examples of the type of material you could collect (or make copies of, or make notes on):

- newspaper articles
- books
- websites/web pages
- magazine articles
- radio programmes
- television programmes/news reports
- records of conversations
- advertisements
- leaflets and brochures
- pictures, photographs and cartoons.

This will be the start of your literature search.

It is important to get organised at this stage, before your filing gets out of control!

1 Put everything together in a file. (Eventually this will be your project file.)

2 Make sure everything you collect has reference details. For websites, this will be the website address and the date you accessed it. (If possible, print a copy of the relevant page.) For newspapers and magazines, record the name of the publication, the date and the page number.

3 Keep an index of all your articles with a quick summary of the contents. This will save you going through lots of paper to find a single fact.

4 Your summary could include marks out of five for how relevant each piece is.

5 Use highlighters and notes on the text to single out the most important points.

6 As you collect more material, arrange it according to sub-topics.

The easiest way to compile a literature file is to do it as part of your everyday life. You will probably want to choose a topic that you are learning about in another unit, and the resources you use for other units could be very useful. Remember to use a variety of sources. Your literature review must include primary and secondary sources, and appropriate graphs and illustrations. Start collecting them now.

22.10 Finding literature

Student Book 1
pp 428–452

In your groups think of as many possible sources of information about your topic as you can, and how you are likely to find them. Record your findings in the table below. The first entry (for textbooks) is an example. Be imaginative!

Source of information	How to find it	Advantages	Drawbacks
Textbooks	Library, bookshops, online bookshops, friends, college department	Relevant, often free to use, easy to find	May be out of date, or too general

22.11 Project checklist

Student Book 1
pp 428–452

This is a checklist of all the tasks you will need to complete for Assessment tasks 2 and 3 (p 319). Please keep the list at the front of your project file and bring it to every session. This will help you keep up to date. You don't have to complete the tasks in order, but you should aim to complete one every week. This unit does involve a lot of work, but spreading it out across the year will make it much easier.

Remember, the work you do in research methodology should give you all the information and skills you need to complete all the basic elements of your project. Use class time wisely to get the help and advice you need and to complete the tasks listed below.

Project checklist

Name: ....

Project title: ....

Task	Grading criteria	Target completion date	Actual completion date	Comments/actions to take
Compile literature file	P3			
Write literature review	P3			
Describe your topic, and explain why you chose it	P3, M1			
Write statement of hypotheses	P3			
Create instrument (questionnaire/interview schedule)	P4			
Pilot instrument	P4			
Update instrument	P4			

Continued overleaf

22.11 Project checklist (*contd*)

Task	Grading criteria	Target completion date	Actual completion date	Comments/actions to take
Distribute questionnaires	P4			
Complete interviews	P4			
Collate questionnaire data	P4			
Analyse data/create graphs etc.	P3			
Write abstract	P5			
Write up method	P5			
Write up findings and conclusion	P5			
Relate findings to hypothesis	P6, M2			
Identify any sources of bias	P7, M3			
Identify any sources of error	P7, M3			
Identify any ethical issues raised by your project	P7, M4			
Create file index and appendices	P5			
Suggest improvements to your project	P7, D1			

Continued overleaf

22.11 Project checklist (*contd*)

Task	Grading criteria	Target completion date	Actual completion date	Comments/actions to take
Discuss how your results could influence practice	M4			
Check completed work against assignment brief	All			
Make any necessary changes, make a copy	All			
Hand in assignment	All			
Celebrate!	All			

22.12 Understanding validity and reliability

Student Book 1
pp 428–452

Researchers need to be sure that their work is both reliable and valid. Completing this worksheet will enable you to define, explain and apply the concepts of validity and reliability.

Validity is

....

....

....

Reliability is

....

....

....

Consider the following cases. Will they provide reliable, valid data? What could you do to make them more reliable and more valid?

1   I want to find out what the parents of a pre-school class of children do for a living, so I decide to ask each child to tell me.

   Reliable   yes/no

   Valid   yes/no

   Comments ....

2   A large soft drink company organises free tickets for students at a popular nightclub. The evening is part of the launch of Munki, a new banana- and peanut-flavoured drink. At the end of the evening the students each fill out a questionnaire on their favourite drinks.

   Reliable   yes/no

   Valid   yes/no

   Comments ....

3   Five different observers are asked to measure the number of anti-social behaviours they see in a shopping mall between 2 p.m. and 3 p.m. on a Saturday.

   Reliable   yes/no

   Valid   yes/no

   Comments ....

Continued overleaf

22.12 Understanding validity and reliability (*contd*)

4 A group of students is given an assignment brief that is confusing and full of errors. The brief is then changed to be clear and easy to understand, and given to a second group. Is this a valid and reliable way to measure achievement for both groups?

Reliable   yes/no

Valid   yes/no

Comments ....

5 A recruitment company gives all candidates a typing test. Those with the highest scores are labelled the best candidates, and given the best-paid assignments.

Reliable   yes/no

Valid   yes/no

Comments ....

6 A local council decide to build new houses on the site of a local play park. They sent observers to the park for three consecutive Tuesday mornings in October, and saw no children playing there.

Reliable   yes/no

Valid   yes/no

Comments ....

7 A well-known film actress recently blamed her increase in weight on the elasticated waists in her favourite skirts. She thought that as long as she could still get into those skirts her weight was not a problem.

Reliable   yes/no

Valid   yes/no

Comments ....

8 I've just written a new intelligence test. How can I check whether it is valid and reliable?

9 Using a questionnaire, I asked people if they liked spinach and Brussels sprout flavoured crisps. A total of 95 per cent said they loved them. I was rather surprised at this result. How can I find out if the question I asked was reliable and valid?

10 How could you measure the average number of cars in the college car park in a way that was reliable and valid?

22.13 Dealing with vulnerable client groups

Student Book 1
pp 428–452

When we conduct research we need to ensure that ethical issues are taken into account, particularly when dealing with vulnerable clients. Consider the following cases. Then, for each one, suggest ways in which you could ensure that people taking part in the research are treated ethically.

1   Samir wants to find out about bullying among young adults with learning difficulties. He has heard from a friend who works in the day-care facility nearby that some of the young people who go there have talked about being abused by others. Samir plans to go and interview them.

2   Rosie and Emily want to find out if older people are more forgetful than younger people. They have set up a fast-moving memory game on the computer. They plan to use it with their classmates at college, and also with the residents of a local care home.

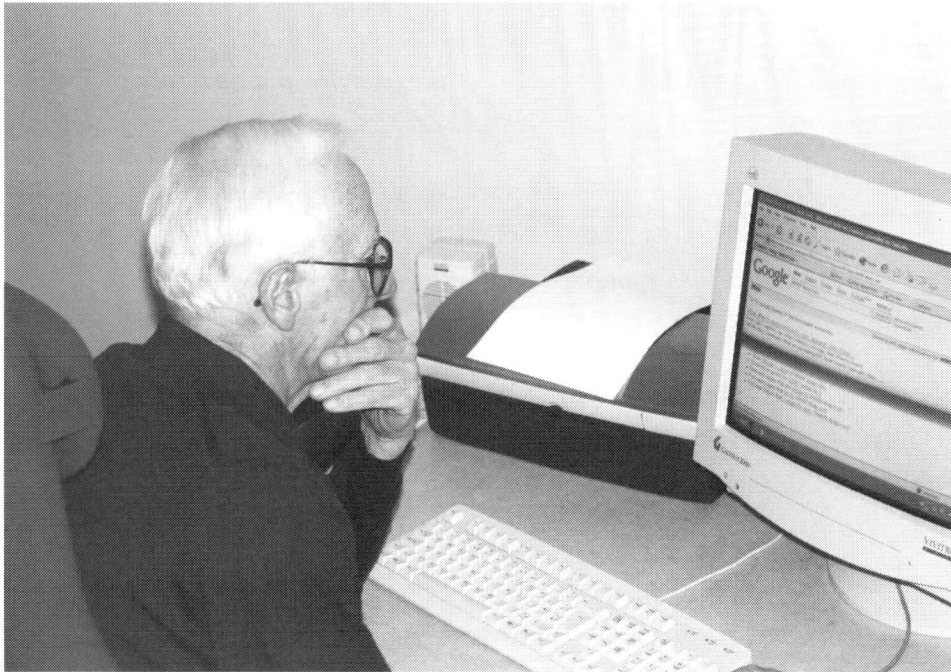

3   To find out about drug use in her area, social worker Amanda has set up some focus groups at her local youth club, involving young people who she knows have experimented with drugs. She plans to use her findings in an article for the local newspaper.

22.14 Applying ethics

Student Book 1
pp 428–452

Consider the cases below. Then, for each one, suggest ways in which you could ensure that people taking part in the research are treated ethically.

Remember the following:

■ consent

■ confidentiality

■ the right to withdraw

■ deception

■ debriefing

■ protection from harm (physical and emotional).

1 During his placement at a primary school, Jamil has been asking children about their experiences in a school with a special needs unit.

2 In her project on depression, Nikki writes about a friend's mother, who has attempted suicide. She includes her age, her profession, the ages of her three children, and a short physical description.

3 To find out how helpful people are in an emergency, a group of college students set up a pretend accident in the town centre. This involves a skateboarder crashing into a mother pushing a pram. The baby (a doll) will be thrown to the ground, and the 'mother' will pretend to be badly hurt.

4 Mrs Hillman completed a questionnaire for a student who comes in to help at her care home. She cannot remember much about it, but is distressed because she knows she answered some personal questions. The student has not been back, and Mrs Hillman does not know what the questionnaire was for.

5 Elliott was running late with his project, so he made up some data. His results now suggest that most students on his course have used abusive language towards service users during their placement. Elliott's tutor is very concerned, and is going to discipline all the students.

22.15 Means, modes and medians

Student Book 1
 pp 428–452

At the end of this activity you will be able to calculate means, modes and medians, and explain when you would use each one.

First, you need to collect a data set. This is a set of measurements or scores. For example, each member of the class could record the number of text messages they have sent in the last week. Here is a data set as an example:

2, 12, 12, 19, 19, 20, 20, 20, 25

Write your own data set in the box below.

> My data set

To calculate the mean:
First, add all the numbers together. For the example data, this would be:

2 + 12 + 12 + 19 + 19 + 20 + 20 + 20 + 25 = 149

Second, divide the total (149) by the number of individual scores (9).

$\frac{149}{9}$ = 16.56   So the example mean is 16.56.

Write your own mean in the box below.

> My calculated mean

Look again at the example mean. Can you suggest a problem with that figure? How would you deal with it?

To calculate the median:
First, rank the data. This means putting the lowest number first, then the next lowest, and so on (in ascending order), and give each number a rank:

2	12	12	19	19	20	20	20	25
1	**2**	**3**	**4**	**5**	**6**	**7**	**8**	**9**

Continued overleaf

22.15 Means, modes and medians (*contd*)

The median is the number with the middle rank. In this case the middle rank is 5, as it is exactly in the middle of 1 and 9. The median is therefore **19**.

```
My median
```

The example above has an odd number of test scores. What if there is an even number of test scores, as in the example below?

Scores:	2	12	12	19	19	20	20	20	25	26
Rank positions:	1	2	3	4	5	6	7	8	9	10

In this case, the median is halfway between the fifth and sixth numbers (19 and 20). The median is therefore **19.5**.

To find the mode:

The mode is simply the score that occurred most often. So, in the example, the mode is **20**.

```
My mode
```

Now compare the three types of averages. In the example they are 16.56, 19 and 20.

```
My three averages
```

Look at your own averages above and answer the following questions:

■ Which is most useful and why?

■ When would you be most likely to use a mean average?

■ When would you be most likely to use a mode average?

■ When would you be most likely to use a median average?

■ Why would you calculate all three?

22.16 Understanding bias and error

Student Book 1
pp 428–452

This is a discussion activity that will help you understand the issues of bias and error. Read the statements and questions, discuss them in small groups and note down your responses.

First, can you define the following three terms?
- bias
- prejudice
- discrimination.

Bias in research

Imagine that I told you about a survey on children's diets. The results of this survey indicate that children who eat fast food once or twice a week are just as healthy as those who never eat fast food.

What do you think about these findings?

What if the survey was sponsored by:
- the government
- a chain of fast-food restaurants
- an organic farmers' association?

In each case, how would your reaction to the results change?

When you read about this type of research, do you ever check who has carried it out?

Biased researchers

We are all biased (yes, even you!) – but some biases are positive. What type of biases do you have that could affect your research?

Biased participants

What if I said to you now: 'Tell me the very worst thing you know about the person sitting next to you'?

Would you tell the truth?

Why not?

Imagine that a fantastically good-looking researcher asks you to answer a questionnaire.

You notice they have a Vegetarian Society badge on.

What do you say if they ask: 'Are you vegetarian?'

Unconscious bias

Often, we don't realise that we are biased.

Think about this question:

'What time should a five-year-old go to bed?'

a) 5–6 p.m.   b) 6–7 p.m.   c) 7–8 p.m.

Where is the bias here?   *Continued overleaf*

[347]

22.16 Understanding bias and error (*contd*)

Expectancy effects

Imagine that you are expecting two parcels for your birthday. One is from your rich caring auntie, the other is from your rather mean, eccentric auntie. Neither parcel is labelled. One is large, and beautifully wrapped in expensive paper. The other is small and has been shoved in a supermarket carrier bag.

Which parcel is from which auntie?

How did you decide?

How could these types of decisions affect research?

If we do not treat participants objectively, we risk expectancy effects having an impact on our results.

These expectancy effects can be reduced by:
- making participants anonymous
- asking someone to check your results
- not using friends and family as participants
- using uniform instruments.

Demand characteristics

People who volunteer to take part in research are generally helpful types. So they help, by trying to give the researcher the responses they think the researcher wants. Others try to guess what the research is about and give the 'right' answers.

Can you give some examples of the sorts of answers people might give?

Types of bias

Researcher expectancy effects: This is when the researcher's biases affect the results

Demand characteristics: This is when the participant does what they believe the researcher wants

Can you think of some more examples of each?

Errors

If you make errors in your other assignments, it's bad news!

But if you make errors doing your research project, it's good news, because you can use them as part of your review and evaluation.

Where do errors come from?
- The maths: Statistics can be tricky, and it's easy to get things wrong. How can you minimise errors in your calculations?
- The instrument: How can you make sure your questionnaire or interview schedule is effective, valid and reliable?
- The planning: What do you need to include in your plan to make sure your research project is a success?

22.17 Using Excel®

Student Book 1
pp 428–452

Although there are many computer packages available to process and present statistical information, the one you are most likely to have access to is Microsoft Excel®. This activity will guide you through the process of producing a bar chart for your project report.

1 First you need a data set. This is a list of your results, like the one below, which records the medical conditions among 50 elderly residents of a care home.

Coronary heart disease	28
Arthritis	31
Hearing loss	19
Loss of limb	2
Diabetes	14
Atherosclerosis	19
Parkinson's disease	12
Depression	6
Senile dementia	34
Asthma	16
Other unspecified	44

2 Next you need to insert your data into Excel®. Open a new file and then you can either type the data in. Or, if you have it in a word processor like Microsoft Word, you can copy and paste it in. It should then look like the one above.

3 Next, select your whole table by right-clicking on the top left-hand corner until a little cross in a box appears. Then drag your cursor over the table until all the cells are selected.

4 Now go to **Chart Wizard**, by clicking on the icon on the toolbar. (The Chart Wizard icon looks like a tiny bar chart.)

5 Select **column,** and check that the top left-hand **chart sub-type** is selected.

6 Click on **Next**. Chart Wizard will show you a small version of the graph, together with the data range and series. Don't worry about these right now.

7 Click **Next** again. The tabs across the top of the window allow you to change the titles and labels on your chart. Add a title, and value and category labels for the Y (upright) and X (horizontal) axes.

8 When you are happy with your labels, click **Next** once more. You can now choose whether to put your graph on a new sheet, or as an object next to your table.

9 Click **Finish**. You should have a bar chart like the one below, which you can copy and paste into other documents, or print on a separate sheet.

10 You can adapt the steps above with new data, or to produce pie charts, etc.

22.17 Using Excel® (*contd*)

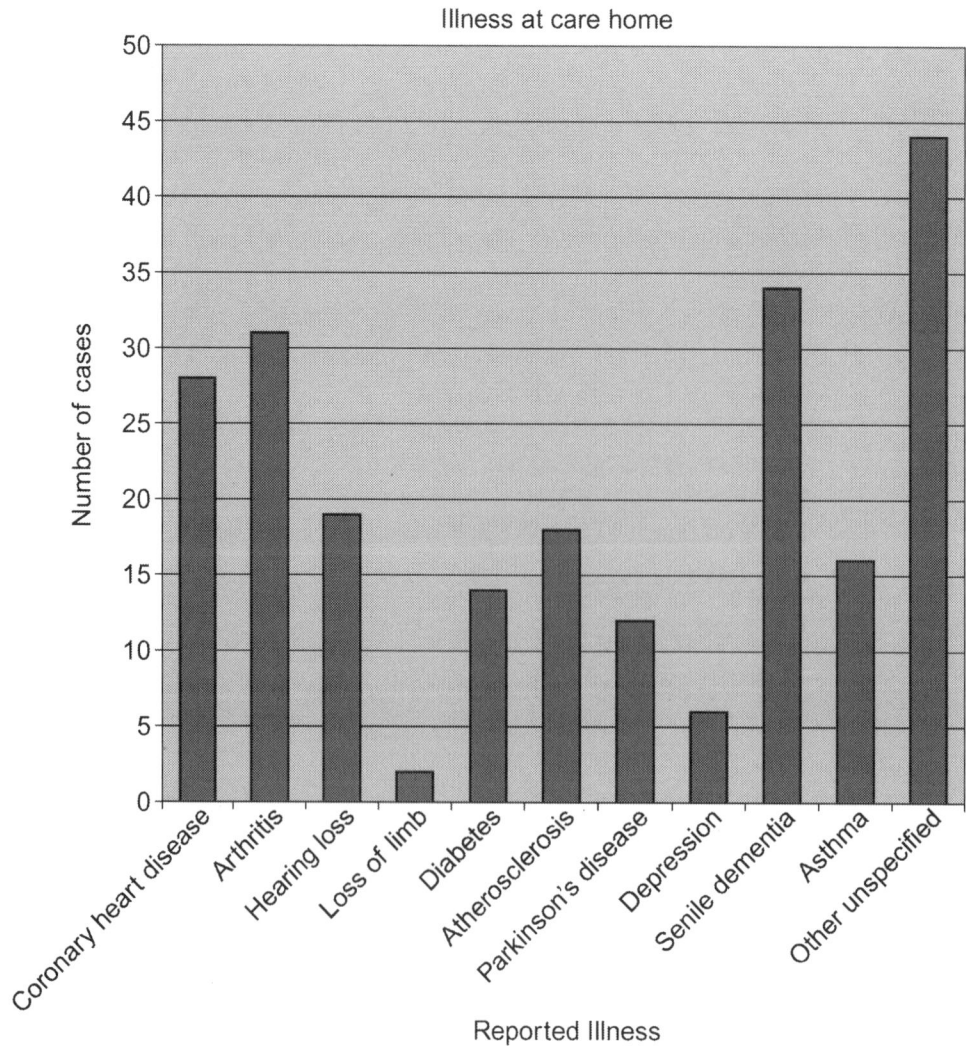

22.18   Drawing conclusions

Student Book 1
pp 452–463

This activity will show you how to interpret your findings, relate them back to your hypothesis and present them clearly.

Sean has just finished gathering the data for his project, and has made the notes below.

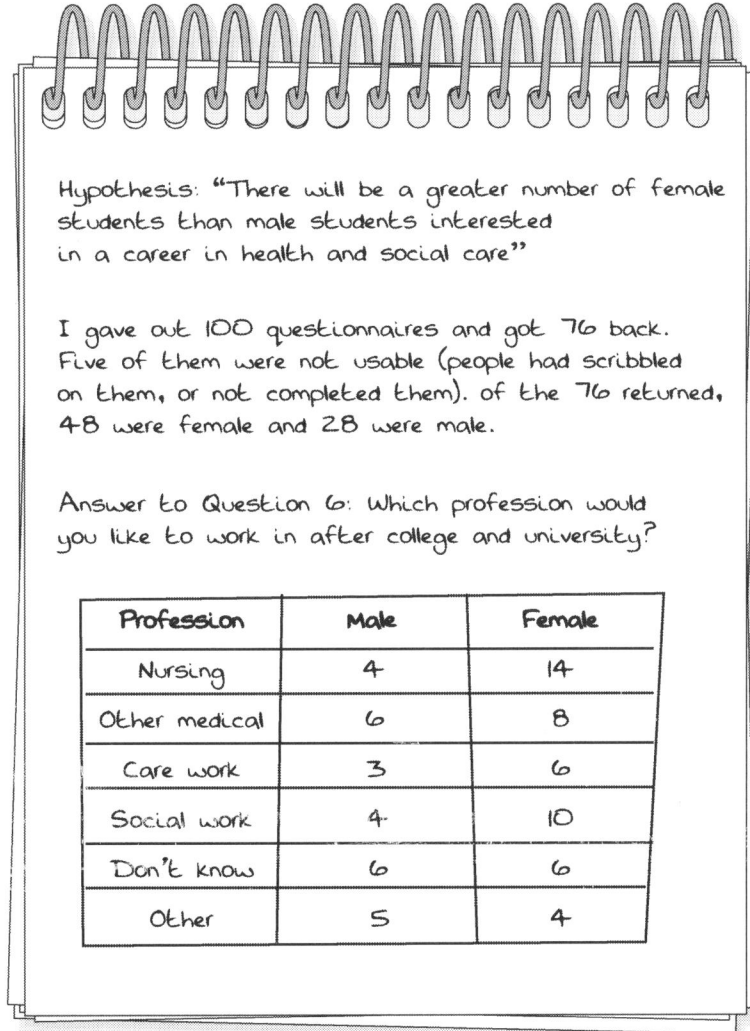

> Hypothesis: "There will be a greater number of female students than male students interested in a career in health and social care"
>
> I gave out 100 questionnaires and got 76 back. Five of them were not usable (people had scribbled on them, or not completed them). Of the 76 returned, 48 were female and 28 were male.
>
> Answer to Question 6: Which profession would you like to work in after college and university?
>
> | Profession | Male | Female |
> |------------|------|--------|
> | Nursing | 4 | 14 |
> | Other medical | 6 | 8 |
> | Care work | 3 | 6 |
> | Social work | 4 | 10 |
> | Don't know | 6 | 6 |
> | Other | 5 | 4 |

Looking at the notes Sean has made, answer the following questions:

1   What was the response rate?

2   What percentage of the respondents were male?

3   What percentage of the respondents were female?

4   What percentage of male respondents were interested in a career in health or social care?

5   What percentage of female respondents were interested in a career in health or social care?

6   What type of chart or graph could Sean use to display the findings in his table?

7   How do these findings relate to Sean's hypothesis?

8   Do you think these findings are valid? (Give reasons for your answer.)

9   Can you suggest at least three ways Sean could have improved his research?

10   What other hypotheses could you test with this research?

22.19 The role of the media

Student Book 1
pp 452–463

This activity will give you a critical insight into the way research is reported in the media. Look through recent newspapers for reports on the results of research. (Hint: you may want to use newspaper websites to search for these stories.) Ideally, you will find several reports of the same piece of research. Then choose two reports to compare: one from a broadsheet newspaper (e.g. *The Times*, the *Guardian* or the *Daily Telegraph*) and another from a tabloid or 'red top' (e.g. the *Sun*, the *Mirror* or the *News of the World*).

Now think about the following questions:

1 Which report includes more detail?

2 Is the type of language used different in each article?

3 Does one article have more of an emotional impact?

4 Which article do you think is more accurate?

5 What do you think each reporter is trying to do?

22.20 Evaluation of research

Student Book 1
pp 452–463

Work in groups of three or four. You will need to choose someone with good handwriting to make notes.

1 Everyone in your group needs to describe the best and worst things that happened during their project. Be as honest as you can.

2 Choose and write down two things that went wrong when you were completing your projects. (You don't have to say whom this happened to!) Explain how things happened – but don't write down how you solved the problems.

3 Next, write down two things that went really well, and try to explain how you felt about them. What do they tell you about current practice?

4 Now, each group should pass their notes to another group.

5 Read the other group's accounts. Are they similar to your own?

6 For the things that went wrong in both groups, discuss and note down answers to the following questions:
 ■ How would you solve the problems?
 ■ What can you learn from this experience?
 ■ How would you do things differently in future?

7 For the things that went well, discuss and note down answers to the following questions:
 ■ Why do you think these things went so well?
 ■ What can you learn from this experience?
 ■ How would this affect the way you plan research in future?

8 Finally, discuss your findings as a whole class.